Current Topics in Microbiology and Immunology

Volume 405

More information about this series at http://www.springer.com/series/82

Natalia Savelyeva · Christian Ottensmeier
Editors

Cancer Vaccines

Responsible Series Editor: Yuri Gleba

Springer

Editors
Natalia Savelyeva
Faculty of Medicine, Cancer Sciences Unit
University of Southampton
Southampton
UK

Christian Ottensmeier
Faculty of Medicine, Cancer Sciences Unit
University of Southampton
Southampton
UK

ISSN 0070-217X ISSN 2196-9965 (electronic)
Current Topics in Microbiology and Immunology
ISBN 978-3-319-23909-5 ISBN 978-3-319-23910-1 (eBook)
DOI 10.1007/978-3-319-23910-1

Library of Congress Control Number: 2017943243

Printed on acid-free paper

This Springer imprint is published by Springer Nature
The registered company is Springer International Publishing AG
The registered company address is: Gewerbestrasse 11, 6330 Cham, Switzerland

Preface

Immunotherapy treatments which harness and enhance the intrinsic powers of the immune system have revolutionised management of solid malignancies. It is extraordinary that over the span of just a few years the way clinicians think about solid tumour management has changed: even in advanced and in rapidly progressive disease like previously fatal cancers such as melanoma, lung cancer or bladder cancers have become treatable. Cautious optimism is emerging that some patients may become long-term disease free and perhaps may be cured.

However, these strategies rely on releasing the pre-existing anti-tumour immune response and only benefit up to 50% of patients. For those patients whose cancers cannot be controlled in this way, induction of immune responses and re-education of T-cells through vaccination can offer a path forward. The concept of boosting insufficient pre-existing responses or priming anti-cancer immune responses using vaccines is gathering pace to provide hope for patients. Developing successful vaccination strategies is crucial and significant advances have already been made in this field.

This book provides an overview of a number of approaches for vaccination, in particular, for lung and head and neck cancers including approaches which are still in preclinical development as well as those which have been already clinically tested. The importance of selection of a vaccine platform to induce successful antigen-specific immune responses has been given attention. The book highlights both laboratory and clinical experience with nucleic acid vaccines including DNA vaccines, which in combination with electroporation have become an effective way of antigen delivery in vivo leading to the successful targeting of the Human Papilloma Virus-driven high-grade cervical dysplasia. In parallel, novel and potent vaccines using mRNA are rapidly being transferred from the laboratory to bedside.

Vaccination approaches for targeting viral oncoantigens in cancers linked to viral aetiology are contrasted with challenges associated with targeting self-cancer antigens in cancer which are not induced by viruses. The need to overcome immunological tolerance to self-cancer antigens by cancer vaccines has been addressed here by two parallel approaches, one based on using chimeric antigens and another on including foreign linked CD4 T-cell help. We share our own clinical experience of using foreign linked T-cell help in DNA vaccines that have also fuelled the development of new generations of cancer vaccines.

Finally, the authors of this book draw attention to the importance of using costimulatory antibodies in combinational strategies as exemplar for new avenues which are opening up for cancer immunotherapy.

This book is aimed at postgraduate students, non-clinical researchers as well as clinicians and all those who aspire to develop novel vaccination approaches for cancer patients with unmet clinical needs.

Southampton, UK

Natalia Savelyeva
Christian Ottensmeier

Contents

New Approaches in Immunotherapy for the Treatment of Lung Cancer

Sonia Quaratino, Ulf Forssmann and Jens-Peter Marschner

Abstract Despite the several advances in the last few years into treatment of advanced lung cancer, the 5-year survival remains extremely low. New therapeutic strategies are currently under investigation, and immunotherapy seems to offer a promising treatment alternative. In the last decade, therapeutic cancer vaccines in lung cancer have been rather disappointing, mainly due to the lack of efficient predictive biomarkers. A better refinement of the patient population that might respond to treatment might finally lead to a success story. For the first time, the immune checkpoint inhibitors are demonstrating sustained antitumor response and improved survival and they may be the first immunotherapeutics available for patients with lung cancer.

Contents

S. Quaratino (✉)
Kymab Ltd, The Bennet Building (B930), Babraham Research Campus, Cambridge CB22 3AT, UK
e-mail: sonia.quaratino@novartis.com

U. Forssmann
Bayer Pharma AG, Müllerstraße 178, 13353 Berlin, Germany

J.-P. Marschner
Affimed Therapeutics AG, Technologiepark, Im Neuenheimer Feld 528, 69120 Heidelberg, Germany

Current Topics in Microbiology and Immunology (2017) 405:1–31
DOI 10.1007/82_2014_428

Published Online: 19 December 2014

1 Introduction—NSCLC and Immunotherapy

Lung cancer is the most common cause of cancer mortality globally, accounting for 1.2 million deaths per year (Ferlay et al. 2010). Non-small cell lung cancer (NSCLC) accounts for 80–85 % of all cases and small cell lung cancer accounts for the remaining 15–20 % (Peters et al. 2012). Within NSCLC, the squamous cell carcinoma accounts for approximately 30 % and the non-squamous NSCLC for the 70 %: the latter group is mainly formed by adenocarcinomas, but it can also include large cell carcinomas and less well-differentiated variants (Goldstraw et al. 2011) (Fig. 1).

Fig. 1 Cellular classification of lung cancer

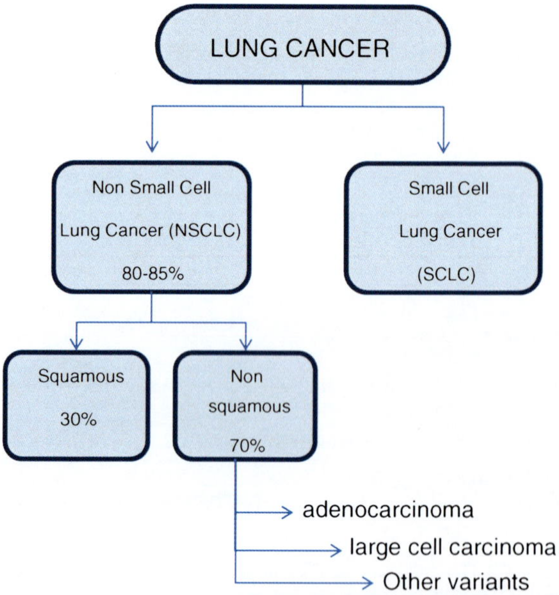

The majority of lung cancer patients present with advanced disease (stage IIIb/IV), and despite targeted therapy has increased the treatment options in the latest years, the overall 5-year survival rate is less than 5 % (Detterbeck et al. 2009).

In first line, the standard of care for stage IV patients consists in the combination of cytotoxic chemotherapy (carboplatin or cisplatin in combination with paclitaxel, gemcitabine, docetaxel, vinorelbine, irinotecan, and pemetrexed) (National Comprehensive Cancer Network (NCCN) 2014).

More recently, targeted therapies have increased the treatment options for patients with certain genetic mutations, opening the path for a more personalized treatment (Blackhall et al. 2013). For instance, epidermal growth factor receptor (EGFR) tyrosine kinase inhibitors (TKIs) such as gefitinib, erlotinib, and afatinib offer a therapeutic window in patients with identified genetic alterations of a key oncogenic driver, the EGFR (Peters et al. 2012). The EML4-ALK fusion gene, resulting from an inversion in chromosome 2, has also been identified as an oncogenic driver in NSCLC (Kwak et al. 2010). It is encountered more frequently in never-smokers, the adenocarcinoma subtype and in younger patients, representing probably ~5 % of adenocarcinoma (Shaw et al. 2009). Patients with ALK mutation can be efficiently treated by the TKI crizotinib (Shaw et al. 2013).

While targeted therapies against driver oncoproteins such as EGFR and ALK have increased the treatment options for patients with non-squamous NSCLC, there are few therapeutic alternatives against tumors without known-driver mutations, and chemotherapy (carboplatin + paclitaxel or pemetrexed) remains the standard of care for squamous NSCLC patients.

The development and implementation of new therapeutic strategies is therefore essential to improve prognosis in lung cancer, and immunotherapy may offer a promising treatment alternative.

Immunotherapy using therapeutic cancer vaccines has shown promise in early clinical trials and has advanced to late-phase development with disappointing results. These include the therapeutic vaccines that target MAGE-3 and MUC1. A promising approach currently in clinical evaluation in NSCLC is the use of immune checkpoint modulators. By blocking inhibitory molecules or, alternatively, activating stimulatory molecules, these treatments are designed to unleash and/or enhance preexisting anticancer immune responses.

2 The Role of the Immune System in NSCLC

The immune system has a complex interaction with the tumor, as it can have either a tumor-promoting or tumor-inhibitory role, depending on the tissue localization, the cell types of the tumor immune infiltrate and the cytokines they secrete. The nature of the immune cells within the tissue can influence tumor progression and has prognostic significance.

An increased tumor infiltration with CD4+ and CD8+ T-helper (Th) 1 cells has been considered a strong favorable prognostic predictor independently associated with improved survival in lung cancer (Kawai et al. 2008). Similarly, a Th1-enriched gene signature in the tumor microenvironment may favor the presence of immune effector cells in the tumor of patients who responded to the MAGE-3 cancer vaccine (Ulloa-Montoya et al. 2013). Conversely, the IL4 gene pathway and other genes associated with a Th2 signature are significantly enriched in the blood of NSCLC patients in tumor progression (Chen et al. 2013). In NSCLC, higher number of cytotoxic T cells (CTL) and Th1 type cells have been associated with survival benefit regardless of the disease subtype (Bremnes 2011; Dieu-Nosjean 2008), whereas a low CTL/Treg ratio and Th2 type cells are a predictor of recurrence and shorter survival (Petersen et al. 2006).

Like the majority of other tumors, also NSCLC uses different strategies to evade the immune system and prevent destruction by effector T cells. Firstly by down-regulating key molecules such as MHC class I molecules and tumor-associated antigens to avoid immune recognition, and secondly preventing T-cell activation by disabling T-cell function or inducing T-cell apoptosis (Schreiber et al. 2011).

In surgically resected specimens, 25–94 % of NSCLCs have down-regulated HLA class I expression (So et al. 2005) and abnormal expression of the β2-microglobulin (Baba et al. 2007), hampering an efficient antigen presentation of tumor-associated epitopes to T cells. Lung cancer cells also express the programmed death ligand-1 (PD-L1) which has been shown to suppress immune responses through engagement with the negative regulator PD-1 expressed on activated T cells and B cells (Konishi et al. 2004; Topalian et al. 2012).

Alternatively, tumor escape may result from an immunosuppressive tumor microenvironment via the production of vascular endothelial growth factor (VEGF), transforming growth factor-β (TGF-β), or indoleamine 2,3-dioxygenase (IDO) and/or the recruitment of regulatory immune cells that function as the effectors of immunosuppression (Schreiber et al. 2011).

Several cellular and soluble suppressive mechanisms have been described in NSCLC. The increased number of M2 macrophages, which secrete IL-8 and IL-10 and inhibit Th1 immune response, is associated with poor prognosis and disease recurrence in NSCLC (Suzuki et al. 2011). Similarly, a tumor accumulation of myeloid-derived suppressor cells (MDSC) and regulatory T cells (Tregs) is associated with unfavorable prognosis in NSCLC patients (Diaz-Montero et al. 2009; Woo et al. 2001).

MDSC can strongly suppress T-cell function via up-regulation of reactive oxygen species (ROS) production (Huang et al. 2013). Tumor-infiltrating Foxp3+ Tregs were positively correlated with intratumoral cyclooxygenase-2 (COX-2) expression and associated with a worse prognosis in resected NSCLC (Shimizu et al. 2010; Hanagiri et al. 2013). Both the inhibition of ROS and COX2 might offer a therapeutic option to counterbalance the effects of these two suppressive regulators.

The immune system plays an active role not only in adenocarcinoma but also in squamous cell carcinoma. For instance, a higher number of infiltrating CD8+ CTL and a significantly lower number of Tregs have been found in squamous than adenocarcinoma (Black 2013; Stinchcombe 2014). However, in squamous cell carcinoma, the favorable CTL/Treg ratio does not correlate with a survival advantage, possibly due to an immunosuppressive tumor environment and other immune-evading strategies (Suzuki et al. 2011; Stinchcombe 2014).

A major component of the adaptive immune response relies on the specific recognition of T-cell antigens. This starts with the T-cell receptor recognizing the antigenic peptide presented by the major histocompatibility complex (MHC) on the antigen-presenting cells (APCs), leading to T-cell activation. Engagement of the co-receptor CD28 with B7-1 (CD80) and B7-2 (CD86) ligands on the APCs provides a stimulatory signal for T cells, sustaining T-cell activation (Chambers and Allison 1997). Subsequent engagement of the cytotoxic T-lymphocyte-associated antigen 4 (CTLA-4) with the same ligands on the APCs results in attenuation of the response (Walunas et al. 1994; Chambers and Allison 1997). Tregs are also known to up-regulate CTLA-4, further contributing to suppressed activation and expansion of CTL (Peggs et al. 2009). Another negative regulator expressed on activated T cells is programmed death 1 (PD1), whose binding with its ligands PD-L1 and PD-L2 on APCs and tumor cells results in down-regulation of T-cell activation (Dong et al. 2002). Tumors are able to up-regulate the PD-L1 ligand expression in order to bind to the PD1 expressed on T cells and thus down-regulating the immune response and promoting T-cell apoptosis (Dong et al. 2002). Blocking the negative T-cell regulators has proven to sustain the T-cell immune response and enhanced antitumor immunity (Leach et al.1996; Brahmer 2014). In NSCLC, elevated PD-L1 levels were positively correlated with increased TILs and associated with better outcome in lung carcinomas (Velcheti et al. 2014). Higher PD-L1 levels were detected in squamous cell carcinomas compared to adenocarcinoma (56.7 % vs. 27.5 %; $P = 0.009$) despite having comparable lymphocytic infiltrates (Velcheti et al. 2014).

The potential to identify subsets of NSCLC patients with an inflammatory tumor microenvironment that predicts for longer survival may also predict for response to immunotherapy and checkpoint inhibitor blockade.

Understanding of the immune evasion mechanisms regulated by tumor cells is necessary for developing more effective immunotherapeutic approaches to lung cancer. Ultimately, it is likely that the success of immune therapy in lung cancer will depend on a particular immune biomarker signature and the integration of strategies that aims to boost the immune response while down-regulating the cancer-induced immune suppression.

3 Vaccines

Vaccines investigated in NSCLC are usually antigen specific and are based on peptides, viral vectors, cell lines, or anti-idiotypic antibodies. Ideally, antigens selected for the immunological approaches should be highly expressed by the tumor but not by healthy tissues and should be immunogenic (Bradbury and Shepherd 2008).

This article will focus on vaccines in advanced stage of clinical development. Table 1 provides a list of vaccines which are currently investigated in phase III clinical trials.

Table 1 Therapeutic cancer vaccines in phase III clinical development in NSCLC

NSCLC stage	Vaccine (*sponsor*)	Mode of action	Antigen	Adjuvant	Phase III trial		
					Design	No. of patients	Trial duration (START data)
Stage Ib/IIIa, adjuvant	GSK1572932A (*GSK*)	Peptide based	MAGE A3	AS15	Double-blind, placebo-controlled, phase III (**14**); *MAGRIT* MAGE-A3 versus placebo after resection ± adjuvant CTX Prim. EP: DFS	2,270	2007–2014 (data available; **14a**)
Stage III, maintenance	L-BLP25; tecemotide (*Merck KGaA*)	Peptide based	MUC1	MPL	Double-blind, placebo-controlled, phase III (**28**); *START* L-BLP25 maintenance versus placebo after CRT Prim. EP: OS	1,513	2007–2012 (data available; **28a**)
					Double-blind, placebo-controlled, phase III (**28b**); *START2* L-BLP25 maintenance versus placebo after concurrent CRT Prim. EP: OS	1,000	2014–2018
	GV1001; tertomotide (*KAEL-GemVax*)	Peptide based	telomerase (hTERT)	GMCSF	Double-blind, placebo-controlled, phase III (**37**); *LucaVax* GV1001 maintenance versus placebo after CRT Prim EP: OS	600	4 years planned (not open)

(continued)

Table 1 (continued)

NSCLC stage	Vaccine (*sponsor*)	Mode of action	Antigen	Adjuvant	Phase III trial		
					Design	No. of patients	Trial duration (START data)
Stage III/IV	Belagenpumatucel-L; Lucanix *(NovaRx)*	Cell based	4 allogeneic NSCLC cell lines	TGF-β antisense	Double-blind, placebo-controlled, phase III (**42**) Lucanix maintenance versus placebo after first line; *STOP* Prim. EP: OS	532	2008–2013 (data available; **45**)
	Racotumomab (*Recombio SL; CIMAB, Cuba*)	Anti-idiotypic	NGc-containing gangliosides	–	Randomized, open-label, phase III (**49**) Racotumomab+BSC versus BSC after first line Prim. EP: OS	1,082	2011–2015
Stage IV[(1)]	TG4010; MVA-MUC1-IL2 *(transgene)*	Viral vector based	MUC1	IL2	Double-blind, placebo-controlled, phase IIb/III (**58a**); *TIME* MUC1 +, % ANK-cells CTX+TG4010 versus CTX +placebo in first line Phase IIb: prim. EP: validation of biomarker Phase III: prim. EP: OS	210 (ph IIb) 800 (ph III)	2012–2015 (ph IIb data available; **58b**)
	CIMAVax–(*CIMAB, Cuba; Bioven*)	rhEGF linked to carrier protein	EGF	Montanide ISA 51	Randomized, open-label, phase III (**68**) CIMAvax versus best supportive care after CTX Prim. EP: OS	579	2006–?
					Randomized, open-label, phase III (**70**) CIMAvax versus BSC first line	?	2011–2015 (trial terminated; **70**)

(continued)

Table 1 (continued)

NSCLC stage	Vaccine (*sponsor*)	Mode of action	Antigen	Adjuvant	Phase III trial		
					Design	No. of patients	Trial duration (START data)
					Prim. EP: OS		
	Talactoferrin alfa (*aggenix*)	Unspecific immune stimulation	–	–	Double-blind, placebo-controlled, phase III (**77**); *FORTIS-M* Talactoferrin+BSC versus placebo+BSC in 3rd+ line Prim. EP: OS	742	2008–2012 (data available; **78**)
					Double-blind, placebo-controlled, phase III (**79**); *FORTIS-C* Talactoferrin+CTX versus placebo+CTX in first line Prim EP: OS and PFS (co-primary)	94 (1,100)	2009–2012 (trial stopped; **80**)
	Tergenpumatucel-L; HyperAcute (*newlink genetics*)	Cell based	3 allogeneic NSCLC cell lines	αGal	Randomized, open-label, phase IIb/III (**87**) Phase IIb: dose schedule finding (2 doses) Phase III: tergenpumatucel-L versus CTX first line; Prim. EP: OS	240	2013–2015

Prim. EP primary endpoint
CTX chemotherapy
PFS progression-free survival
BSC best supportive care
ANK activated NK-cells
1 Includes stage IIIB (wet)

3.1 Melanoma-Associated Antigen 3 (MAGE-A3, GSK1572932A)

The MAGE-A3 antigen is expressed by various tumors. It is not expressed in normal tissue except testis and placenta; however, testis and placenta lack the presentation by HLA molecules (De Plaen et al. 1994). MAGE-A3 is expressed in 35–50 % of NSCLC tumors (Van den Eynde BJ 1997; Sienel 2004; Vansteenkiste et al. 2007), and its expression seems to be a prognostic factor for the clinical outcome in NSCLC (Brichard 2007).

Consequently, MAGE-A3 is a tumor specific antigen which makes it unique for the development of an antigen-specific cancer immunotherapy (ASCI). The MAGE-A3 immunotherapeutic GSK1572932A consists of the MAGE-A3 peptide in combination with an adjuvant. The peptide used in newer clinical trials is produced by recombinant technology (Tyagi and Mirakhur 2009). In earlier clinical trials, the adjuvant $AS02_B$ was used, including the phase II study in NSCLC. However, compared to $AS02_B$, the adjuvant AS15 resulted in an increased clinical activity as demonstrated in a melanoma trial (Kruit 2008). Therefore, the AS15 immunostimulant was chosen for all further trials (MAGRIT).

Phase II trial in adjuvant NSCLC This was a randomized, double-blind, placebo-controlled trial in completely resected MAGE-A3 positive-stage IB or II NSCLC patients (Vansteenkiste et al. 2013). 33 % of the 1,089 screened patients were MAGE-A3 positive, 183 patients were enrolled, and 122 patients were assigned to MAGE-A3, 60 to placebo.

After a median observation period of 44 months, the hazard ratio for the primary endpoint disease-free interval (DFI) was 0.75 (95 % CI, 0.46–1.23; $p = 0.254$) in favor of the MAGE-A3 treatment. This effect was not statistically significant. Similar results have been observed for the secondary endpoints disease-free survival (DFS) and overall survival (OS). After 70 weeks of median observation, the effect for the primary endpoint DFI was almost the same with $HR = 0.78$ (95 % CI, 0.49–1.24; $p = 0.259$). In addition, this effect was consistent for all stratification factors (disease stage, histology, and resection technique). However, after 70 months of median observation, the treatment effect on the secondary endpoint DFS was weaker and did even no longer exist for OS.

A total of 117 of 119 MAGE-A3-treated patients who were eligible for immune response assessment developed anti-MAGE-A3 IgG antibodies after four doses of the vaccine. The remaining two patients developed an immune response after six and nine doses. No induction of immune response was observed in 57 placebo-treated patients. There was no correlation between immune response and DFI.

MAGE-A3 immunotherapeutic treatment was safe with no relevant difference in terms of grade 3/4 AES compared to placebo. Local reactions were more frequently observed in the MAGE-A3 arm and were all of mild-to-moderate intensity.

Gene signature (GS) was investigated in tumor samples in a phase II trial in melanoma (Kruit et al. 2013). 84 genes, mainly immune related, were identified as potentially predictive for the efficacy of MAGE-A3. This GS was then prospectively investigated in the phase II trial in NSCLC (Ulloa-Montoya et al. 2013). 61 (39 %) of 157 tested NSCLC patients were GS positive. Comparing the effect of the vaccine with placebo for the primary endpoint DFI, hazard ratio was 0.42 (95 % CI, 0.17–1.03; $p = 0.06$) for the GS-positive patients and hazard ratio was 1.17 (95 % CI, 0.59–2.31; $p = 0.65$) for the GS-negative patients. Also, for OS, where no clinical effect was seen after 70 months of median observation in the whole population, hazard ratio was 0.63 (95 % CI, 0.22–1.78; $p = 0.81$) in favor of MAGE-A3 vaccination in patients with positive GS.

Phase III trial in NSCLC: MAGRIT A randomized, double-blind phase III trial in patients with resected stage IB/II/IIIA NSCLC was initiated based on the phase II data. Patients were eligible if they were MAGE-A3 positive, underwent surgery with or without standard adjuvant chemotherapy. 13 intramuscular injections are scheduled over 27 months. The primary endpoint was DFS, and the secondary endpoint was prospective validation of GS (Tyagi and Mirakhur 2009).

MAGRIT started in October 2007 and aimed to recruit 2,270 patients from around 400 sites in 33 countries (clinicaltrials.gov). On April 2, 2014 GlaxoSmithKline announced its decision to stop the MAGRIT trial, after establishing that it will not be possible to identify a subpopulation of gene signature-positive NSCLC patients that may benefit from the treatment (GSK press release). Data showed that MARGIT did not meet its first or second co-primary endpoints as it did not significantly extend disease-free survival when compared to placebo in either the overall MAGE-A3-positive population or in those MAGE-A3-positive patients who did not receive chemotherapy.

In summary, although the phase II trial indicated a clinical benefit of MAGE-A3 immunotherapy in patients with completely resected stage IB/II NSCLC, an effect which was even more pronounced in patients with positive GS, the phase III trial MARGIT failed to demonstrate a clinical benefit for the patients.

3.2 L-BLP25 (Tecemotide, Formerly Stimuvax)

The mucinous glycoprotein MUC1, a member of a family of mucins, is an integral membrane protein with extracellular, transmembrane, and cytoplasmic domains. MUC1 has a broad distribution in a variety of normal tissues and tumor tissues (Zotter et al. 1988; Ho et al. 1993; Kufe 2009). MUC1 has oncogenic potential and is able to confer resistance to genotoxic agents (Agrawal et al. 1998). Further, MUC1 seems to play a role in tumor progression, because it can stimulate cell proliferation through growth factor receptor, β-catenin, and ERα, and also suppresses apoptosis through the regulation of JNK, NF-kB, HSP90, and extrinsic apoptotic pathways (Bafna et al. 2010). MUC1 also alters various signaling pathways (Zhao et al. 2009; Raijna et al. 2011). In contrast to normal tissue, MUC1 is aberrantly glycosylated in tumors which makes it a unique target for cancer treatment. Furthermore, underglycosylated MUC1 primes class I-restricted CTL more efficiently than glycosylated MUC1 (Hiltbold 1999). MUC1 is expressed in >90 % of early-stage NSCLC independent of histology. MUC1 expression is generally maintained in paired primary/nodal tumor samples (Mitchell et al. 2013).

Tecemotide is a peptide-based vaccine consisting of BLP25 lipopeptide, immunoadjuvant monophosphoryl lipid A (MPL), and three lipids forming a liposomal product (Butts et al. 2005). Three days after a low-dose intravenous cyclophosphamide administration, tecemotide is administered subcutaneously weekly over 8 weeks, followed by administration every 6 weeks until disease progression.

Phase II trials in stage III/IV NSCLC Tecemotide was investigated as maintenance treatment in a randomized phase IIB trial in stage IIIB/IV NSCLC (Butts et al. 2005). Patients were eligible if they did not progress after initial therapy, i.e. chemoradiotherapy or chemotherapy. They were randomly assigned to tecemotide plus best supportive care (BSC) or BSC alone. The primary endpoint was OS. 171 patients were accrued, 65 with stage III disease, and 106 with stage IV disease. The median OS time was 17.4 months for patients in the tecemotide arm and 13 months in the BSC arm with a hazard ratio of 0.739 (95 % CI, 0.509–1.073; $p = 0.112$) in favor of tecemotide. This effect was even more pronounced in the subgroup of patients with stage IIIB locoregional disease; the hazard ratio was 0.524 (95 % CI, 0.261–1.052; $p = 0.069$). An updated survival analysis revealed that patients with stage IIIB locoregional disease had a median OS of 30.6 months in the tecemotide arm versus 13.3 months in the BSC arm with a 45 % reduced risk to die [HR 0.548, 95 % CI 0.301–0.999 (Butts et al. 2011)].

Comparable survival data, observed in a single-arm phase II trial in stage III locoregional NSCLC patients ($n = 22$), provided some consistency (Butts et al. 2010). Long-term observation data of this trial indicated a median OS of 51.9 months (Butts et al. 2012).

Phase III trial START Encouraged by the phase II data, a randomized, double-blind phase III trial was conducted in stage III locoregional NSCLC (Butts et al. 2013, 2014). 1,513 patients that did not progress after chemoradiotherapy were randomized to tecemotide or placebo in a 2:1 manner. Chemoradiotherapy was given concurrently or sequentially and consisted of a platinum-based chemotherapy and at least 50 Gy of radiotherapy. Caused by a clinical hold, the primary analysis cohort consisted of 1,239 patients. Median OS was 25.6 months in the tecemotide arm versus 22.3 months in the placebo arm (HR 0.88, 95 % CI, 0.75–1.03, $p = 0.123$). A subgroup analysis for the strata of START revealed a more pronounced treatment effect in patients with prior concurrent chemoradiotherapy ($n = 806$). The median OS in this subgroup was 30.8 months for patients in the tecemotide arm and 20.6 months for patients in the placebo arm (HR 0.78, 95 % CI, 0.64–0.95, $p = 0.016$). Tecemotide was well tolerated with no safety concerns.

Based on the subgroup finding of START, the START2 trial was initiated. START2 is a phase III, multicenter, 1:1 randomized, double-blind, placebo-controlled clinical trial designed to assess the efficacy, safety, and tolerability of tecemotide in patients suffering from unresectable, locally advanced (stage III) NSCLC who have had a response or stable disease after at least two cycles of platinum-based concurrent chemoradiotherapy (CRT). The study is expected to recruit about 1,000 patients. The study's primary endpoint is OS. Secondary end-points include time to symptom progression, progression-free survival, and time to progression (Merck KGaA press release, clinicaltrials.gov NCT02049151). The trial has been stopped in September 2014 (press release Merck KGaA).

In summary, the phase III trial could not demonstrate a survival benefit for patients treated with tecemotide. However, subgroup analyses indicate that patients with prior concurrent chemoradiotherapy may benefit from tecemotide treatment. The value of this subgroup finding is currently investigated in another phase III trial.

3.3 GV1001 (Telomerase Vaccine, Tertomotide)

The reverse transcriptase subunit of telomerase (hTERT) is overexpressed in the majority of tumors and, under normal conditions, by embryonic cells and bone marrow stem cells (Kim et al. 1994). It is absent in most adult tissues. Therefore, it is an attractive target for antigen-specific cancer immunotherapy.

GV1001 is a 16-mer peptide vaccine which is injected intradermally 10–15 min after the administration of the adjuvant GM-CSF. It induces both, $CD4^+$ and $CD8^+$, responses and may cause epitope spreading (Inderberg-Suso EM et al. 2012). The administration schedule consists of 3 injections in the first week, followed by injections in weeks 2, 3, 4, 6, 10, and then booster injections every 4 weeks. GV1001 was investigated in several tumor entities such as breast and prostate cancer, melanoma, and other solid tumors; however, most data were generated in pancreatic cancer and NSCLC. Based on phI/II data in a trial in patients with pancreatic cancer (Bernhardt et al. 2006; Kyte et al. 2009), two phase III trials have been initiated in this indication. One was stopped early because a lack of efficacy (press release), the second failed to demonstrate evidence for efficacy (Middleton et al. 2013).

Phase I/II trials in NSCLC In the trial CTN-2006, 23 unresectable stage III NSCLC patients were vaccinated after the initial treatment with radiotherapy plus weekly docetaxel. Specific T-cell response was shown in 16 of 20 eligible patients. Survival was longer in patients with immune response. The treatment was well tolerated (Brunsvig et al. 2011).

A phase I/II trial, CTN 2000, investigated the vaccination in 26 patients, most of them in stage IV disease. Immune responses were detected in 11 out of 24 eligible patients (Brunsvig et al. 2006). An 8-year update of this trial revealed that OS was significantly increased in immune responders compared to non-responders with a median survival of 19 and 3.5 months, respectively (Brunsvig et al. 2011). Four patients were long-term survivors, two of them received vaccinations still 9 years after start of vaccination. All four long-term survivors exhibited strong and durable T-cell responses.

Phase III trial LucaVax A phase III trial was planned investigating the effect of GV1001 in stage III NSCLC. Patients with unresectable disease who got chemoradiotherapy with curative intent are eligible. Chemoradiotherapy has to consist of platinum-based doublets which must not contain gemcitabine and radiotherapy with a dose of up to 66 Gy. Patients are randomized in a double-blind manner to either GV1001 or placebo. The trial was planned to start in April 2012 but is not recruiting, yet (clinical trials.gov, NCT01579188).

In summary, there is some evidence for immunological responses after vaccination of patients with GV1001. GV1001 seems to be well tolerated and showed some efficacy in early trials. However, ongoing phase III trials in pancreatic cancer are failed, while the phase III trial in NSCLC did not start recruitment. It is open if the development of GV1001 will be continued.

3.4 Belagenpumatucel-L (TGF-β Antisense Gene-Modified Allogeneic Tumor Cell Vaccine, Lucanix^{TM})

Belagenpumatucel-L is a cell-based vaccine which consists of four human NSCLC cell lines: two adenocarcinomas, one squamous cell carcinoma, and one large cell carcinoma. All cell lines were transfected with an antisense gene for TGF-β (Nemunaitis et al. 2006). Using defined human cancer cell lines presenting antigens for vaccination of NSCLC patients is a reasonable approach, because data from gene expression profiling in adenocarcinomas indicate that the majority of tumor-related genes are co-expressed by different lung tumor subtypes (Hayes et al. 2006). In addition, this approach has the advantage that the vaccine can be used "off the shelf."

TGF-β has a broad variety of effects on tumors, which may be even controversial (Katz et al. 2013). TGF-β signaling can result in tumor promotion by several modes of action. Immune evasion is one of them, and blocking it may be a useful tool to increase the effect of a vaccine. There are other direct effects of TGF-β which promote tumors, for example promotion of invasion and angiogenesis and development of metastases.

Belagenpumatucel-L is administered intradermally (2.5×10^7 cells in a volume of 0.4 mL) monthly for 18 months and then once at 21 and 24 months in the absence of disease progression (clinical trial.gov, NCT00676507).

Phase II trials Belagenpumatucel-L was investigated in an open-label, three-arm phase II trial (Nemunaitis et al. 2006). Three doses of the vaccine were investigated: 1.25, 2.5, and 5×10^7 cell/injection (cohorts 1, 2, and 3, respectively). Patients were eligible if they had a confirmed stage II (n = 2), IIIA (n = 12), IIIB (n = 15) or IV (n = 46) NSCLC. Treatment with belagenpumatucel-L was started after at least 30 days following the initial cytotoxic therapy.

The treatment was safe with no difference in serious adverse events across dose cohorts. All but two-grade 3/4 adverse events were attributed to disease progression.

Dose-related survival results were observed. Cohorts 2 and 3 were significant different compared to cohort 1 (p = 0.0069). Also 1- and 2-year survival probability was higher for cohorts 2 and 3 compared to cohort 1: 68 and 52 % compared to 39 and 20 %, respectively. The median survival time was 581 days in dose cohorts 2 and 3, i.e., significantly higher than in cohort 1 (252 days, p = 0.0186).

In PBMC of all patients, an increased intracellular cytokine production was measured at week 8 compared to base line. Further, patients with stable disease (SD) or better had higher frequencies of IFN-γ, IL-6 and IL4. Seven of nine patients with negative ELISPOT at baseline developed a response at week 12. The majority of stage IIIB/IV NSCLC patients with SD or better produced a markedly elevated ELISPOT response. With regard to the humoral immune response, a correlation of positive response and clinical outcome was described.

The clinical data were confirmed in a smaller phase II study in 21 patients with advanced stage NSCLC (Nemunaitis et al. 2009). In addition, further immunological tests were performed in late-stage NSCLC patients of phase II patients (Fakhari et al. 2009). According to these data, immune responders survived 32.5 months compared to 11.6 months for non-responders.

Phase III trial An international multicenter, randomized, double-blind, placebo-controlled study of Lucanix™ maintenance therapy for stages III/IV NSCLC subjects who have responded to or have stable disease following one regimen of front-line, platinum-based combination chemotherapy was initiated in 2008 (STOP; Clinicaltrials.gov, NCT00676507). Primary endpoint was overall survival.

STOP did not meet its predefined primary endpoint in the entire patient population (Giaccone 2013); median OS was 20.3 months with the vaccine compared to 17.8 months with placebo (HR 0.94; p = 0.594).

However, prognostic factors for improved outcome were identified in subgroup analyses. The OS was shown to be significantly impacted by the time interval between randomization and the end of frontline chemotherapy (p = 0.002). The OS was improved by 7.3 months with belagenpumatucel-L in 305 stage IIIB/IV patients who were randomised within 12 weeks of chemotherapy completion. In this cohort, the median OS was 20.7 months with belagenpumatucel-L compared to 13.4 months with placebo (HR 0.75; p = 0.083).

Other factors prognostic of better outcome were disease stage, whether prior radiation was received and histology. The patients with confirmed pretreatment radiation showed optimally improved median OS of 29.8 months difference between the treatments; patients receiving belagenpumatucel-L following radiation showed median OS of 40.1 months compared to 10.3 months with placebo (HR 0.45; p = 0.014).

In summary, despite encouraging data from early clinical trials, the phase III trial failed to demonstrate efficacy of belagenpumatucel-L for the intent to treat population. However, subgroup analyses revealed that defined patient populations may benefit from the vaccination. Further studies are warranted to confirm this data.

3.5 *Racotumomab (Anti-idiotypic NeuGc-GM3 mAb, 1E10 Antibody)*

NGcGM3 ganglioside is expressed by many tumors and seems to be practically undetectable in healthy human tissue (Fernandez et al. 2010; Gomez and Ardigo 2012). GM3 is expressed in >90 % of NSCLC tumors and is involved in tumor induced dentritic cell suppression (van Cruijsen et al. 2009).

Racotumomab is an IgG1 anti-idiotypic monoclonal antibody developed by the Center of Molecular Immunology, Havana, Cuba (Vázquez et al. 2012). Racotumomab is administered intradermally (1 mg/ml) five times every 2 weeks during the induction period followed by monthly vaccinations (clinicaltrials.gov, NCT01460472).

Phase I trials were performed in different tumor types including melanoma, breast cancer, SCLC, and NSCLC (Vázquez et al. 2012). It was found that the administration is safe and that it resulted in a strong and specific immune response against NeuGc containing gangliosides (Hernández et al. 2008).

Phase II trials A multicenter, randomized, placebo-controlled, double-blind trial in patients with advanced NSCLC (stage IIIB/IV) who had achieved stable disease or better after initial onco-specific treatment was conducted (Macías et al. 2012). 176 patients were randomized to the vaccine or placebo. Moderate-to-mild local injection site reaction has been observed in the vaccination arm; otherwise, no difference was seen between both arms. The median OS was 8.3 months in the racotumomab arm and 6.3 months in the placebo arm. The OS rate at 1 and 2 years was 38 and 17 % in the racotumomab arm and 24 and 7 % in the placebo arm, respectively. For patients who received >5 vaccinations/placebo administrations (n = 135), this effect was more pronounced.

In another open, non-randomized phase II trial, patients with advanced NSCLC (stage IIIB/IV) who did progress following initial onco-specific treatment were treated with racotumomab (Gomez et al. 2013). Most of the patients had received 4–6 cycles of cisplatin plus vinblastine. 180 patients were accrued. Median survival was 8.06 months, and the OS rate at 2 years was 21 %. Compared to the abovementioned trial, a comparable OS was observed for patients who received the vaccine.

Phase III trial A prospective, randomized multicenter, open-label phase III study of racotumomab plus BSC versus BSC in patients with advanced NSCLC was initiated in 2010 (clinicaltrials.gov, NCT01460472). The primary endpoint is OS, secondary endpoints are safety, PFS and immunology. 1,082 patients will be enrolled, and data are expected in September 2015. Patients are eligible if they suffer from stage III or IV NSCLC and did not progress after standard one line treatment. The trial is conducted in Argentina, Brazil, Cuba and Singapore.

In summary, racotumomab was well tolerated and showed efficacy immunological response in phase II trials and no details on data have been published so far. Obviously, the ganglioside seems to be an interesting target and the phase III trial may provide more information on this vaccine.

3.6 TG4010 (MVA-MUC1-IL2)

TG4010 is an antigen-specific vaccine targeting MUC1 (for MUC1, see also chapter about tecemotide). TG4010 is based on a viral vector, a modified vaccinia of Ankara (MVA), which, in addition to MUC1, expresses interleukin 2. TG4010 is administered subcutaneously at a dose of 108 pfu weekly for 6 weeks and then every 3 weeks (Limacher and Quoix 2012).

Two small phase I trials in 13 patients with MUC1 positive metastatic solid tumors were conducted (Rochlitz et al. 2003). The trials showed that the administration of TG4010 is well tolerated with injection site reactions and flulike symptoms only. It was further observed, that four patients had disease stabilization. One patient with NSCLC, who initially progressed, developed a long lasting response. In addition, some T-cell proliferative immune responses were observed.

Phase II studies A phase II study was conducted in 65 patients randomized to either chemotherapy (cisplatin plus vinorelbine) plus TG4010 (arm 1) or to TG 4010 alone (arm 2) for first-line therapy of stage IIIB/IV NSCLC (Ramlau et al. 2008a). All patients had MUC1-positive tumors as assessed by IHC. The stronger clinical effect was observed in 44 patients randomized to arm 1. 33 of these 44 patients were evaluable for response, 13 achieved a partial response with a response rate of 35.1 %.12 other patents (27.3 %) achieved stabilization of disease. Immunological data (T-cell proliferation test and ELISPOT) were not conclusive. Immunological responses were seen as well before (baseline) as after vaccination. Actually, positive ELISPOTs at any time during the trial correlated with a better survival.

Based on these data, another randomized, open-label phase IIb trial investigated the effect of TG4010 in first-line therapy for stage IV NSCLC which was tested MUC1 positive (Quoix et al. 2011; Ramlau et al. 2008b). 148 patients were recruited, 74 patients were randomized to the combination therapy group (cisplatin plus gemcitabine plus TG4010), and the remaining patients were randomized to the chemotherapy alone group. Progression-free survival (PFS) at 6 months was the chosen primary endpoint. In the combination group, 43.2 (95 % CI 33.4–53.5) were progression free at 6 months, while only 35.1 % (95 % CI 25.9–45.3) were progression free at 6 months in the chemotherapy group. Objective response rate was 41.9 (95 % CI 30.5–53.9) and 28.4 (95 % CI 18.5–40.1) for combination therapy and chemotherapy, respectively. There was no difference in overall survival. A pre-specified analyses revealed that the percentage of activated natural killer cells (CD16+, CD56+, and CD69+) had predictive value. Patient with normal percentage of activated natural killer cells (73.2 % of patients) benefited more from TG4010 treatment, and this included also median OS which was 17.1 months for the combination group and 11.3 months for the chemotherapy group. The interaction between pretreatment percentage of activated natural killer cells and treatment group was significant for OS ($p = 0.0023$). Overall TG4010 was well tolerated with fever, abdominal pain, and injection site pain as site effects which occurred more frequently in the combination group. While the incidence of serious adverse events was similar in both treatment groups of the ITT population, there was a significantly higher incidence for these events in the combination group for the subpopulation with higher percentage of activated natural killer cells.

Phase IIb/III trial TIME This is a double-blind trial comparing the combination of first-line chemotherapy with TG4010 or placebo in stage IV NSCLC with MUC1 expressing tumor (Quoix et al. 2012). The phase IIb part ($n = 210$) aimed at prospectively validating the level of activated NK-cells, the so-called triple-positive activated lymphocyte levels (CD16+, CD56+, CD69+; TrPAL), as predictive marker with PFS as primary endpoint. In contract to the originally planned approach, recently communicated data indicated that a PFS analysis using a quartile approach for the TrPAL lead to predictive threshold for the phase III part of the trial (press release 2014). The quartile analysis showed that in the 75 % of patients having the lower baseline level of TrPAL and who received TG4010, there was a clinically meaningful improvement in PFS, as indicated by a >25 % reduction in the risk of progression or death compared to placebo. Conversely, in the 25 % of patients with the higher level of TrPAL (highest quartile) and who received TG4010, there was no improvement in PFS. Additionally, in subgroup analyses using the quartile approach, an even larger improvement in PFS was obtained in patients with non-squamous tumors not treated with bevacizumab (73 % of initial study population). The design of the phase III part is now under discussion with regulatory authorities. The study started in 2012 with an estimated primary completion date end of 2015 (clinicaltrials.gov, NCT01383148).

In summary, TG4010 is well tolerated and showed clinical efficacy in combination with chemotherapy in metastatic NSCLC in a randomized phase II trial. A biomarker was identified (activated NK-cells, TrPAL). Data of the phase IIb part of the registration trial will be discussed with regulatory authorities in order to design the phase III part.

3.7 EGF Vaccine (CimaVax)

The epidermal growth factor (EGF) plays an important role in tumor growth, mitosis, and metastasis. The EGF receptor (EGFR) is expressed in NSCLC (Salomon et al. 1995), and two types of anti-EGF receptor approaches have been investigated in NSCLC: tyrosine kinase inhibitors and monoclonal antibodies (Ciardello and Tortora 2008; Pirker 2013).

An EGF vaccine was developed in Cuba with recombinant human EGF linked to a carrier protein (P64k Neisseria Meningitidis recombinant protein). A pilot trial in 10 patients with solid tumors indicated that this approach is immunologically effective and tolerable (González et al. 1998).

Two pilot trials were performed in 40 stage IIIB/IV NSCLC patients after onco-specific treatment in order to investigate the effectiveness of two different adjuvants in combination with the vaccine. Based on the antibody responses measured, Montanide ISA 51 was chosen for future clinical trials (Gonzáles et al. 2003). Another analysis using pooled data of the pilot trials showed clinical efficacy, in particular in seroconverted patients (Gonzáles et al. 2007).

Phase II trial 80 patients with stage IIIB/IV NSCLC who received first-line treatment were randomized to the vaccine plus supportive care versus supportive care (Neninger Vinageras et al. 2008; García et al. 2008). About 30 % of these patients had progressive disease at the time of randomization. In the treatment arm, patients received a low-dose cyclophosphamide administration 3 days prior to vaccination, then 4 weekly intra-muscular injections of 50 μg EGF followed by monthly injections.

The median OS was 6.47 months in the vaccine arm and 5.33 months in the control arm ($p = 0.098$). This effect was more pronounced in patients younger than 60 years with a median OS of 11.57 versus 5.33 months in the vaccination and control arm, respectively. Antigen responses and EGF concentration were measured in 42 patients (26 vaccinated and 16 controls) only. Data showed that patients with good antibody response had the better survival benefit with a median OS of 11.7 months compared to 3.6 months in patients with poor antibody response. Further, an inversed correlation between EGF concentration and survival was demonstrated. Vaccination was safe with mild-to-moderate-related adverse events only.

Phase III trial In 2006, a phase III trial was initiated at 18 sites in Cuba which is still ongoing. 579 patients are randomized 2:1 to vaccine or control (Rodríguez et al. 2010). The therapeutic schedule for the vaccine is the same as in the phase II study; however, the vaccine is administered in four injection sites resulting in a four times higher dose. Patients are stratified for age: >60 years versus ≤60 years. Preliminary results of 160 patients show a trend toward a delayed separation of the survival curves in favor of the vaccine arm (Rodríguez et al. 2010).

A total of 40 patients of this phase III trial who received the high-dose regimen were compared to 40 patients of the phase II trial who received the lower-dose regimen (Rodríguez et al. 2011). The patient groups from both trials were balanced in terms of baseline and tumor characteristics. Both regimens were well tolerated with only grade 1- and grade 2-related adverse events. The humoral response was more pronounced in the high-dose group with an antibody titer of 1:7328 (geometric mean) compared to 1:3160 in the control group. In the high-dose group, the rate of good antibody responders was 54.8 % and the rate of "super good responders" was 30.8 %. In the phase II trial, the respective rates are 52.8 and 10 %. The median OS in high-dosed patients was 13.57 months compared to 6.47 months in low-dosed patients.

Another phase III open-label, randomized trial in stage III/IV NSCLC patients is ongoing and finished recruitment. Patients in the age of 20–65 years were eligible and randomized to the vaccine or BSC as first-line therapy. According to changes in clinicaltrials.gov (March 2014), the trial has been terminated in order to initiate a new phase III design including biomarker to enrich the patient population and to further strengthen OS benefit (clinicaltrials.gov, NCT01444118). The level of circulating EGF is used as biomarker and a minimum threshold level has been set as inclusion criterion for the trial.

In summary, phase II data on safety, efficacy, and immunology are encouraging. First data of an ongoing phase III trial suggest that an increased dose of the vaccine may have a stronger effect in terms of immunology and efficacy without an increasing risk for the patients. The phase III trial was terminated, and the outcome has not been made public so far. CimaVax was licensed in Cuba for the treatment of adult patients with stage IIIB/IV NSCLC (Rodríguez et al. 2010). Bioven has licensed in the rights on the EGF vaccine developed in Cuba. Bioven names this product EGF *P*athway-*T*argeted Immunization, PTI, instead of vaccine in order to make clear distinction between classical vaccines targeting tumor antigens such as MUC1, MAGE 3, L-BLP-25 presented here, and the PTI approach.

3.8 Talactoferrin Alfa

Talactoferrin alfa is a recombinant human lactoferrin (Kelly and Giaccone 2010). It is structurally and functionally similar to native human lactoferrin as it can be purified from human milk. Lactoferrin has multiple known biological effects such as anti-inflammatory effects or anti-tumor effects. In addition, there are different immune modulatory effects. After oral administration, talactoferrin recruits dentritic cells in the Peyer's patches of the intestine. These dentritic cells present (tumor associated) antigens and initiate an immune stimulatory cascade in the gut associated lymphoid tissue (GALT).

The anti-tumor effect of talactoferrin was demonstrated in mouse models. It was shown that oral talactoferrin induces mucosal IFN-gamma production as well as expansion of CD8+ T lymphocytes and NK-cells and enhancement of CD8+ cytotoxicity (Spadaro et al. 2007).

A phase I trial was conducted in patients with solid tumors. Ten patients who had failed conventional chemotherapy were recruited in the first part of the trial which was intended to escalate the dose and to identify the maximum-tolerated dose (MTD) (Hayes et al. 2006b). Talactoferrin was well tolerated, an MTD was not defined. Talactoferrin induced an increase in circulating IL18. Five patients had stable disease after 2 months of treatment, seven patients showed a reduction in tumor growth rate. In the second part, further 26 patients were recruited that received the two highest daily doses tested in part one (4.5 or 9 g/day) (Hayes and Falchook 2010). 12 of the total 36 patients suffered from NSCLC. 11 of them have received prior CTX or radiochemotherapy. Out of the 12 patients, seven had SD. The median PFS was 4.3 months, the median OS was 8.8 months. The substance was well tolerated.

Phase II trials Two randomized, double-blind, placebo-controlled phase II studies have been initiated: one in stage IV NSCLC patients that progressed after CTX and one in previously untreated stage IV NSCLC patients.

In the first trial, 100 patients were included of which 81 patients received at least one dose (evaluable population) (Parikh et al. 2011). The majority of patients received one prior therapy, about 1/4 received two or more prior therapies. Talactoferrin was dosed 1.5 mg twice daily for 12 weeks followed by 2 weeks off for a maximum of three cycles until progression. The median OS was 6.1 months in the talactoferrin arm and 3.1 months in the placebo arm and the primary endpoint was met ($p = 0.05$). The 1-year survival rates were 29 and 16 %, respectively.

The second trial recruited 110 stage IV NSCLC patients who did not receive prior therapy for NSCLC (Digumarti et al. 2011). Patients were randomized to CTX plus talactoferrin or CTX plus placebo. Patients in the talactoferrin arm received 1.5 mg twice daily for three 6-week cycles (5 weeks on, 1 week off the drug) until progression. Primary endpoint was response rate (RR). In the evaluable population, RR was 47 % in the talactoferrin arm and 29 % in the placebo arm ($p = 0.05$). Median PFS was 7.0 and 4.2 months (HR = 0.85; $p = 0.24$), and median OS was 10.4 and 8.5 months (HR = 0.87; $p = 0.26$), respectively.

In both phase II trials, talactoferrin was well tolerated with grade 3 and 4 events occurring slightly more frequent in the placebo arms.

Phase III trials Based on the phase II data, two phase III trials were initiated: FORTIS-M and FORTIS-C.

FORTIS-M was a randomized, double-blind, placebo-controlled trial which compared the clinical effect of talactoferrin-alfa plus BSC with placebo plus BSC in patients with stage IV NSCLC who have failed two or more prior treatment regimens (clinicaltrials.gov, NCT00707304). The study did not meet the primary endpoint, i.e., to demonstrate a significant survival benefit for talactoferrin compared to placebo (aggenix press release). 742 patients were enrolled globally at 160 sites. Patients in the talactoferrin arm had a median OS of 7.5 months compared with 7.7 months for the placebo arm (HR = 1.04, $p = 0.66$).

FORTIS-C was a randomized, placebo-controlled study of talactoferrin-alfa in combination with carboplatin and paclitaxel as first-line therapy in patients with stage IV NSCLC. Co-primary endpoints were OS and PFS (clintrials.gov NCT00706862). This trial was stopped early because of the negative results from FORTIS-M (press release). At this time, 94 of the planned 1,100 patients were enrolled in the US. For the 94 enrolled patients, median PFS was 5.8 months in the talactoferrin arm and 5.6 months in the placebo arm (HR = 0.97; $p = 0.89$). Median OS was 11.4 versus 12.7 months (HR = 1.25; $p = 0.36$), respectively.

In summary, despite encouraging phase II data, talactoferrin-alfa failed to demonstrate clinical efficacy in late-stage NSCLC. The question was raised if this very late stage of disease, i.e., stage IV NSCLC with several previous lines of chemotherapy, is the right candidate for immunotherapy (Madan et al. 2013).

3.9 Tergenpumatucel-L (HyperAcute)

The α(1,3)galactosyl (αGal) gene is functional in mammalian species but inactive in humans (Joziasse and Orial 1999). Due to continuous presentation of the antigen αGal by intestinal and pulmonal bacteria, the human immune system develops specific antibodies recognizing αGal. These antibodies are responsible for a hyperacute reaction to cells expressing αGal, e.g., after xenotransplantation.

Already more than a decade ago, the approach of eliciting hyperacute xenograft response to treat cancer was described (Link et al. 1998). In animal models, it was shown that immunity against αGal can induce antitumor activity (Rossi et al. 2008).

Tergenpumatucel-L is a cell-based vaccine consisting of genetically modified allogeneic NSCLC cells bearing αGal moieties (Morris et al. 2013). Tergenpumatucel is administered intradermally.

Phase II trial 28 patients with metastatic or recurrent NSCLC were recruited into a single-arm phase II trial prior to systemic therapies (Morris et al. 2012, 2013). Patients received eight doses of 300×10^6 cells every 2 weeks. The median OS was 11.3 months. Eight patients had stable disease over more than 16 weeks. Nine out of 16 patients who received follow-up chemotherapy developed a response according to RECIST criteria. The vaccine was well tolerated. All patients showed increased anti-αGal antibody levels and 61 % of patients showed increased interferon-gamma levels (ELISPOT, no details described). These patients were characterized by a longer median OS of 21.9 months compared to 5.5 months for patients with lower IFN-gamma levels (Morris et al. 2012). The authors concluded that, compared to historical controls, the observed survival duration is encouraging. Further, due to the responses seen in the follow-up chemotherapies, the authors concluded that the vaccination has a chemosensitizing effect.

Phase IIb/III trial Based on the phase II data, an open-label, randomized, multi-institutional adaptive design phase IIb/III trial was initiated in January 2013 (clintrials.gov, NCT01774578). Patients are eligible if they have stage IIIB/IV NCSLC and received prior line(s) of chemotherapy. In the phase IIb part, two dosing schedules will be investigated either 300×10^6 cells weekly for 11 weeks and then every 2 months for five additional doses or 300×10^6 cells every 2 weeks for six doses followed by additional 10 monthly doses. In both groups, a total of 16 immunizations is planned. The phase III part will then further investigate the clinical effect of Tergenpumatucel-L administering the selected dose from phase IIb part. 240 patients will be enrolled and randomized to either the vaccine or to chemotherapy. Primary endpoint is overall survival; results are expected in July 2015.

In summary, data from the phase II study indicate some clinical efficacy, although this trial was not randomized and no details have been published so far.

3.10 Summary—Vaccines

Several vaccines have been/are in phase III clinical development in NSCLC. To date, there is no evidence from phase III trials that vaccines can cause a clinically meaningful benefit in patients suffering from NSCLC. All finished trials did not meet the primary endpoint: MAGRIT (MAGE-A3), START (tecemotide), STOP (Lucanix), FORTIS M and FORTIS C (talactoferrin alpha) and probably also the CIMAVax trial (EGF vaccine). In addition, the LucaVax trial (GV1001) is not followed up and the START2 (tecemotide) follow-up trial was discontinued due to disappointing phase II data from a Japanese study in the same setting. Overall, the results of vaccinations in NSCLC are disappointing so far.

However, there are trials ongoing which can tell us more about the value of vaccinations in NSCLC. TIME (TG4010) as well as the phase III trials with racotumomab and tergenpumatucel-L will generate further data over the next years. Also, new phase III trials with belagenpumatucel-L (Lucanix) and CIMAVax may be initiated based on further analyses of the data.

Outlook: In addition to the development of vaccines as single immunological treatment approach, the combination of vaccines with non-specific immune stimulators, in particular checkpoint inhibitors, seems to be a promising approach which may strengthen the specific immunological effects of vaccines (Rangachari and Brahmer 2013). We are still in an early phase of investigating vaccines. Further understanding of the mode of action and in particular combination therapies may help to make vaccines more successful in NSCLC.

4 Immune Checkpoint Blockers

Since the mechanism of action of immune checkpoint blockers is not dependent on the expression of specific antigens in contrast to the vaccination approach, a broad application in different tumor types is conceivable. The strategy to augment antitumor responses through the blockade of immune checkpoint pathways has only recently been started to be explored for lung cancer, especially in NSCLC, and therefore, this part is not reporting the very limited experience in SCLC which has recently been summarized by Spiegel and Socinski (2013). Two pathways, the CTLA-4:B7-1/-2 and the PD-1:PD-L1/-L2 axis, are clinically investigated, and the current status is described below.

4.1 CTLA-4 Blockade

Positive phase III results in metastatic melanoma (Hodi et al. 2010; Robert et al. 2011) have stimulated the exploration of the anti-CTLA-4 monoclonal antibody ipilimumab in lung cancer. Thus, ipilimumab was evaluated in combination with paclitaxel and carboplatin (PC) in a randomized, double-blind, phase II, first-line clinical study in patients with locally advanced or metastatic NSCLC, or extended SCLC (phase II study for previously untreated subjects with non-small cell lung cancer (NSCLC) or small cell lung cancer (SCLC) (clinicaltrials.gov NCT00527735). Since the optimal sequence of chemo- and immunotherapy is challenging, two schedules, i.e., concurrent or phased, were explored. The study met its primary endpoint (defined as significant improvement in immune-related (ir)PFS) for phased treatment versus control (HR 0.72; $p = 0.05$), but not for concurrent treatment (HR 0.81; $p = 0.13$). The median irPFS/PFS/OS for phased, concurrent, and control treatments (i.e., PC only) were 5.7/5.1/12.2; 5.5/4.1/9.7 and 4.6/4.2/8.3 months, respectively (Lynch et al. 2010). Observed incidences of grade 3/4 treatment-related adverse events were similar: 39, 41, and 37 % for patients in the phased, concurrent and control groups, respectively. However, the rate of grade 3/4 immune-related AEs were differing as could be expected: 15 % in the phased-group, 20 % in the concurrent-group, and 6 % in the control-group patients. In addition, a trend for greater clinical activity was observed in patients with squamous histology (Lynch et al. 2010). Overall, these results triggered the initiation of a phase III trial in patients with stage IV squamous cell NSCLC to investigate ipilimumab plus PC versus placebo plus PC in August 2011 (clinicaltrials.gov NCT01285609).

Tremelimumab, another monoclonal anti-CTLA-4 antibody was explored in phase II in the maintenance setting after first-line chemotherapy for advanced NSCLC, where it did not improve PFS (Brahmer 2013). Up to date, no further trials have been initiated.

4.2 PD-1/PD-L1 Blockade

While CTLA-4 primarily regulates early stages of T-cell activation at their initial response to antigen as a signal dampener, the role of PD-1 is to limit the activity of T cells in peripheral tissues, especially in inflammatory situations (Pardoll 2012).

The first trial using a blocker of the PD-1/PD-L1 pathway, i.e., nivolumab/BMS-936558 an anti-PD-1 antibody, was a first-in-man single-agent dose-escalation trial. In this trial, one durable complete response (CR) (colorectal carcinoma, CRC) and two partial responses (PR) (melanoma and renal cell carcinoma, RCC) were observed in 39 patients. Two additional patients (melanoma, NSCLC) had significant lesional tumor regressions not meeting PR criteria. The initial safety profile was favorable in comparison with ipilimumab (Brahmer et al. 2010). These promising results boosted the clinical development activities on this specific immune checkpoint. The consequent multiple-dose-escalation trial with nivolumab containing several expansion cohorts recruited 296 patients overall (Topalian et al. 2012). Remarkably, 14 of 76 (18 %) advanced NSCLC patients evaluable for efficacy displayed an objective response (or) and five additional patients a stable disease (SD) for more than 24 weeks. The RR was higher in the squamous (6/18, 33 %) compared to the non-squamous subtype (7/56, 12 %). Again, the safety profile in the overall study population was favorable with a 14 % rate of grade 3/4 treatment-related adverse events, while 3 deaths from pulmonary toxicity were reported. Nivolumab monotherapy follow-up data presented at ASCO 2013 reported an overall RR of 17 % (22 responses in 129 patients; squamous vs. non-squamous: 17 vs. 18 %), a median PFS of 2.3 months, and a median OS of 9.6 months (Brahmer et al. 2013). This cohort was also investigated for the association of tumor PD-L1 expression with clinical activity. The tumors were defined as PD-L1 (PD-L1+) positive when ≥5 % of the tumor cells had membrane staining at any intensity. Using this cutoff, 5 of 31 patients defined as PD-L1+ had an OR, while 4 of 32 patients defined as PD-L1− had an OR as well (Antonia et al. 2013). Hence, further evaluation of PD-L1 as a molecular marker of nivolumab therapy is required.

First preliminary data in NSCLC have also been reported recently for lambrolizumab/MK-3475, which is another anti-PD-1 antibody. Thirty-eight patients (19/38) previously treated with two systemic regimens had been enrolled. The ORR (confirmed and unconfirmed using RECIST 1.1) was 21 % applying an independent central images review and 24 % using investigator-assessed irRC. The median duration of response by irRC had not been reached, with a median follow-up of 9 months (minimum 6 months). Pretreatment tumor PD-L1 expression was a statistically significant predictor of response. In patients with evaluable tumor PD-L1 expression, all confirmed responses by RECIST v 1.1 (and irRC) occurred in patients with tumors strongly positive for PD-L1. Fifty percent of the patients had drug-related adverse events, and there was only one case of a grade 3 (pulmonary edema), but no higher drug-related adverse events (Garon et al. 2013). Follow-up data presented at AACR 2014 reported a median PFS of 9 weeks, and a median OS of 51 weeks. PD-L1 IHC score was above a potential cut point in nine patients and below a potential cut point in 22 patients (seven patients could not be evaluated), and significant associations between tumor PD-L1 expression and ORR (57 vs. 5 %) were observed (Gandhi et al. 2014).

BMS-936559, an anti-PD-L1 antibody was explored in a multiple-dose-escalation phase I trial in 207 patients covering 49 advanced NSCLC patients evaluable for efficacy (Brahmer et al. 2012). RR for squamous and non-squamous subtypes were similar (1/13, 8 vs. 4/36, 11 %; all patients 5/49, 10 %) and not that impressive. However, as for nivolumab, a dose dependency in NSCLC patients could clearly be observed showing activity at 3 and 10 mg/kg. Grade 3/4 treatment-related adverse events were observed in only 9 % of the overall trial population.

Another anti-PD-L1 antibody, MPDL3280A, is also explored in phase I (Spiegel and Socinski 2013). The NSCLC expansion cohort (locally advanced or metastatic disease) was reported to display an impressive overall RR of 24 % (9 of 37 patients with both squamous and non-squamous histology). The incidence of grade 3/4 treatment-emergent adverse events in the NSCLC safety cohort was 34 %. Interestingly, no grade 3–5 pneumonitis or diarrhea was reported. Biomarker analyses from archival tumor showed a correlation between PD-L1 status and efficacy. Latest analyses revealed that patients with PD-L1-positive tumors showed an ORR of 100 % (4/4), while patients who were PD-L1 tumor status negative had an ORR of 15 % (4/26). Further, it was concluded that MPDL3280A is probably the first targeted agent showing more activity in smoking patients than in never-smokers. Moreover, the 24-week PFS was reported to be 46 % (Soria et al. 2013).

Several trials have recently been initiated with nivolumab in NSCLC: two open-label randomized phase III trials comparing nivolumab versus docetaxel in previously treated advanced or metastatic NSCLC, one trial in squamous and the other trial in non-squamous histology (clinicaltrials.gov NCT01642004, NCT01673867). An open-label phase III safety trial of nivolumab in subjects with advanced or metastatic NSCLC who have progressed during or after receiving at least one prior systemic regimen to estimate the incidence and characterize the outcome of high-grade, select adverse events has also been recently initiated (clinicaltrials.gov NCT02066636). Additional phase II trials are actively recruiting or ongoing (clinicaltrials.gov NCT02041533, NCT01721759).

A phase I trial in stage IIIB/IV NSCLC patients is exploring different combinations of nivolumab with (a) gemcitabine/cisplatin, (b) pemetrexed/cisplatin, (c) carboplatin/paclitaxel, (d) erlotinib, (e) ipilimumab, (f) bevacizumab maintenance, (g) switch maintenance, or (h) as monotherapy in first-line patients with brain metastases (clinicaltrials.gov NCT01454102). In addition, a randomized phase II trial in subjects with recurrent metastatic NSCLC exploring epigenetic priming with azacitidine and entinostat or oral azacitidine alone prior to nivolumab treatment has been initiated (clinicaltrials.gov NCT01928576). Priming with these methylation blockers holds promise as DNA demethylation may contribute to PD-1 overexpression. Another anti-PD-1 antibody, lambrolizumab/MK-3475, is also put forward to phase II/III: A randomized trial is exploring its efficacy and safety versus docetaxel in previously treated subjects with NSCLC (clinicaltrials.gov NCT01905657). A phase I study of lambrolizumab is investigating the combination with cisplatin/pemetrexed or carboplatin/paclitaxel in patients with advanced NSCLC (clinicaltrials.gov NCT01840579). Further, phase I and II trials with MK-3475 in NSCLC in monotherapeutic setting and in combination settings with paclitaxel, carboplatin, pemetrexed, bevacizumab, ipilimumab, and erlotinib have been initiated (clinicaltrials.gov NCT02039674). The anti-PD-L1 antibody MPDL3280A is also further explored in one phase III and three phase II trials in advanced NSCLC (clinicaltrials.gov NCT02008227, NCT01846416, NCT02031458,). Moreover, a phase III trial with the anti-PD-L1 antibody MEDI4736 as sequential therapy in patients with locally advanced, unresectable NSCLC (stage III) who have not progressed following definitive, platinum-based, concurrent chemoradiation therapy has been initiated (clinicaltrials.gov NCT02087423).

5 Conclusion

Lung cancer has for a long time not been considered to be a very immunogenic tumor type such as melanoma or renal cancer. This perception has nowadays changed. Several vaccines are in phase III clinical development in NSCLC. Only few data are available so far, and no evidence for the clinical efficacy of vaccines could be demonstrated, yet. Recently, a phase III trial of talactoferrin alfa did not meet the primary endpoint (not described here because the development was stopped). Also, for tecemotide and Lucanix, a clinical benefit in terms of OS could not be demonstrated in large phase III trials. The appropriate patient selection, either with gene signature or using the optimal combination treatment, may help yield the survival improvement with vaccines. Over the next few years, we will get a clearer picture about the role of vaccines in the treatment of NSCLC. Currently, the most promising results in NSCLC have been observed in early clinical trials using immune checkpoint inhibitors which led to an accelerated clinical development. If the promises of the initial results prove true, the first approval of an immune checkpoint blocker for NSCLC can be expected around 2016.

References

Agrawal B et al (1998) The biological role of mucins in cellular interactions and immune regulation: prospects for cancer immunotherapy. Mol Med Today 4:397–403

Fernandez LE et al (2010) NGcGM3 ganglioside: a privileged target for cancer vaccines. Clin Dev Immunol, Article ID 814397

Soria JC et al (2013) Clinical activity, safety and biomarkers of PD-L1 blockade in non-small cell lung cancer (NSCLC): additional analyses from a clinical study of the engineered antibody MPDL3280A (anti-PDL1). European cancer congress 2013 (ECCO-ESMO-ESTRO), Abstract 3408. http://eccamsterdam2013.ecco-org.eu/Scientific-Programme/Abstract-search.aspx#

Gandhi L et al (2014) MK-3475 (anti-PD-1 monoclonal antibody) for non-small cell lung cancer (NSCLC): antitumor activity and association with tumor PD-L1 expression. Abstract CT105. AACR annual meeting

Antonia SJ et al (2013) Association of PD-L1 tumor expression and immune biomarkers with clinical activity in patients with non-small cell lung cancer (NSCLC) treated with nivolumab (anti-PD-1; BMS-936558;Ono-4538). J Thorac Oncol 8(Suppl 2):S907–S908

Baba T et al (2007) Lack and restoration of sensitivity of lung cancer cells to cellular attack with special reference to expression of human leukocyte antigen class I and/or major histocompatibility complex class I chain related molecules A/B. Cancer Sci 98:1795–1802

Bafna S et al (2010) Membrane-bound mucins: the mechanistic basis for alterations in the growth and survival of cancer cells. Oncogene 29:2893–2904

Bernhardt SL et al (2006) Telomerase peptide vaccination of patients with non-resectable pancreatic cancer: a dose escalating phase I/II study. Br J Cancer 95:1474–1482

Black CC et al (2013) Adenocarcinoma contains more immune tolerance regulatory T-cell lymphocytes (versus squamous carcinoma) in non-small-cell lung cancer. Lung 191(3):265–270

Blackhall F et al (2013) The impact on the multidisciplinary teams of molecular profiling for personalized therapy in non-small cell lung cancer. Lung Cancer 79:101–103

Bradbury PA, Shepherd F (2008) Immunotherapy for lung cancer. J Thorac Oncol 3(Suppl 2): S164–S170
Brahmer J (2013) Harnessing the immune system for the treatment of non-small-cell-lung cancer. J Clin Oncol 31:1021–1028
Brahmer JR (2014) Immune checkpoint blockade: the hope for immunotherapy as a treatment of lung cancer? Semin Oncol 41:126–132
Brahmer J et al (2010) Phase I study of single-agent anti-programmed death-1 (MDX-1106) in refractory solid tumors: safety, clinical activity, pharmacodynamics, and immunologic correlates. J Clin Oncol 28:3167–3175
Brahmer J et al (2012) Safety and activity of anti-PD-L1 antibody in patients with advanced cancer. N Engl J Med 366:2455–2465
Brahmer J et al (2013) Survival and long-term follow-up of the phase I trial of nivolumab (Anti-PD-1; BMS-936558; ONO-4538) in patients (pts) with previously treated advanced non-small cell lung cancer (NSCLC). J Clin Oncol 31(Suppl):8030
Bremnes RM et al (2011) The role of tumor-infiltrating immune cells and chronic inflammation at the tumor site on cancer development, progression, and prognosis: emphasis on non-small cell lung cancer. J. Thorac Oncol 6:824–833
Brichard VG (2007) GSK's antigen-specific cancer immunotherapy program: pilot results leading to phase III clinical development. Vaccine 25(Suppl 2):B61–B71
Brunsvig P et al (2006) Telomerase peptide vaccination: a phase I/II study in patients with non-small cell lung cancer. Cancer Immunol Immunother 55:1553–1564
Brunsvig P et al (2011) Telomerase peptide vaccination in NSCLC: a phase II trial in stage III patients vaccinated after chemoradiotherapy and an 8-year update on a phase I/II trial. Clin Cancer Res 17:6847–6857
Butts C et al (2005) Randomized phase IIB trial of BLP25 liposome vaccine in stage IIIB and IV non-small cell lung cancer. J Clin Oncol 23:6674–6681
Butts C et al (2010) A multicenter open-label study to assess the safety of a new formulation of BLP25 liposome vaccine in patients with unresectable stage III non-small-cell lung cancer. Clin Lung Cancer 11:391–395
Butts C et al (2011) Updated survival analysis in patients with stage IIIB or IV non-small-cell lung cancer receiving BLP25 liposomal vaccine (L-BLP25): phase IIB randomized, multicenter, open-label trial. J Cancer Res Clin Oncol 137:1337–1342
Butts C et al (2012) Long-term efficacy and safety of L-BLP25 vaccine in a multi-center open-label study of patients with unresectable stage III NSCLC. Annals of Oncol 23(Suppl 9, ix):395
Butts C et al (2013) START: a phase III study of L-BLP25 cancer immunotherapy for unresectable stage III non-small cell lung cancer. J Clin Oncol 31:7500
Butts C et al (2014) Tecemotide (L-BLP25) versus placebo after chemoradiotherapy for stage III non-small-cell lung cancer (START): a randomised, double-blind, phase 3 trial. Lancet Oncol 15(1):59–68
Chambers CA, Allison JP (1997) Co-stimulation in T cell responses. Curr Opin Immunol 9:396–404
Chen YC et al (2013) Peripheral immune cell gene expression changes in advanced non-small cell lung cancer patients treated with first line combination chemotherapy. PLoS One 8:e57053
Ciardiello F, Tortora G (2008) EGFR antagonists in cancer treatment. N Engl J Med 358:1160–1174
De Plaen E et al (1994) Structure, chromosomal location, and expression of 12 genes of the MAGE family. Immunogenetics 40:360
Detterbeck FC, Boffa DJ, Tanoue LT (2009) The new lung cancer staging system. Chest 136:260–271
Diaz-Montero CM et al (2009) Increased circulating myeloid-derived suppressor cells correlate with clinical cancer stage, metastatic tumor burden, and doxorubicin-cyclophosphamide chemotherapy. Cancer Immunol Immunother 58:49–59
Dieu-Nosjean MC et al (2008) Long term survival for patients with non-small cell lung cancer with intratumoral lymphoid structures. J Clin Oncol 26:4410–4417

Digumarti R et al (2011) A randomized, double-blind, placebo-controlled, phase II study of oral talactoferrin in combination with carboplatin and paclitaxel in previously untreated locally advanced or metastatic non-small cell lung cancer. J Thorac Oncol 6:1098–1103
Dong H et al (2002) Tumor-associated B7-H1 promotes T-cell apoptosis: a potential mechanism of immune evasion. Nat Med 8:793–800 Erratum in: Nat Med 8(9):1039
Fakhari H et al (2009) Correlation of immune responses and survival in a phase II study of belagenpumatucel-L in non-small cell lung cancer. J Clin Oncol 27(Suppl):3013
Ferlay J et al (2010) Estimates of worldwide burden of cancer in 2008: GLOBOCAN 2008. Int J Cancer 127:2893–2917
García B et al (2008) Effective inhibition of the epidermal growth factor/epidermal growth factor receptor binding by anti-epidermal growth factor antibodies is related to better survival in advanced non-small cell lung cancer patients treated with epidermal growth factor cancer vaccine. Clin Cancer Res 14:840–846
Garon EB et al (2013) Preliminary clinical safety and activity of MK-3475 monotherapy for the treatment of previously treated patients with non-small cell lung cancer. J Thorac Oncol 8 (Suppl 2):S364–S365
Giaccone G (2013) Late breaking abstract: a phase III study of belagenpumatucel-L therapeutic tumor cell vaccine for non-small cell lung cancer (NSCLC). Abstract search—European cancer congress 2013. http://eccamsterdam2013.ecco-org.eu/Scientific-Programme/Abstract-search.aspx?abstractid=8961
Goldstraw P et al (2011) Non-small-cell lung cancer. Lancet 378:1727–1740
Gomez RE, Ardigo ML (2012) Anti-idiotype antibodies in cancer treatment: the pharmaceutical industry perspective. Frontiers Oncol 2, Article 147
Gomez RE et al (2013) Active immunotherapy in patients with progressive disease (PD) after first line therapy: Racotumomab experience. J Clin Oncol 31(Suppl):3086
González G et al (1998) A novel cancer vaccine composed of human-recombinant epidermal growth factor linked to a carrier protein: report of a pilot clinical trial. Ann Oncol 9:431–435
González G et al (2003) Epidermal growth factor-based cancer vaccine for non-small cell lung cancer therapy. Ann Oncol 14:461–466
González G et al (2007) Therapeutic vaccination with epidermal growth factor (EGF) in advanced lung cancer. Human Vaccines 3:8–13
Hanagiri T et al (2013) Clinical significance of the frequency of regulatory T cells in regional lymph node lymphocytes as a prognostic factor for non-small-cell lung cancer. Lung Cancer 81:475–479
Hayes TG, Falchook GS (2010) Phase IB of oral talactoferrin in the treatment of patients with metastatic solid tumors. Invest New Drugs 28:156–162
Hayes DN et al (2006a) Gene expression profiling reveals reproducible human lung adenocarcinoma subtypes in multiple independent patient cohorts. J Clin Oncol 24:5079–5090
Hayes TG et al (2006b) Phase I trial of oral talactoferrin alfa in refractory solid tumors. Invest New Drugs 24:233–240
Hernández AM et al (2008) Characterization of the antibody response against NeuGcGM3 ganglioside elicited in non-small cell lung cancer patients immunized with an anti-idiotypic antibody. J Immunol 181:6625–6634
Hiltbold EM (1999) Presentation of MUC1 tumor antigen by class I MHC and CTL function correlate with the glycosylation state of the protein taken up by dendritic cells. Cell Immunol 194:143–149
Ho SB et al (1993) Heterogeneity of mucin gene expression in normal and neoplastic tissues. Cancer Res 53:641–651
Hodi SF et al (2010) Ipilimumab plus dacarbacine for previously untreated metastatic melanoma. N Engl J Med 363:711–723
Huang A et al (2013) Increased CD14+HLA-DR-/low myeloid-derived suppressor cells correlate with extrathoracic metastasis and poor response to chemotherapy in non-small cell lung cancer patients. Cancer Immunol Immunother 62:1439–1451

Inderberg-Suso E-M et al (2012) Widespread CD4[+] T-cell reactivity to novel hTERT epitopes following vaccination of cancer patients with single hTERT peptide GV1001. Oncoimmunology 1:670–686

Joziasse DH, Orial R (1999) Xenotransplantation: the importance of the Galalpha1,3Gal epitope in hyperacute vascular rejection. Biochim Biophys Acta 1455:403–418

Katz LH et al (2013) Targeting TGF-β signaling in cancer. Expert Opin Ther Targets 17:743–760

Kawai O et al (2008) Predominant infiltration of macrophages and CD8(+) T cells in cancer nests is a significant predictor of survival in stage IV non-small cell lung cancer. Cancer 113:1387–1395

Kelly RJ, Giaccone G (2010) The role of talactoferrin alfa in the treatment of non-small cell lung cancer. Expert Opin Biol Ther 10:1379–1386

Kim NW et al (1994) Specific association of human telomerase activity with immortal cells and cancer. Science 266:2011–2015

Konishi J et al (2004) B7-H1 expression on non small cell lung cancer cells and its relationship with tumor infiltrating lymphocytes and their PD-1 expression. Clin Cancer Res 10:5094–5100

Kruit WH (2008) Immunization with recombinant MAGE-A3 protein combined with adjuvant systems AS15 or AS 02B in patients with unresectable and progressive metastatic cutaneous melanoma: a randomized open-label Phase II study of the EORTC Melanoma Group (16032–18031). J Clin Oncol 26(Suppl):9065

Kruit WH et al (2013) Selection of immunostimulant AS15 for active immunization with MAGE-A3 protein: results of a randomized phase II study of the European Organization for Research and Treatment of Cancer Melanoma Group in metastatic melanoma. J Clin Oncol 31:2413–2420

Kufe DW (2009) Mucins in cancer: function, prognosis and therapy. Nature Reviews 9:874–885

Kwak EL, Bang YJ, Camidge DR et al (2010) Anaplastic lymphoma kinase inhibition in non-small-cell lung cancer. N Engl J Med 363:1693–1703

Kyte JA (2009) Cancer vaccination with telomerase peptide GV1001. Expert Opin Investig Drugs 18:687–694

Leach DR, Krummel MF, Allison JP (1996) Enhancement of antitumor immunity by CTLA-4 blockade. Science 271:1734–1736

Limacher J-M, Quoix E (2012) TG4010. A therapeutic vaccine against MUC1 expressing tumors. Oncoimmunology 1:791–792

Link CR Jr et al (1998) Eliciting hyperacute xenograft response to treat human cancer: alpha (1,3) galactosyltransferase gene therapy. Anticancer Res 18:2301–2308

Lynch TJ et al (2010) Phase II trial of ipilimumab (IPI) and paclitaxel/carboplatin (P/C) in first line stage IIIb/IV non-small cell lung cancer (NSCLC). J Clin Oncol 28(Suppl):7531

Macias A et al (2012) Active specific immunotherapy with racotumomab in the treatment of advanced non small cell lung cancer (NSCLC). Ann Oncol 23(Suppl 9, ix):406

Madan RA et al (2013) Effect of talactoferrin alfa on the immune system in adults with non-small cell lung cancer. The Oncologist 18:821–822

Middleton GW et al (2013) A phase III randomized trial of chemoimmunotherapy comprising gemcitabine and capecitabine with or without telomerase vaccine GV1001 in patients with locally advanced or metastatic pancreatic cancer. J Clin Oncol 31(Suppl):LBA4004

Mitchell PL et al (2013) Mucin 1 (MUC1) expression in patients (pts) with early stage non-small cell lung cancer (NSCLC): relationship between immunohistochemistry (IHC), tumor characteristics, and survival. J Clin Oncol 31(Suppl):3011

Morris J-C et al (2012) Correlation of interferon-g (γ) response with survival in a phase II hyperacute (HAL) immunotherapy trial for non-small cell lung cancer (NSCLC). J Clin Oncol 30(Suppl):2571

Morris JC et al (2013) Potential chemo-sensitization effect of tergenpumatucel-L immunotherapy in treated patients with adjuvant non-small cell lung cancer (NSCLC). J Clin Oncol 31 (Suppl):8094

National Comprehensive Cancer Network (NCCN) (2014) Clinical Practice Guidelines in Oncology. Non-small cell lung cancer, version 3.2014. Accesses 22 April 2014

Nemunaitis J et al (2006) Phase II study of belagenpumatucel-L, a transforming growth factor beta-2 antisense gene-modified allogeneic tumor cell vaccine in non-small cell lung cancer. J Clin Oncol 24:4721–4730

Nemunaitis J et al (2009) Phase II trial of belagenpumatucel-L, a TGF-beta2 antisense gene modified allogeneic tumor vaccine in advanced non small cell lung cancer (NSCLC) patients. Cancer Gene Ther 16:620–624

Neninger Vinageras E et al (2008) Phase II randomized controlled trial of an epidermal growth factor vaccine in advanced non-small cell lung cancer. J Clin Oncol 26:1452–1458

Pardoll DM (2012) The blockade of immune checkpoints in cancer immunotherapy. Nat Rev Cancer 12:252–264

Parikh PM et al (2011) Randomized, double-blind, placebo-controlled phase II study of single-agent oral talactoferrin in patients with locally advanced or metastatic non-small cell lung cancer that progressed after chemotherapy. J Clin Onc 29:4129–4136

Peggs KS et al (2009) Blockade of CTLA-4 on both effector and regulatory T cell compartments contributes to the antitumor activity of anti-CTLA-4 antibodies. J Exp Med 206(8):1717–1725

Peters S et al (2012) Metastatic non-small-cell lung cancer (NSCLC): ESMO clinical practice guidelines for diagnosis, treatment and follow-up. Ann Oncol 23(Suppl 7):vii56–vii64

Petersen RP et al (2006) Tumor infiltrating FOXP3 regulators T cells associated with recurrence in pathologic stage I NSCLC patients. Cancer 107:2866–28762

Pirker R (2013) EGFR-directed monoclonal antibodies in non-small cell lung cancer. Targ Oncol 8:47–53

Quoix E et al (2011) Therapeutic vaccination with TG4010 and first-line chemotherapy in advanced non-small cell lung cancer: a controlled phase IIb trial. Lancet Oncol 12:1125–1133

Quoix E et al (2012) TIME: a phase IIb/III randomized, double-blind, placebo-controlled study comparing first-line therapy with or without TG4010 immunotherapy product inn patients with stage IV non-small cell lung cancer (NSCLC). J Clin Oncol 30(Suppl):TPS7610

Raijna D et al (2011) Dependence on the MUC1-C oncoprotein in non–small cell lung cancer cells. Mol Cancer Ther 10:806–816

Ramlau R et al (2008a) Randomized phase IIB trial evaluating the therapeutic vaccine TG4010 (MVA-MUC1-IL2) as an adjunct to chemotherapy in patients with advanced non-small cell lung cancer (NSCLC). J Clin Oncol 26(Suppl):8023

Ramlau R et al (2008b) A phase II study of Tg4010 (Mva-Muc1-Il2) in association with chemotherapy in patients with stage III/IV non-small cell lung cancer. J Thor Oncol 3:735–744

Rangachari D, Brahmer JR (2013) Targeting the immune system in the treatment of non-small cell lung cancer. Curr Treat Options Oncol 14(4):580–594

Robert C et al (2011) Improved survival with ipilimumab in patients with metastatic melanoma. N Engl J Med 364:2517–2526

Rochlitz C et al (2003) Phase I immunotherapy with a modified vaccinia virus (MVA) expressing human MUC1 as antigen-specific immunotherapy in patients with MUC1-positive advanced cancer. J Gene Med 5:690–699

Rodríguez PC et al (2010) Clinical development and perspectives of CIMAvax EGF, Cuban vaccine for non-small cell lung cancer therapy. MEDICC Review 12:17–23

Rodríguez PC et al (2011) Safety, immunogenicity and preliminary efficacy of multiple-site vaccination with an epidermal growth factor (EGF) based cancer vaccine in advanced non small cell lung cancer (NSCLC) patients. J Immune Based Ther Vaccines 9:1–6

Rossi G et al (2008) Allogeneic melanoma vaccine expressing aGal epitopes induced antitumor immunity to autologous antigen in mice without signs of toxicity. J Immunother 31:545–554

Salomon DS et al (1995) Epidermal growth factor-related peptides and their receptors in human malignancies. Cir Rev Oncol Hematol 19:183–232

Schreiber RD et al (2011) Cancer immunoediting: integrating immunity's roles in cancer suppression and promotion. Science 331:1565–1570

Shaw AT et al (2009) Clinical features and outcome of patients with non-small-cell lung cancer who harbor EML4-ALK. J Clin Oncol 27:4247–4253

Shaw AT et al (2013) Crizotinib versus chemotherapy in advanced ALK-positive lung cancer. N Engl J Med 368:2385–2394

Shimizu K et al (2010) Tumor infiltrating Foxp3+ regulatory T cells are correlated with cyclooxygenase-2 expression and are associated with recurrence in resected non-small cell lung cancer. J Thorac Oncol 5:585–590

Sienel W et al (2004) Melanoma associated antigen (MAGE)-A3 expression in stages I and II non-small cell lung cancer: results of a multicenter study. Eur J Cardiothorac Surg 25:131–134

So T et al (2005) Haplotype loss of HLA class I antigen as an escape mechanism from immune attack in lung cancer. Cancer Res 65:5945–5952

Spadaro M et al (2007) Requirement for INF-γ, CD8+ T Lymphocytes, and NKT cells in talactoferrin-induced inhibition of neu+ tumors. Cancer Res 67:6425–6432

Spiegel R, Socinski M (2013) Rationale for chemotherapy, immunotherapy, and checkpoint blockade in SCLC. J Thorac Oncol 8:587–589

Stinchcombe TE (2014) Unmet needs in squamous cell carcinoma of the lung: potential role for immunotherapy. Med Oncol 31:960

Suzuki K et al (2011) Prognostic immune markers in non-small cell lung cancer clin. Cancer Res 17:5247–5256

Topalian SL et al (2012) Safety, activity, and immune correlates of anti-PD-1 antibody in cancer. N Engl J Med 366:2443–2454

Tyagi P, Mirakhur B (2009) MAGRIT: the largest-ever phase III lung cancer trial aims to establish a novel tumor-specific approach to therapy. Clin Lung Cancer 10:371–374

Ulloa-Montoya F et al (2013) Predictive gene signature in MAGE-A3 antigen-specific cancer immunotherapy. J Clin Oncol 31:2388–2395

Van Cruijsen H et al (2009) Tissue micro array analysis of ganglioside N-glycolyl GM3 expression and signal transducer and activator of transcription (STAT)-3 activation in relation to dendritic cell infiltration and microvessel density in non-small cell lung cancer. BMC Cancer 9:180–189

Van den Eynde BJ et al (1997) T cell defined tumor antigens. Curr Opin Immunol 9:684–693

Vansteenkiste J et al (2007) Final results of a multi-center, double blind, randomized placebo controlled phase II study to assess the efficacy of MAGE-A3 immunotherapeutic as adjuvant therapy in stage IB/II non-small cell lung cancer (NSCLC). J Clin Oncol 25(Suppl):7554

Vansteenkiste J et al (2013) Adjuvant MAGE-A3 immunotherapy in resected non-small cell lung cancer: phase II randomized study results. J Clin Oncol 31:2396–2403

Vázquez AM et al (2012) Racotumomab: an anti-idiotype vaccine related to N-glycolyl-containing gangliosides—preclinical and clinical data. Frontiers Oncol 2:150

Velcheti V et al (2014) Programmed death ligand-1 expression in non-small cell lung cancer. Lab Investig 94:107–116

Walunas TL et al (1994) CTLA-4 can function as a negative regulator of T cell activation. Immunity 5:405–413

Woo EY et al (2001) Regulatory CD4+CD25+ T cells in tumors from patients with early-stage non-small cell lung cancer and late-stage ovarian cancer. Cancer Res 61:4766–4772

Zhao Q et al (2009) Circulating galectin-3 promotes metastasis by modifying MUC1 localization on cancer cell surface. Cancer Res 69:6799–6806

Zotter S et al (1988) Tissue and tumor distribution of human polymorphic epithelial mucin. Cancer Rev 11–12:55–101

Novel Approaches for Vaccination Against HPV-Induced Cancers

Emma King, Christian Ottensmeier and Kevin G.J. Pollock

Abstract To date, more than 5 % of all cancers are as a result of human papillomavirus (HPV) infection, and this incidence is increasing. Early recognition of disease is associated with good survival, but late presentation results in devastating consequences. Prevention is better than cure, and there are now successful prophylactic vaccination programmes in place. We discuss these and the prospect of therapeutic vaccinations in the near future to address a growing need for improved therapeutic options.

Contents

E. King (✉) · C. Ottensmeier
University of Southampton, Southampton, UK
e-mail: e.king@soton.ac.uk

K.G.J. Pollock (✉)
Health Protection Scotland, Glasgow, Scotland
e-mail: kevin.pollock@nhs.net

Current Topics in Microbiology and Immunology (2017) 405:33–53
DOI 10.1007/82_2015_430

Published Online: 04 March 2015

1 HPV Lifecycle—Exposure, Infection and Clearance

Infections cause more than 15 % of human cancers, and approximately one-third of these are as a result of human papillomavirus (HPV). HPV is a ubiquitous double-stranded DNA virus, and it is estimated that there are more than 100 different HPV types that can infect humans. They are subdivided into low and high risk (HR), pertaining to their malignant potential. It is estimated that a third of all primary school children are infected with low-risk HPV, resulting in cutaneous warts (Bruggink et al. 2012). Cervical smear samples in unvaccinated women suggest that approximately half of women aged 20–21 carry an infection with HR HPV types and 58 % are infected with any HPV type (Kavanagh et al. 2014). Prevalence studies using oral swabbing and testing for HPV suggest that 37–60 % of people are infected, although there are a number of caveats to consider with such prevalence studies (Steinau et al. 2014). Given that oropharyngeal and cervical cancers are relatively rare (although the former are increasingly incident), it is evident that most people who are exposed to HPV through sexual contact will clear the virus via cell-mediated immunity (Stern et al. 2000).

The HPV virus contains both 'early' and 'late' genes: the early genes, E1 and E2, are virus-encoded replication factors; E4 and E5 act to regulate late viral functions by mechanisms that are not yet well understood. Interestingly, E3 exists in only a few papillomavirus types, but not HPV16 (the HR subtype that is responsible for more than 97 % of HPV-driven malignancy in head and neck squamous cell carcinoma): the gene is not expressed as a protein and has no known function. Late genes L1 and L2 are synthesised following amplification and produce capsid proteins, which the virus needs for full assembly and release of infectious virions (Shulzhenko et al. 2014).

In the cervix (where most extensively studied), HPV virions infect the basal cell layer, as a result of microwounds that expose the basal layer. Viral capsids bind initially to the basement membrane and then to keratinocytes, as they move into the wound (Kines et al. 2009). Both Annexin A2 and S100 calcium-binding protein A10 are integral but with separate roles during HPV16 binding, entry and trafficking of HPV16 (Dziduszko and Ozbun 2013). Following cellular entry and uncoating, HPV is replicated in the nucleus to about 100 episomal copies per cell. This phase is orchestrated by the early genes, E1, E2, E6 and E7. E1 and E2 initiate viral DNA replication, and E6 and E7 maintain long-term replication competence (Frattini and Laimins 1994; Sedman and Stenlund 1995). In undifferentiated basal cells, the viral proteins are expressed at very low levels, favouring immune evasion. As the basal cells divide, each daughter cell contains HPV within the nucleus: E2 is central to this process as it binds to specific ACCN6GGT motifs in the viral genome and attaches it to mitotic chromosomes, tethering the virus genome to the host chromosomes during meiosis (Mcbride et al. 2006). In addition, E2 maintains a stable viral copy number, essential to allow continued persistence in basal cells; it can both positively and negatively regulate the early viral promoter that regulates E1, E6 and E7 as well as E2 itself (Steger and Corbach 1997).

Although the undifferentiated basal cells contain very low levels of viral proteins, as the infected host cell leaves the basal layer and differentiates, high levels of protein synthesis are induced. This delayed expression of viral proteins undoubtedly delays expression of viral antigens until they are in a less immune-competent compartment. However, sustaining long-term viral infection is a strategy not without problems: the virus does not produce its own replicative enzymes, host cell replication is required, and as the host cell differentiates, replication stops. To overcome this problem, the virus forces the differentiated cell to continue to replicate, largely under the control of E7 and its ability to inactivate retinoblastoma (Rb) protein (Felsani et al. 2006). The late viral promoter increases the copy numbers from hundreds to thousands, and then, the capsid proteins are produced. L1 and L2 are considered highly immunogenic, but are not expressed until the most differentiated strata, minimising immune impact. The virions are shed into the environment without lysis or necrosis, avoiding an inflammatory response. Thus, HPV infection is entirely intraepithelial with only limited transfer of antigen to adjacent lymph nodes, minimising an adaptive immune response.

The entry of HPV into epithelial cells is best documented in cervical cells. Data relating to HPV infection in the oropharynx and other genital areas are poorly documented.

Dependent upon type, HPV infection ranges from benign cutaneous warts (primarily due to HPV 1, HPV 2, HPV 27 and HPV 57) (Bruggink et al. 2012), to genital warts, recurrent respiratory papillomatosis (HPV 6 and HPV 11) and some HR 'oncogenic' HPV types can precipitate cancers; notably the majority of cervical cancers, 75 % of oropharyngeal cancer, 90 % of anal cancers and 40 % of vulval, vaginal and penile cancers are as a result of HR HPV (Anantharaman et al. 2013; Jemal et al. 2013).

Viral infection of the host can have several outcomes. Acute infection may develop, which is followed by recovery from the virus and total elimination of the virus mediated by cellular immunity. Alternatively, a chronic infection may persist, with prolonged carriage of the virus with or without further relapses of acute disease. Instead of immune-mediated clearance following infection, a latent stage may develop, during which clinical signs of disease are absent and new virions are not produced and released. It is possible that such latent infections may undergo subsequent reactivation leading to new virion synthesis, with or without the re-emergence of clinical disease: this late re-emergence may underlie disease recurrence including genital warts and may also contribute to the development of the aforementioned cancers (Maglennon and Doorbar 2012).

2 Malignant Transformation

In most patients, the host immune system prevails and the HPV infection resolves. However, in a significant minority, the infection is present for long periods allowing additional cellular changes and mutations to occur, leading to cancer. The ancient relationship between HPV and its host relies on productive infection to maintain a continued viral existence: under this perspective, induction of malignant transformation is beneficial to neither host nor virus, but undoubtedly occurs. Although the role of E6 and E7 in the basal layer is uncertain during infection, it is crucial in malignant transformation. During malignant progression, the HPV genome can integrate into a host cell chromosome and as a result, E6 and E7 were thought to remain the only viral proteins that continue to be expressed. HPV genome integration is a terminal event and not a manifestation of the normal viral life cycle. Interestingly, viral integration is not a prerequisite for malignant transformation and episomal persistence can also result in malignant transformation (Olthof et al. 2014): It is likely that both episomal and integrated virus exists in the same cell. In anogenital carcinoma, there is a significant correlation between the frequency of integrated viral DNA and progression of dysplastic lesions to malignancy (Vinokurova et al. 2008). In addition, integration appears to be influenced by the subtype: in cervical malignancy, 55 % of HPV16 and 92 % of HPV18 cases have viral integration. Finally, in 39 % of oropharyngeal malignancies, viral integration was detected. Interestingly, in the latter cohort, there was no significant difference in the viral copy numbers of E2, E6 or E7 in either integrated or episomal cases (Olthof et al. 2014).

HPV-induced malignant transformation has been most extensively studied in the cervix: levels of both E6 and E7 increase in parallel to the increases in degree of dysplaia, i.e. cervical intraepithelial neoplasia 1(CIN) to CIN3. In CIN1 lesions, the virus can typically complete its life cycle and produce viral particles: clinically, patients have flat cervical warts. CIN2 lesions have elevated levels of E6 and E7 compared to CIN1, predisposing them to the accumulation of genetic changes as a result of diminished tumour suppressor gene (TSG) activity. Specifically, E6 downregulates p53, and E7 downregulates Rb.

Cancers arise secondary to the action of E6 and E7 oncoprotiens, and only HR HPVs harbour significant malignant potential. Both E6 and E7 lack intrinsic enzymatic activity and function by associating with, and functionally reprogramming key components of the host cellular signal transduction networks. The E6 protein most frequently interacts with an E3 ubiquitin ligase, E6-associated protein (E6AP) (Huibregtse et al. 1991). The 'ubiquitin cascade' adds multiple ubiquitin monomers to the protein, destined to be degraded by proteosomal degradation, and this includes p53 (Scheffner et al. 1993). When p53 is bound by E6 and E6AP, it is unable to induce apoptosis and is degraded. E6 can also inhibit p53 activation by blocking the alternate reading frame p14 pathway and by interacting with histone acetyltransferase, hADA3 (Khoronenkova and Dianov 2011; Kumar et al. 2002). In addition, E6 in combination with E6AP can promote telomerase activity, via E6AP (Klingelhutz et al. 1996). Finally, HR E6 proteins (and not low-risk E6 proteins) can interact with PDZ domain-containing proteins (including hDIg) (Kiyono et al. 1997), MAGI-1 (Glaunsinger et al. 2000), hScrib (Nakagawa and Huibregtse 2000), MUPP1 (Lee et al. 2000) and PTPN3 (Jing et al. 2007) affecting epithelial cell polarity (McLaughlin-Drubin and Munger 2009; Muench et al. 2009) [ref].

Interestingly, E7 is considered the 'main' HPV oncoprotein and at low frequency is able to immortalise human epithelial cells. HPV16 E7, from both HR and LR HPV, binds the cullin 2 ubiquitin ligase complex and silences pRB and associated proteins (p105, p107, p130). The HR HPV E7 binds with much greater affinity than LR E7 (Munger et al. 2001). This binding results in E2F transcription factor repression, allowing entry into S-phase. pRb degradation results in p16 upregulation encoded by the sequence on the CDKN2a gene (Khleif et al. 1996). This results in high p16 expression in HPV-driven malignancy. Interestingly, p16 is a potent TSG, but E7 also directly activates cyclins A and E downstream of p16, negating the TSG effect (Zerfass et al. 1995). However, increased expression of p16 acts as a good biomarker for HPV-driven malignancy.

There are many additional host cell factors that HR E7 proteins bind to including HDACs 1, 2 and 3, p21, p27 (cell cycle inhibitory functions), ATM (DNA damage sensor) and p600 (anoikis). Interestingly, abrogation of pRb function by HR E7 protein leads to increased stabilisation of p53 potentially leading to increased apoptosis. As a result, the HR E6 proteins have evolved to induce degradation of p53 to block apoptosis (Howie et al. 2009). E5, E6 and E7 oncoproteins are all considered anti-apoptotic, and the main contributors to malignant transformation, E2 and E7 are also pro-apoptotic proteins, and a balance therefore exists (Garnett and Duerksen-Hughes 2006).

Interestingly, E6 and E7 also act as potent mitotic mutators, thereby increasing the occurrence of mutations that contribute to carcinogenic progression (McLaughlin-Drubin and Munger 2009). The E6 and E7 genes are located in the same open reading frame and are transcribed as a single transcript. E2 protein differentially regulates E6/E7 expression: the transcription of E6/E7 is controlled by E2. E2 binds to its promoter which upregulates p97, which in turn activates the transcription of E6. Interestingly, E2 protein stabilises p53 and maintains apoptosis in HeLa cells (Webster et al. 2000). HPV 16 and HPV 18 E2 proteins have been shown to activate transcription of HPV 16 E6 and E7 oncogenes (Bouvard et al. 1994); however, there are numerous other factors that affect the repression and activation of E6 and E7 oncoproteins. When HPV integrates into the host genome, E2 is inhibited, resulting in a loss of E2 apoptosis and E2-mediated regulation of E6 and E7 (Arisa-Pulido et al. 2006). Clearly, episomal virus does not lose E2-mediated regulation.

Although E6 and E7 are cited as the main oncogenes, E5 also has a role to play. E5 is the smallest HPV oncoprotein and in HPV16, E5 is primarily localised within the endoplasmic reticulum (ER) (Conrad et al. 1993; Borzacchiello et al. 2010). E5 expression in oropharynx malignancy is associated with high EGFR expression, which is linked with poor outcome (Um et al. 2014). E5 protects against apoptosis through inhibition of death receptor apoptosis and ER stress-induced apoptosis (Jiang and Yue 2014). E5 protein may cooperate with E6 and E7 to immortalise cells, and play an inhibitory role in apoptosis (Jiang and Yue 2014). E5 may contribute to the early stages of cancer initiation, but in integrated viruses, E5 is often lost and is not necessary for the maintenance of the transformed phenotype.

Interestingly, in low-risk subtypes, E5 is missing or lacks an ORF and/or a translation start codon (Schiffman et al. 2005).

We understand now that the host immune system is central to survival in many solid tumours, including HPV-induced head and neck malignancy (Ward et al. 2014a). It is likely that it is also important during the early stages of malignant transformation: in order to restrict an immune response, it is probable that both the adaptive and innate immune systems are affected by HPV-infected cells. Healthy keratinocytes constitutively express low levels of interferon-inducible genes in the absence of added interferon. However, cells infected by high-risk HPV E6 and E7 proteins repress the transcription of many interferon target genes including Stat-1, IRF-1 and IRF-3. In addition, both E6 and E7 can minimise the expression of TLR-9, important to sense double-stranded DNA (Ghittoni et al. 2010). Furthermore, keratinocytes constitutively express low levels of several proteins that are upregulated following viral infection. HPV infection does not result in upregulation of key pro-inflammatory cytokines including IL-1, IL-6, TNFa and TGFb, but does upregulate anti-inflammatory IL-10 (Alcocer-González et al. 2006). Clearance of HPV-infected lesions is via cell-mediated responses and cytolysis, and dendritic cells are central to this process. HPV L2 proteins have been shown to suppress maturation, migration and cytokine secretion by dendritic cells (Fahey et al. 2009). MHC class I is downregulated as a result of E6, E7 or E5. In addition, E7 has been reported to downregulate TAP, interfering with antigen presentation via MHC class I (O'Brien and Saveria Campo 2002). Clinically, immunosuppressed patients are at increased risk of both benign and malignant HPV infections. Rates of anal HPV infection are extremely high in HIV-positive patients, especially in those men that have sex with men, resulting in high rates of anal intraepithelial neoplasia (AIN) and anal cancer (Gami et al. 2014).

3 HPV-Related Cancer

The World Health Organization (WHO) published their 'position paper' on HPV in 2009. It identified that in 2005, there were 500,000 cases of cervical cancer and 260,000 related deaths worldwide. The rates were variable from 1 to 50 per 100,000 females, higher in Latin America and the Caribbean, sub-Saharan Africa and Asia. Most were diagnosed when older than 40 years. Up to 80 % can be prevented by screening programmes, and mortality rates remain significantly higher in the developing world.

Vulvar, vaginal, penile, anal and oropharyngeal cancers, and their precancerous lesions are all relatively rare, and most of these cancers occur in adults aged more than 50 years. HPVs are estimated to cause at least 80 % of anal cancer, 75 % of oropharyngeal cancer and 40–60 % of vulvar, vaginal and penile cancers, though prevalence rates do vary.

The estimated burden of non-cervical HPV-related cancers in Europe is higher in men than in women and is driven primarily by head and neck cancers. It has been estimated that 17,403 cancer cases attributable to HPV (15,497 attributable to HPV 16/18) occur each year in *men* in Europe. This compares with an estimated 9,308 non-cervical cancer cases attributable to HPV 16/18 each year in *women* in Europe (Hartwig et al. 2012).

3.1 Cervical Cancer

HPV infections in the genital tract are the most common sexually transmitted infections. Although progression to malignancy is rare, the high prevalence of the virus makes HPV-related cancers among the most common malignancies. In the UK, cervical cancer is the second most common cancer in women under 35 years [1]. HPV types 16 and 18 are essential precipitants in at least 70 % of cervical cancers (Smith et al. 2007) but may contribute in excess of 80 % of cervical cancers in particular geographic areas, such as Scotland (Cuschieri et al. 2010). Worldwide, 0.5 million new cases of cervical cancer are reported with 274,000 associated deaths annually, making it the second most prevalent cancer in women (Brotherton et al. 2011). Certain HR HPV types, recognised as class I carcinogens by the WHO, are necessary risk factors for the development of cervical cancer.

Not all cervical precancers progress to an invasive cancer: Approximately 25 % of CIN2 and 3 lesions completely regress within a short time frame (4 months) (Trimble et al. 2005). Detection of antibodies against E6 and E7 in serum does not predict which lesions will regress (Trimble et al. 2009a). However, the presence of CD8+ T cells in cervical dysplastic lesions does predict dysplasia regression (Trimble et al. 2010).

High-risk viruses in the cervix include HPV 16, HPV 18, HPV 31, HPV 33 and HPV 45, and together they cause 97 % of cervical cancers worldwide. By contrast, HPV 6 and HPV 11 frequently infect the genital tract, but are rarely detected in malignancy (Lorincz et al. 1992). In all, there are more than 40 HPV subtypes frequently detected within the female genital tract (Schiffman et al. 2005): Schiffman et al. prospectively followed 10,000 women and identified HPV16 as uniquely likely to both persist and to cause neoplastic progression when it persisted. Remarkably, 20 % of HPV16-infected women were either diagnosed with CIN3 or cancer either at enrolment or within 5 years. Other carcinogenic types were not as persistent, but could induce malignancy at a less frequent rate, and many were persistent, without significant malignant potential. Most women clear the infection within 12–18 months. However, a 10 % minority fail to clear the infection, resulting in a persistent infection: if this is HR HPV, there is a risk of malignant progression.

HPV is not only implicated in squamous cell carcinoma (SCC). In the cervix, HPV DNA is detected in most adenocarcinomas, adenosquamous carcinomas and carcinomas with neuroendocrine differentiation (Howley and Lowy 2007). HPV16 is most commonly associated with squamous cell carcinomas, while HPV18 is the predominant type found in adenocarcinomas and neuroendocrine carcinomas.

The Papanicolaou (Pap) smear allows the recognition of cellular abnormalities in HPV-infected cells, and screening has reduced the number of cervical cancers by 80 % in the USA, over the past 50 years. Early stages (I–IIa) of cervical cancer can be treated successfully, but locally advanced cancers are characterised by high recurrence rates and a poor prognosis. The standard therapy of locally advanced cervical cancer is a combination of radiotherapy and cisplatin-based chemotherapy with an overall 5-year survival of less than 50 %. Patients with stage IV or recurrent cervical cancer treated with cisplatin alone or in combination with topotecan only have a median survival of less than 1 year [57].

3.2 Anogenital Cancer

Anogenital malignancies include those arising from the vulva, vagina, penis, scrotum and anus. The majority (90 %) of vulval carcinomas are SCC, representing 4–5 % of malignancies in women (Dittmer et al. 2012). The majority of these are in older women and not related to HPV. However, there is an increasing incidence in younger (<50) women, and 43 % are related to HPV 16 and HPV 18. Early lymph node spread is frequent due to the prominent lymphatic supply, and surgery is the primary mode of treatment. Survival varies from early- to late-stage disease from 90 to 18 %.

Vaginal cancer is rare with under 260 new cases diagnosed in the UK each year (CRUK), less than 1 out of every 600 cancers diagnosed in women. Seventy percentage of vaginal cancers are caused by HPV, the majority HPV16. Treatment is radiotherapy (with or without chemotherapy) and salvage surgery if required.

Penile cancer is rare in men in developed countries, but common in underdeveloped countries. Risk factors include non-circumcision and HPV infection. HPV DNA has been identified in both benign and malignant penile lesions including condylomata acuminate, Bowens disease and SCC (Schoeneich et al. 1999). Lymphadenopathy is present between 28 and 64 % of cases at presentation. Surgery is the main form of treatment.

Scrotal carcinoma is also associated with HPV, predominately subtype 18. In a recent study, 40 % of patients had HPV-driven scrotal SCC (Matoso et al. 2014). It is again treated surgically with wide local excision, and survival is related to stage at presentation.

Anal carcinoma is an uncommon malignancy. In the general population, the incidence is between 0.8 and 1.4 cases per 100,000 people-years. This rises to 35 and 128 cases per 100,000 in men practicing anal intercourse and those HIV-positive patients practicing anal intercourse, respectively. Risk groups include HPV16 infection and high-grade AIN. Most AIN is associated with HPV (6, 11, 16 and 18). The risk for progression to malignancy from AIN is 10 % at 5 years (Scholefield et al. 2011). HPV is responsible for approximately 3,000 anal cancer cases in the USA per year (Markowitz et al. 2007).

3.3 Oropharynx Cancer

Head and neck SCC is the sixth leading incident cancer worldwide. In the USA, there were 11,500 deaths in 2012 from this malignancy (Siegel et al. 2012). Of these, HPV is responsible for approximately 3,500 of the cases (Markowitz et al. 2007). There has been a significant increase (225 %) in HPV-driven head and neck malignancy over the past 15–20 years, and this is predicted to continue to rise (Chaturvedi et al. 2011), especially in the Western world, where smoking is in decline. By 2020, the number of HPV head and neck cancers will exceed cervical cancers if this trend continues. Compared to HPV-independent head and neck cancer, HPV-driven patients are younger, frequently white males, non- or light-smokers and with only moderate or light alcohol consumption. It is likely that HPV head and neck cancer is a sexually transmitted disease (Gillison et al. 2008). HPV-driven cancer in the head and neck is predominantly related to the oropharynx. The oropharynx is an anatomical subsite that includes both palatine and lingual tonsils, soft palate and lateral pharyngeal wall. Both distinct sets of tonsillar tissue consist of organised lymphoid tissue, surrounded by stratified squamous epithelium. The surface area is significantly increased due to multiple crypts, facilitating antigen capture and immunosurveillance. This epithelium has an incomplete basal cell layer and basement membrane (to facilitate antigen trafficking), dispensing with the need for microtrauma for viral access (Pai and Westra 2009).

Traditional risk factors for head and neck cancer were smoking and alcohol. This cohort of patients have a significantly worse prognosis than those with HPV-driven malignancy (Ward et al. 2014b). Treatment includes surgery, chemotherapy or radiotherapy, either alone or in combination. In the HPV-driven group, survival does not depend on treatment type, instead on the infiltration of lymphocytes into the tumour (Ward et al. 2014a, b).

4 Prophylactic Vaccination—Cohorts Vaccinated, Uptake, Serological Evaluation

Both the prophylactic bivalent (Cervarix [HPV16 and 18]) and quadrivalent (Gardasil [HPV 6, HPV 11, HPV 16 and HPV 18]) vaccines prevent infection using L1 virus-like particles (VLP). Both prevent cervical HPV 16 and HPV 18 infection and confer protection against subsequent virally induced CIN (Paavonen et al. 2009; Brotherton et al. 2011; Pollock et al. 2014). Low levels of neutralising antibodies against L1 are detectable in 50–70 % of patients, 6–18 months following HPV infection (Viscidi et al. 1997; Carter et al. 2000; Safaeian et al. 2010). E1, E2, E6 and L2 do not evoke any measurable antibody response following natural infection (Mariani and Venuti 2010).

Although it is assumed that that the HPV vaccine protects via neutralising antibody, this mechanism has only ever been demonstrated in a preclinical model using passive transfer of serum immunoglobulins (Suzich et al. 1995). More recent evidence suggests that AS04-adjuvanted vaccines (such as Cervarix) stimulate NF-κB with increased cytokine production as a result of increased numbers of activated, antigen-loaded dendritic cells and monocytes in the lymph nodes draining the injection site, further increasing the activation of antigen-specific T cells (Didierlaurent et al. 2009). Systemic immunisations with L1 VLP generates antibody concentrations fourfold higher than following a natural infection, as a result of both route of administration and concentration of antigen (Harro et al. 2001). Although the commercial HPV vaccines have proven efficacy, the correlation between either antibody levels or B-cell memory has not been established (Stanley et al. 2012). Animal models suggest that only very low levels of antibody are required to be protective (Day et al. 2010).

Although both Gardasil and Cervarix use L1 VLP, quadrivalent vaccine produces neutralising antibodies to HPV L1, which are type restricted and possess limited cross-reactivity. However, bivalent vaccine confers a degree of cross-protection against some phylogenetically related types including HPV 31, HPV 33 and HPV 45 (Kavanagh et al. 2014). While L2 does not produce a neutralising antibody response in natural infections (it is not highly immunogenic, unlike L1), following deliberate immunisation with L2 protein, neutralising antibodies were protective against viral challenge in cows and rabbits. Strikingly, these antibodies could cross-neutralise a broad range of HPV subtypes (Karanam et al. 2009). However, this vaccine remains poorly immunogenic, consistent with other protein vaccines, compared to the L1 VLP. Attempts to improve its immunogenicity are currently being tested in animal models (Tyler et al. 2014).

Population-based surveillance data from countries such as Australia, Denmark and the United Kingdom provides early encouragement that prophylactic HPV vaccination is significantly associated with a reduction in both low- and high-grade cervical abnormalities (CIN1-3) in young women (Brotherton et al. 2011; Crowe et al. 2014; Baldur-Felskov et al. 2014; Pollock et al. 2014). Furthermore, the quadrivalent vaccine, which additionally includes HPV types 6 and 11 that are associated with 85–95 % of genital warts, has also been shown to be strongly associated with a reduction in genital warts in both females and heterosexual males (Ali et al. 2013). In Australia, the decrease in genital warts in heterosexual men was observed prior to the implementation of vaccination of boys and is likely due to herd immunity.

In the Western world, cancers of the anus, penis, scrotum, vagina and vulva (henceforth described as non-cervical genital cancers) are increasing in incidence (Parkin and Bray 2006). The increase in non-cervical genital cancers may be associated with a concomitant rise in HR oncogenic HPV infections, with HPV 16 and HPV 18 estimated to contribute between 74–93 % of these cancers (Olsen et al. 2012). Autoinoculation of HPV occurs both from cervix to anus and from anus to cervix in the same woman, and it appears to be relatively common (Moscicki et al. 2012). Although no natural history studies of anal intra-epithelial neoplasia (AIN) are available in women, women with other HPV-associated lesions, including high-grade CIN and vulvar cancer, have higher rates of anal cancer. Therefore, it seems biologically plausible that girls vaccinated with the HPV vaccine will have a significantly reduced propensity in developing non-cervical genital cancers and oropharyngeal malignancy (Garland et al. 2009; Giuliano et al. 2011; Kreimer et al. 2011; Olsen et al. 2012; Herrero et al. 2013) with a successful prophylactic vaccination programme.

While the benefits of the HPV vaccine are now being realised (Crowe et al. 2014; Ali et al. 2013; Pollock et al. 2014), efficacy is dependent on a number of critical factors. National vaccine programmes, which target preadolescent girls through school-based delivery, are likely to be more successful in preventing HPV infection and disease (Sinka et al. 2014; Pollock et al. 2014). However, such coordinated programmes require a robust and well-governed infrastructure and tend only to be a feature of affluent countries. In spite of this, a high HPV vaccine uptake has been achieved in Rwanda, showing what can be achieved (Hopkins and Wood 2013). Nevertheless, the burden of disease attributable to HPV infection is significantly greater in deprived countries, where recognised barriers such as high vaccine cost must be overcome if global burden of disease is to be reduced (Campo and Roden 2010).

Gender-neutral vaccination has been recommended in the USA, Canada, Austria and Australia. Considered cost-effective modelling has preceded such decisions suggesting that when the burden of disease in men is included in the models, depending upon vaccine price and vaccine uptake as well as other factors, male vaccination can become cost-effective (Stanley 2014). Although the HPV vaccine is not currently offered to boys within the United Kingdom, the UK Joint Committee on Vaccination and Immunisation is appraising the evidence as to whether vaccination of boys would be cost-effective. In a recent Norwegian analysis, public health priority and cost-effectiveness appears to be directed towards increasing vaccine uptake in girls rather than expanding vaccination coverage to boys, but this is crucially dependent upon vaccine tender price (Burger et al. 2014).

There are indirect benefits of the HPV vaccine. Achieving high HPV vaccine uptake may reduce inequalities in cervical cancer prevention by mitigating inequalities observed in the cervical screening programme. Knowledge and awareness of HPV infection, cervical cancer and screening in young girls who have been vaccinated against the virus is surprisingly low (Bowyer et al. 2013). Thus, it may be assumed that in older women knowledge and awareness of the virus and its association with cervical cancer will be even lower. By having a high-profile HPV vaccine campaign with prompt dissemination of the realised benefits, it provides an opportunity to emphasise the importance of attendance at cervical screening for both vaccinated women and older, unvaccinated women. Given that there is a small minority of mothers and daughters from disadvantaged backgrounds who do not participate in either cervical screening or HPV vaccination, it is imperative that awareness of HPV is raised through targeted efforts to reach these deprived groups (Spencer et al. 2014).

4.1 Prophylactic Vaccines for Established Lesions

Although both licensed HPV vaccines are most effective in individuals with no prior exposure to HPV, there are reports of vaccination after HPV DNA was demonstrated in cervical specimens (Hildesheim et al. 2007). They demonstrated that the bivalent vaccine did not improve the clearance rate of the virus. In addition, there are reports of resolution of HPV-induced warts after quadrivalent HPV vaccination (Silling et al. 2014; Kreuter et al. 2010). These studies enrolled patients who were immunocompromised and suggest that there may be clinical benefit in post-exposure treatment of persistent warts. However, in a recent case series, there was no clinical improvement in immunocompetent patients with HPV 6-positive condylomatas who received quadrivalent vaccine (Kreuter and Wieland 2013). It is likely that the decreased expression of L1 in chronic premalignant lesions and loss of L1 expression in SCC (and the infected basal cells) is responsible for the unsuccessful outcome of prophylactic vaccine for established malignant disease (Yoshida et al. 2008). The majority of healthy controls and cervical cancer patients are able to mount a systemic Th1 response against L1 (van Poelgeest et al. 2006). Well-designed clinical trials are required to elucidate the immunological mechanisms required for wart clearance.

5 Therapeutic Vaccines

HPV-driven malignancy unlocks a unique opportunity for cancer immunotherapy. For this patient cohort, the viral oncoproteins (E5, E6 and E7) responsible for malignant transformation and progression are known, permitting targeted treatment. In addition, there is a known immunosuppressive environment that cancer 'creates' and this must also be overcome to permit an effective immune response following vaccination. Recently, regulatory T cells (Tregs) within head and neck cancer were shown to express more immunosuppressive molecules compared to circulating Tregs (Jie et al. 2013): These molecules included cytotoxic T lymphocyte-associated antigen 4 (CTLA-4), T-cell immunoglobulin and mucin protein 3 (TIM-3) and programmed cell death ligand-1 (PD-1). In addition to the checkpoint receptors, cancer visibility to the immune system can also be lessened due to reduced expression of HLA I molecules and also transporters associated with antigen processing (TAP) (Li et al. 2010).

5.1 Proteins and Peptides

There are data to show the likely benefit of immunotherapy in HPV-driven lesions. In a small study, a HPV16 E6/E7-based peptide vaccine caused regression of

HPV-associated premalignant vulvar lesions (Kenter 2009). In addition, a second study in patients with vulval intraepithelial neoplasia (VIN) showed that using an E6E7L2 fusion protein, efficacy was associated with the induction of HPV-specific CD4 and CD8 T cells (Daayana et al. 2010; Welters et al. 2010). A number of other trials with a range of vaccines have shown variable clinical results, but none have shown a convincing correlation between clinical outcome and immunogenicity (Ressing et al. 2000; Baldwin et al. 2003; Smyth et al. 2004; Trimble et al. 2009b; Santin et al. 2008; Frazer et al. 2004; Matijevic et al. 2011; Brun et al. 2011; Maciag et al. 2009).

Current trials evaluating alternative peptide vaccines include a phase I/II study to determine the safety and immune modulating effects of the therapeutic HPV16 E6/E7 long-peptide vaccine (ISA101). This vaccine will be used at different doses with or without IFNα as combination therapy with carboplatin and paclitaxel in women with HPV16-driven advanced or recurrent cervical cancer (NCT02128126). In addition, another phase 1 trial is evaluating the treatment of high-grade squamous intraepithelial neoplasia of the cervix using a vaccine consisting of four HPV16 E6 peptides in combination with Candin® (NCT01653249). Candin is a yeast extract and has anti-HPV effects; it has been used to treat common warts caused by LR HPV. Furthermore, synthetic peptides (SLP-HPV-01® with or without interferon-α injections) are being evaluated in men with AIN (NCT01923116).

In addition, protein vaccines using HPV16-derived peptides presented as a Trojan-type construct to prevent proteolysis and facilitate HLAI processing have been trialled in head and neck patients (Voskens et al. 2012). They were combined with MAGE-A3 proteins (HLA restricted), and although a peripheral blood response could be detected (PBMCs from 4 of the 5 patients were able to recognise both the full Trojan constructs and constituent HLA-II peptides), there was no clinical response in any of the 5 patients with advanced cancer. In a study with vulval lesions, vaccination of HPV16 E6 and E7 long peptides with incomplete Freund's adjuvant in 20 women with VIN reported 50 % complete response and 75 % having a durable clinical response (Kenter et al. 2009). Unfortunately, when these long peptides were trialled in patients with high-grade CIN, the trial was terminated early due to unacceptable side effects including flu-like symptoms and injection site morbidity (de Vos van Steenwijk et al. 2012).

5.2 Viral Vectors

A modified vaccinia virus (TG4001), designed to express HPV16 E6 and E7 and IL2, was shown to induce a clinical response in 10 patients (48 %) with CIN 2 and 3 lesions following 3 weekly subcutaneous injections (Brun et al. 2011). A collaboration between transgene and EORTC was announced with a view to trial this vaccine in head and neck patients (EORTC: transgene collaborates with EORTC on phase 2b trial with TG4001 in head and neck cancer).

5.3 DNA Vaccines

DNA vaccines remain attractive due to their stability, ease of production and high expression of antigen in transfected cells, but their limited immunogenicity remains problematic (Huang et al. 2010). However, advances in delivery, including electroporation, are likely to significantly impact on immunogenicity (Sardesai and Weiner 2011). In a completed phase I trial, a microencapsulated DNA vaccine (ZYC-101) consisting of multiple HLA-A2-restricted E7 epitopes was evaluated in women with high-grade CIN. Thirty-three percentage of the patients had a complete response (Sheets et al. 2003). There is also a phase I trial currently recruiting head and neck patients testing pNGVL4a-CRT/E7 (Detox) DNA vaccine in combination with cyclophosphamide (NCT01493154). This same vaccine is being used in combination with topical imiquimod in a phase I trial for CIN 3 patients (NCT00788164). Another study (NCT00988559) is evaluating the efficacy and safety of different routes of administration of the same DNA vaccine [pNGVL4a-CRT/E7(detox)] in patients with HPV16+ CIN2/3. Patients will be enrolled in one of six treatment groups including intradermal vaccination (with a needle-free delivery device, a gene gun), intramuscular and intralesional vaccination.

NCT02172911 is an open-label study to evaluate the safety, tolerability and immunogenicity of VGX-3100 (2 separate DNA plasmids encoding E6 and E7 proteins of HPV 16 and HPV 18) and INO-9012 (DNA plasmid encoding human interleukin 12) delivered by electroporation (EP) in patients with biopsy-proven HPV 16 or HPV 18 cervical SCC.

5.4 Bacterial Vector Vaccines

Bacterial vector vaccines have been investigated, with *Listeria monocytogenes* generating the most interest due to its ability to infect APCs in the cytosolic compartment, permitting both MHC class I and II presentation (Wood and Paterson 2014). ADXS11-001 (ADXS-HPV) is a live-attenuated *L. monocytogenes* (Lm)-LLO immunotherapy in trial for the treatment of head and neck cancer HPV-associated dysplasia and malignancy as a window study prior to surgical resection (NCT02002182). This American study is due to complete recruitment ($n = 30$) in January 2015. A second study evaluating the same vaccine in CIN has just been terminated due to lack of enrolment (NCT01116245). Unfortunately, the UK head and neck trial REALISTIC has recently been terminated due to patient infection with Listeria resulting in a serious adverse reaction and withdrawal of the study by the sponsor (NCT01698792). In addition, there are 2 studies looking at the dose range (NCT01356823), efficacy and immunogenicity (NCT01735006) of recombinant HPV 16/18 bivalent vaccine expressed in *Escherichia coli* in vaginal–intraepithelial, vulval–intraepithelial, cervical–intraepithelial neoplasia and cervical cancer. Both trials are reported as ongoing but not recruiting.

For completeness, tumour cell and dendritic cell vaccines have been explored for HPV-driven disease, but production problems (including purity) and administration have remained problematic and will not be discussed further.

6 Summary

It is clear that HPV has relied on its host for both replicative machinery and productive infection for many generations. In the majority of cases, the host's immune system can clear the infection with limited morbidity. In a significant minority, a HR infection remains, providing the initial platform for malignant transformation. We do not yet understand what predisposes individual patients to harbour rather than clear the infection, but it is intriguing to understand which part of the virus/host interaction influences this outcome. It is apparent that this group of malignancies will provide insight into both prophylactic and therapeutic vaccination strategies and hopefully provide understanding that can be transferred to other solid malignancies where the obvious treatment target is not as clear-cut. It will also be interesting to observe what 'help' the immune system requires in addition to the vaccination model: whether in the form of an adjunct or discrete immunostimulatory molecules (i.e. anti-CD40 monoclonal antibodies). It is clear that this is a rapidly emerging field and data generated will facilitate our understanding of the host–tumour interaction.

Conflicts of Interest None declared.

References

Alcocer-González JM, Berumen J, Taméz-Guerra R et al (2006) In vivo expression of immunosuppressive cytokines in human papillomavirus-transformed cervical cancer cells. Viral Immunol 19:481–491

Ali H, Donovan B, Wand H et al (2013) Genital warts in young Australians five years into national human papillomavirus vaccination programme: national surveillance data. BMJ 346:f2032

Anantharaman D, Gheit T, Waterboer T et al (2013) Human papillomavirus infections and upper aero-digestive tract cancers: the ARCAGE study. J Natl Cancer Inst 17:536–545

Arisa-Pulido H, Peyton CL, Joste NE et al (2006) Human papillomavirus type 16 integration in cervical carcinoma in situ and in invasive cervical cancer. J Clin Microbiol 44:1755–1762

Baldur-Felskov B, Dehlendorff C, Munk C et al (2014) Early impact of human papillomavirus vaccination on cervical neoplasia—nationwide follow-up of young Danish women. J Natl Cancer Inst 106:djt460

Baldwin PJ, van der Burg SH, Boswell CM et al (2003) Vaccinia-expressed human papillomavirus 16 and 18 e6 and e7 as a therapeutic vaccination for vulval and vaginal intraepithelial neoplasia. Clin Cancer Res 9:5205–5213

Borzacchiello G, Roperto F, Campo MS et al (2010) 1st international workshop on papillomavirus E5 oncogene—a report. Virology 408:135–137

Bouvard V, Storey A, Pim D et al (1994) Characterization of the human papillomavirus E2 protein: evidence of trans-activation and trans-repression in cervical keratinocytes. EMBO J 13:5451–5459

Bowyer HL, Marlow LA, Hibbitts S et al (2013) Knowledge and awareness of HPV and the HPV vaccine among young women in the first routinely vaccinated cohort in England. Vaccine 31:1051–1056

Brotherton JML, Fridman M, May CL et al (2011) Early effect of the HPV vaccination programme on cervical abnormalities in Victoria, Australia: an ecological study. Lancet 377:2085–2092

Bruggink SC, de Koning MN, Gussekloo J et al (2012) Cutaneous wart-associated HPV types: prevalence and relation with patient characteristics. J Clin Virol 55:250–255

Brun JL, Dalstein V, Leveque J et al (2011) Regression of high-grade cervical intraepithelial neoplasia with TG4001 targeted immunotherapy. Am J Obstet Gynecol 204:169 [e161–e168]

Burger EA, Sy S, Nygard M et al (2014) Prevention of HPV-related cancers in Norway: cost-effectiveness of expanding the HPV vaccination program to include pre-adolescent boys. PLoS One 9:e89974

Campo MS, Roden RBS (2010) Papillomavirus prophylactic vaccines: established successes, new approaches. J Virol 84:1214–1220

Carter JJ, Koutsky LA, Hughes JP et al (2000) Comparison of human papillomavirus types 16, 18, and 6 capsid antibody responses following incident infection. J Infect Dis 181:1911–1919

Chaturvedi AK, Engels EA, Pfeiffer RM et al (2011) Human papillomavirus and rising oropharyngeal cancer incidence in the United States. J Clin Oncol 29:4294–4301

Conrad M, Bubb VJ, Schlegel R (1993) The human papillomavirus type 6 and 16 E5 proteins are membrane-associated proteins which associated with the 16-kilodalton pore-forming protein. J Virol 67:6170–6178

Crowe E, Pandeya N, Brotherton JML et al (2014) Effectiveness of quadrivalent human papillomavirus vaccine for the prevention of cervical abnormalities: case-control study nested within a population based screening programme in Australia. BMJ Open 348:g1458

Cuschieri K, Brewster DH, Williams ARW et al (2010) Distribution of HPV types associated with cervical cancers in Scotland and implications for the impact of HPV vaccines. Br J Cancer 102:930–932

Daayana S, Elkord E, Winters U et al (2010) Phase II trial of imiquimod and HPV therapeutic vaccination in patients with vulval intraepithelial neoplasia. Br J Cancer 102:1129–1136

Day PM, Kines RC, Thompson CD et al (2010) In vivo mechanisms of vaccine-induced protection against HPV infection. Cell Host Microbe 8:260–270

de Vos van Steenwijk PJ, Ramwadhdoebe TH, Lowik MJ et al (2012) A placebo controlled randomized HPV16 synthetic long-peptide vaccination study in women with high-grade cervical squamous intraepithelial lesions. Cancer Immunol Immunother CII 61:1485–1492

Didierlaurent AM, Morel S, Lockman L (2009) AS04, an aluminum salt- and TLR4 agonist-based adjuvant system, induces a transient localized innate immune response leading to enhanced adaptive immunity. J Immunol 183:6186–6197

Dittmer C, Fischer D, Diedrich K et al (2012) Diagnosis and treatment options of vulvar cancer: a review. Arch Gynecol Obstet 285:183–193

Dziduszko A, Ozbun MA (2013) Annexin A2 and S100A10 regulate human papillomavirus type 16 entry and intracellular trafficking in human keratinocytes. J Virol 87:7502–7515

Fahey LM, Raff AB, Da Silva DM et al (2009) A major role for the minor capsid protein of human papillomavirus type 16 in immune escape. J Immunol 183:6151–6156

Felsani A, Mileo AM, Paggi MG (2006) Retinoblastoma family proteins as key targets of the small DNA virus oncoproteins. Oncogene 25(38):5277–5285

Frattini MG, Laimins LA (1994) Binding of the human papillomavirus E1 origin-recognition protein is regulated through complex formation with the E2 enhancer-binding protein. Proc Natl Acad Sci USA 91:12398–12402

Frazer IH, Quinn M, Nicklin JL et al (2004) Phase 1 study of HPV16-specific immunotherapy with E6E7 fusion protein and ISCOMATRIX adjuvant in women with cervical intraepithelial neoplasia. Vaccine 23:172–181

Gami B, Kubba F, Ziprin P (2014) Human papilloma virus and squamous cell carcinoma of the anus. Clin Med Insights Oncol 8:113–119
Garland SM, Steben M, Sings HL et al (2009) Natural history of genital warts: analysis of the placebo arm of 2 randomized phase III trials of a quadrivalent human papillomavirus (types 6, 11, 16, and 18) vaccine. J Infect Dis 199(6):805–814
Garnett TO, Duerksen-Hughes PJ (2006) Modulation of apoptosis by human papillomavirus (HPV) oncoproteins. Arch Virol 151:2321–2335
Ghittoni R, Accardi R, Hasan U et al (2010) The biological properties of E6 and E7 oncoproteins from human papillomaviruses. Virus Genes 40:1–13
Gillison ML, D'Souza G, Westra W et al (2008) Distinct risk factor profiles for human papillomavirus type 16-positive and human papillomavirus type 16-negative head and neck cancers. J Natl Cancer Inst 100:407–420
Giuliano AR, Palefsky JM, Goldstone S et al (2011) Efficacy of quadrivalent HPV vaccine against HPV infection and disease in males. N Engl J Med 364(5):401–411
Glaunsinger BA, Lee SS, Thomas M et al (2000) Interactions of the PDZprotein MAGI-1 with adenovirus E4-ORF1 and high-risk papillomavirus E6 oncoproteins. Oncogene 19:5270–5280
Harro CD, Pang YY, Roden RB et al (2001) Safety and immunogenicity trial in adult volunteers of a human papillomavirus 16 L1 virus-like particle vaccine. J Natl Cancer Inst 93:284–492
Hartwig S, Syrjänen S, Dominiak-Felden G et al (2012) Estimation of the epidemiological burden of human papillomavirus-related cancers and non-malignant diseases in men in Europe: a review. BMC Cancer 12:30
Herrero R, Quint W, Hildesheim A (2013) Reduced prevalence of oral human papillomavirus (HPV) 4 years after bivalent HPV vaccination in a randomized clinical trial in Costa Rica. PLoS One 8(7):e68329
Hildesheim A, Herrero R, Wacholder S et al (2007) Effect of human papillomavirus 16/18 L1 viruslike particle vaccine among young women with preexisting infection: a randomized trial. JAMA 298(7):743–753
Hopkins TG, Wood N (2013) Female human papillomavirus (HPV) vaccination: global uptake and the impact of attitudes. Vaccine 31:1673–1679
Howie HL, Katzenellenbogen RA, Galloway DA (2009) Papillomavirus E6 proteins. Virology 384:324–334
Howley PM, Lowy DR (2007) Papillomaviruses. In: Knipe DM, Howley PM (eds) Fields virology, vol 2. Wolters Kluwer/Lippincott Williams &Wilkins, Philadelphia, pp 2299–2354
Huang CF, Monie A, Weng WH et al (2010) DNA vaccines for cervical cancer. Am J Transl Res 2:75–87
Huibregtse JM, Scheffner M, Howley PM (1991) A cellular protein mediates association of p53 with the E6 oncoprotein of human papillomavirus type 16 or 18. EMBO J 10:4129–4135
Jemal A, Simard EP, Dorell C et al (2013) Annual report to the nation on the status of cancer, 1975–2009, featuring the burden and trends in human papillomavirus (HPV)—associated cancers and hpv vaccination coverage levels. J Natl Cancer Inst 105:175–201
Jiang P, Yue Y (2014) Human papillomavirus oncoproteins and apoptosis (review). Exp Ther Med 7:3–7
Jie HB, Gildener-Leapman N, Li J et al (2013) Intratumoral regulatory T cells upregulate immunosuppressive molecules in head and neck cancer patients. Br J Cancer 109(10): 2629–2635
Jing M, Bohl J, Brimer N et al (2007) Degradation of tyrosine phosphatase PTPN3 (PTPH1) by association with oncogenic human papillomavirus E6 proteins. J Virol 81:2231–2239
Karanam B, Jagu S, Huh WK et al (2009) Developing vaccines against minor capsid antigen L2 to prevent papillomavirus infection. Immunol Cell Biol 87:287–299
Kavanagh K, Pollock KGJ, Potts A et al (2014) Introduction and sustained high coverage of the HPV bivalent vaccine leads to a reduction in prevalence of HPV 16/18 and closely related HPV types. Br J Cancer doi:10.1038/bjc.2014.198 (epub ahead of print)
Kenter GG, Welters MJ, Valentijn AR et al (2009) Vaccination against HPV-16 oncoproteins for vulvar intraepithelial neoplasia. N Engl J Med 361:1838–1847

Khleif SN, DeGregori J, Yee CL et al (1996) Inhibition of cyclin D-CDK4/CDK6 activity is associated with an E2F-mediated induction of cyclin kinase inhibitor activity. Proc Natl Acad Sci USA 93:4350–4354

Khoronenkova SV, Dianov GL (2011) The emerging role of Mule and ARF in the regulation of base exicision repair. FEBS Lett 585:2831–2835

Kines RC, Thompson CD, Lowy DR et al (2009) The initial steps leading to papillomavirus infection occur on the basement membrane prior to cell surface binding. Proc Natl Acad Sci USA 106:20458–20463

Kiyono T, Hiraiwa A, Fujita M et al (1997) Binding of high-risk human papillomavirus E6 oncoproteins to the human homologue of the Drosophila discs large tumor suppressor protein. Proc Natl Acad Sci USA 94:11612–11616

Klingelhutz AJ, Foster SA, McDougall JK (1996) Telomerase activation by the E6 gene product of human papillomavirus type 16. Nature 380:79–82

Kreimer AR, González P, Katki HA et al (2011) Efficacy of a bivalent HPV 16/18 vaccine against anal HPV 16/18 infection among young women: a nested analysis within the Costa Rica vaccine trial. Lancet Oncol 12(9):862–870

Kreuter A, Wieland U (2013) Lack of efficacy in treating condyloma acuminate and preventing recurrences with the recombinant quadrivalent human papillomavirus vaccine in a case series of immunocompetent patients. J Am Acad Dermatol 68:179–180

Kreuter A, Waterboer T, Wieland U (2010) Regression of cutaneous warts in a patient with WILD syndrome following recombinant quadrivalent human papillomavirus vaccination. Arch Dermatol 146:1196–1197

Kumar A, Zhao Y, Meng G et al (2002) Human papillomovirus oncoperotein E6 inactivates the transcriptional coactivator human ADA3. Mol Cell Biol 22:5801–5812

Lee SS, Glaunsinger B, Mantovani F et al (2000) Multi-PDZ domain protein MUPP1 is a cellular target for both adenovirus E4-ORF1 and high-risk papillomavirus type 18 E6 oncoproteins. J Virol 74:9680–9693

Li W, Deng XM, Wang CX et al (2010) Down-regulation of HLA class I antigen in human papillomavirus type 16 E7 expressing HaCaT cells: correlate with TAP-1 expression. Int J Gynecol Cancer Off J Int Gynecol Cancer Soc Feb 20:227–232

Lorincz AT, Reid R, Jenson AB et al (1992) Human papillomavirus infection of the cervix: relative risk associations of 15 common anogenital types. Obstet Gynecol 79:328–337

Maciag PC, Radulovic S, Rothman J (2009) The first clinical use of a live attenuated Listeria monocytogenes vaccine: a phase I safety study of Lm-LLO-E7 in patients with advanced carcinoma of the cervix. Vaccine 27:3975–3983

Maglennon GA, Doorbar J (2012) The biology of papillomavirus latency. Open Virol J 6:190–197

Mariani L, Venuti A (2010) HPV vaccine: an overview of immune response, clinical protection, and new approaches for the future. J Transl Med 8:105

Markowitz LE, Dunne EF, Saraiya M et al (2007) Quadrivalent human papillomavirus vaccine: recommendations of the advisory committee on immunization practices (ACIP). MMWR Recomm Rep 56:1–24

Matijevic M, Hedley ML, Urban RG et al (2011) Immunization with a poly (lactide co-glycolide) encapsulated plasmid DNA expressing antigenic regions of HPV 16 and 18 results in an increase in the precursor frequency of T cells that respond to epitopes from HPV 16, 18, 6 and 11. Cell Immunol 270:62–69

Matoso A, Ross HM, Chen S et al (2014) Squamous neoplasia of the scrotum: a series of 29 cases. Am J Surg Pathol 38:973–981

McBride AA, Oliveira JG, McPhillips MG (2006) Partitioning viral genomes in mitosis: same idea, different targets. Cell Cycle 5:1499–1502

McLaughlin-Drubin ME, Munger K (2009) Oncogenic activities of human papillomaviruses. Virus Res 143:195–208

Moscicki AB, Schiffman M, Burchell A et al (2012) Updating the natural history of human papillomavirus and anogenital cancers. Vaccine 30:24–33

Muench P, Hiller T, Probst S et al (2009) Binding of PDZ proteins to HPV E6 proteins does neither correlate with epidemiological risk classification nor with the immortalization of foreskin keratinocytes. Virology 387:380–387

Münger K, Basile JR, Duensing S et al (2001) Biological activities and molecular targets of the human papillomavirus E7 oncoprotein. Oncogene 20:7888–7898

Nakagawa S, Huibregtse JM (2000) Human scribble (Vartul) is targeted for ubiquitinmediated degradation by the high-risk papillomavirus E6 proteins and the E6AP ubiquitin-protein ligase. Mol Cell Biol 20:8244–8253

O'Brien PM, Saveria Campo M (2002) Evasion of host immunity directed by papillomavirus-encoded proteins. Virus Res 88:103–117

Olsen J, Jørgensen TR, Kofoed K et al (2012) Incidence and cost of anal, penile, vaginal and vulvar cancer in Denmark. BMC Public Health 12:1082

Olthof NC, Speel EJ, Kolligs J et al (2014) Comprehensive analysis of HPV16 integration in OSCC reveals no significant impact of physical status on viral oncogene and virally disrupted human gene expression. PLoS One 9:e88718

Paavonen J, Naud P, Salmeron J et al (2009) Efficacy of human papillomavirus (HPV)-16/18 AS04-adjuvanted vaccine against cervical infection and precancer caused by oncogenic HPV types (PATRICIA): final analysis of a double-blind, randomised study in young women. Lancet 374:301–314

Pai SI, Westra WH (2009) Molecular pathology of head and neck cancer: implications for diagnosis, prognosis, and treatment. Annu Rev Pathol 4:49–70

Parkin DM, Bray F (2006) The burden of HPV-related cancers. Vaccine 24(Suppl 3):11–25

Pollock KG, Kavanagh K, Potts A (2014) Reduction of low- and high-grade cervical abnormalities associated with high uptake of the HPV bivalent vaccine in Scotland. Br J Cancer Sep 2. doi:10.1038/bjc.2014.479. [Epub ahead of print]

Ressing ME, van Driel WJ, Brandt RM et al (2000) Detection of T helper responses, but not of human papillomavirus-specific cytotoxic T lymphocyte responses, after peptide vaccination of patients with cervical carcinoma. J Immunother 23:255–266

Safaeian M, Porras C, Schiffman M et al (2010) Epidemiological study of anti-HPV16/18 seropositivity and subsequent risk of HPV16 and -18 infections. J Natl Cancer Inst 102 (21):1653–1662

Santin AD, Bellone S, Palmieri M et al (2008) Human papillomavirus type 16 and 18 E7-pulsed dendritic cell vaccination of stage IB or IIA cervical cancer patients: a phase I escalating-dose trial. J Virol 82:1968–1979

Sardesai NY, Weiner DB (2011) Electroporation delivery of DNA vaccines: prospects for success. Curr Opin Immunol 23(3):421–429

Scheffner M, Huibregtse JM, Vierstra RD et al (1993) The HPV-16 E6 and E6-AP complex functions as a ubiquitin-protein ligase in the ubiquitination of p53. Cell 75:495–505

Schiffman M, Herrero R, Desalle R et al (2005) The carcinogenicity of human papillomavirus types reflects viral evolution. Virology 337:76–84

Schoeneich G, Perabo FGE, Muller SC (1999) Squamous cell carcinoma of the penis. Andrologia 31(Suppl 1):17–20

Scholefield JH, Harris D, Radcliffe A (2011) Guidelines for management of anal intraepithelial neoplasia. Colorectal Dis 13(Suppl 1):3–10

Sedman J, Stenlund A (1995) Co-operative interaction between the initiator E1 and the transcriptional activator E2 is required for replicator specific DNA replication of bovine papillomavirus in vivo and in vitro. EMBO J 14:6218–6228

Sheets EE, Urban RG, Crum CP et al (2003) Immunotherapy of human cervical highgrade cervical intraepithelial neoplasia with microparticle-delivered human papillomavirus 16 E7 plasmid DNA. Am J Obstet Gynecol 188(4):916–926

Shulzhenko N, Lyng H, Sanson GF et al (2014) Ménage à trois: an evolutionary interplay between human papillomavirus, a tumor, and a woman. Trends Microbiol 22(6):345–353

Siegel R, Naishadham D, Jemal A (2012) Cancer statistics, 2012. CA Cancer J Clin 62:10–29

Silling S, Wieland U, Werner M et al (2014) Resolution of novel human papillomavirus-induced warts after HPV vaccination. Emerg Infect Dis 20:142–145

Sinka K, Kavanagh K, Gordon R et al (2014) Introduction, high and equitable coverage of adolescent HPV vaccine in Scotland. J Epidemiol Community Health 68:57–63

Smith JS, Lindsay L, Hoots B et al (2007) Human papillomavirus type distribution in invasive cervical cancer and high-grade cervical cervical lesions: a meta-analysis update. Int J Cancer 21:621–632

Smyth LJ, Van Poelgeest MI, Davidson EJ et al (2004) Immunological responses in women with human papillomavirus type 16 (HPV-16)-associated anogenital intraepithelial neoplasia induced by heterologous prime-boost HPV-16 oncogene vaccination. Clin Cancer Res 10:2954–2961

Spencer AM, Roberts SA, Brabin L, Patnick J, Verma A (2014) Sociodemographic factors predicting mother's cervical screening and daughter's HPV vaccination uptake. J Epidemiol Community Health 68:571–577

Stanley M (2014) HPV vaccination in boys and men. Hum Vaccin Immunother 10:7

Stanley M, Pinto LA, Trimble C et al (2012) Human papillomavirus vaccines–immune responses. Vaccine 30(Suppl 5):F83–F87

Steger G, Corbach S (1997) Dose-dependent regulation of the early promoter of human papillomavirus type 18 by the viral E2 protein. J Virol 71:50–58

Steinau M, Saralya M, Goodman T et al (2014) HPV prevalence in oropharyngeal cancer before vaccine introduction, United States. Emerg Infect Dis 20:822–828

Stern PL, Brown M, Stacey SN et al (2000) Natural HPV immunity and vaccination strategies. J Clin Virol 19(1–2):57–66

Suzich JA, Ghim SJ, Palmer Hill FJ et al (1995) Systemic immunization with papillomavirus L1 protein completely prevents the development of viral mucosal papillomas. Proc Natl Acad Sci USA 92:11553–11557

Trimble CL, Piantadosi S, Gravitt P et al (2005) Spontaneous regression of high-grade cervical dysplasia: effects of human papillomavirus type and HLA phenotype. Clin Cancer Res 11:4717–4723

Trimble CL, Peng S, Thoburn C et al (2009a) Naturally occurring systemic immune responses to HPV antigens do not predict regression of CIN2/3. Cancer Immunol Immunother 59(5):799–803

Trimble CL, Peng S, Kos F et al (2009b) A phase I trial of a human papillomavirus DNA vaccine for HPV16+ cervical intraepithelial neoplasia 2/3. Clin Cancer Res 15(1):361–367

Trimble CL, Clark RA, Thoburn C et al (2010) Human papillomavirus 16-associated cervical intraepithelial neoplasia in humans excludes CD8 T cells from dysplastic epithelium. J Immunol 185:7107–7114

Tyler M, Tumban E, Dziduszko A et al (2014) Immunization with a consensus epitope from human papillomavirus L2 induces antibodies that are broadly neutralizing. Vaccine 32 (34):4267–4274

Um SH, Mundi N, Yoo J et al (2014) Variable expression of the forgotten oncogene E5 in HPV-positive oropharyngeal cancer. J Clin Virol 61(1):94–100

van Poelgeest MI, Nijhuis ER, Kwappenberg KM et al (2006) Distinct regulation and impact of type 1 T-cell immunity against HPV16 L1, E2 and E6 antigens during HPV16-induced cervical infection and neoplasia. Int J Cancer 118(3):675–683

Vinokurova S, Wentzensen N, Kraus I et al (2008) Type-dependent integration frequency of human papillomavirus genomes in cervical lesions. Cancer Res 68:307–313

Viscidi RP, Kotloff KL, Clayman B et al (1997) Prevalence of antibodies to human papillomavirus (HPV) type 16 virus-like particles in relation to cervical HPV infection among college women. Clin Diagn Lab Immunol 4:122–126

Voskens CJ, Sewell D, Hertzano R et al (2012) Induction of mage-A3 and HPV-16 immunity by Trojan vaccines in patients with head and neck carcinoma. Head Neck 34(12):1734–1746

Ward MJ, Thirdborough SM, Mellows T et al (2014a) Tumour-infiltrating lymphocytes predict for outcome in HPV-positive oropharyngeal cancer. Br J Cancer 110(2):489–500

Ward MJ, Mellows T, Harris S et al (2014b) Staging and treatment of oropharyngeal cancer in the human papillomavirus era. Head Neck (epub ahead of print)
Webster K, Parish J, Pandya M et al (2000) The human papillomavirus (HPV) 16 E2 protein induces apoptosis in the absence of other HPV proteins and via a p53-dependent pathway. J Biol Chem 275:87–94
Welters MJ, Kenter GG, de Vos van Steenwijk PJ et al (2010) Success or failure of vaccination for HPV16-positive vulvar lesions correlates with kinetics and phenotype of induced T-cell responses. Proc Natl Acad Sci USA 107(26):11895–11899
Wood LM, Paterson Y (2014) Attenuated Listeria monocytogenes: a powerful and versatile vector for the future of tumor immunotherapy. Front Cell Infect Microbiol 12(4):51
Yoshida T, Sano T, Kanuma T et al (2008) Immunochemical analysis of HPV L1 capsid protein and p16 protein in liquid-based cytology samples from uterine cervical lesions. Cancer 114 (2):83–88
Zerfass K, Schulze A, Spitkovsky D et al (1995) Sequential activation of cyclin E and cyclin A gene expression by human papillomavirus type 16 E7 through sequences necessary for transformation. J Virol 69:6389–6399

Tapping the Potential of DNA Delivery with Electroporation for Cancer Immunotherapy

Kimberly A. Kraynyak, Angela Bodles-Brakhop and Mark Bagarazzi

Abstract Cancer is a worldwide leading cause of death, and current conventional therapies are limited. The search for alternative preventive or therapeutic solutions is critical if we are going to improve outcomes for patients. The potential for DNA vaccines in the treatment and prevention of cancer has gained great momentum since initial findings almost 2 decades ago that revealed that genetically engineered DNA can elicit an immune response. The combination of adjuvants and an effective delivery method such as electroporation is overcoming past setbacks for naked plasmid DNA (pDNA) as a potential preventive or therapeutic approach to cancer in large animals and humans. In this chapter, we aim to focus on the novel advances in recent years for DNA cancer vaccines, current preclinical data, and the importance of adjuvants and electroporation with emphasis on prostate, melanoma, and cervical cancer.

Contents

K.A. Kraynyak · A. Bodles-Brakhop · M. Bagarazzi (✉)
Inovio Pharmaceuticals, 660 W. Germantown Pike, Suite 110, Plymouth Meeting, PA 19462, USA
e-mail: mbagarazzi@inovio.com

Current Topics in Microbiology and Immunology (2017) 405:55–78
DOI 10.1007/82_2015_431

Published Online: 15 February 2015

1 Introduction

Cancer, a growing global problem, is a group of diseases described by the uncontrolled growth and spread of abnormal cells which can result in death. Cancer accounts for approximately one in eight deaths worldwide and is a growing problem for low- and middle-income countries that lack the funds and/or medical capability to prevent or treat the disease. Both external factors, such as tobacco, infectious organisms, chemicals, and radiation, and internal factors, such as inherited mutations, hormones, immune conditions, and mutations, that occur from metabolism can cause cancer. According to the American Cancer Society in 2014, about 585,720 Americans are expected to die of cancer, almost 1,600 people per day. Cancer is the second most common cause of death in the USA, exceeded only by heart disease, accounting for nearly 1 of every 4 deaths. However, it is estimated that nearly 14.5 million Americans with a history of cancer were alive on January 1, 2014 and by January 1, 2024, that number will increase to nearly 19 million (DeSantis et al. 2014) demonstrating the need for improved treatment options that are financially feasible.

The initial work of Wolff et al. showed that DNA plasmids injected intramuscularly could generate long-term gene expression in vivo and set the stage for the role of plasmid DNA (pDNA) in the scientific and medical fields (Wolff et al. 1990). DNA vaccines are plasmids that encode for parts of a pathogen (antigens) to induce a pathogen-specific immune response in the immunized host. This prophylactic vaccination serves to prevent infection altogether or lessen the disease burden caused by that pathogen. DNA immunotherapies consist of plasmid-encoding antigens to induce an antigen-specific immune response to help fight an existing condition. Enhancing the immune response is one strategy currently being investigated as a means to effectively recognize and kill transformed cells in order to overcome cancer. In this chapter, we aim to discuss the potential of DNA vaccines and delivery with electroporation (EP) in the prevention and treatment of cancer-related disease, concentrating on melanoma, prostate, telomerase reverse transcriptase (TERT), and human papillomavirus (HPV)-related cancers. First generation DNA vaccines have been notoriously ineffective at generating potent immune responses in large animals and humans. However, the efficacy of DNA vaccines was dramatically improved when combined with EP delivery. Accordingly, we will focus on EP delivery as well as molecular adjuvants to boost the immune response. Moreover, the utilization of effective pDNA vaccines delivered by EP could prevent further tumor recurrences, due to the establishment of persistent immune memory. The overwhelming impact of cancer necessitates the need for a novel solution to this serious and fatal multifaceted disease. The combination of naked pDNA with an adjuvant and the delivery method of EP has produced encouraging positive results (Flingai et al. 2013) and may someday provide possibility and hope for many suffering from cancer.

1.1 Current Cancer Treatments

The treatment for cancer is as diverse as the disease itself. Each type of cancer has its own set of treatments with an assorted arsenal that has been approved and can be utilized. There are approximately six broad treatment options including watchful waiting or active surveillance, surgery, radiation therapy, hormone therapy, chemotherapy, and biologic therapy. While chemotherapy remains the mainstay of current cancer treatment, it has a limited therapeutic benefit, is significantly toxic, and can lead to severe side effects and often resistance. Overall survival is not always dramatically improved. Novel therapeutic alternatives and techniques are therefore required.

Prostate cancer is the most common type of cancer in men, and it is estimated that there will be 233,000 new cases in 2014 with approximately 30,000 deaths in the USA alone. There are over 25 approved drugs for the treatment of prostate cancer according to the National Cancer Institute. The last several years have seen the arrival of novel therapeutic agents for prostate cancer (Abdulla and Kapoor 2011; Adamo et al. 2012). Numerous recently approved immunotherapeutics such as sipuleucel-T, androgen axis inhibitors including abiraterone acetate and enzalutamide, a chemotherapeutic agent, cabazitaxel, and a radiopharmaceutical, radium-223, have resulted in positive results with increased survival for patients with castration-resistant prostate cancer (Agarwal et al. 2014). However, there is controversy over the clinically relevant therapeutic improvement (Jacobs et al. 2014) leaving an opening for the development of novel therapeutics such as DNA-based vaccines.

Skin cancer is in the top five of common types of cancers diagnosed in the USA, with an estimated 76,000 new cases annually. For melanoma patients, there are roughly 20 drug treatments available that have been approved by the FDA; however, these therapies, overall, have been demonstrated to be only marginally successful as metastatic melanoma is resistant to native apoptotic and anti-growth signals, is highly metastatic and deploys several local immune evasion mechanisms. Since 2011, 4 new agents have been approved for the treatment of patients with metastatic melanoma (ipilimumab, vemurafenib, dabrafenib, and trametinib), and several new agents are currently in phase 3 trials with hopes of even more agents, including DNA-based vaccines, being approved for this fatal disease (Saranga-Perry et al. 2014).

Breast cancer is a heterogeneous complex of diseases, a spectrum of many subtypes with distinct biological features that lead to differences in response patterns to various treatment modalities and clinical outcomes, making it difficult to develop a successful therapeutic strategy (Yersal and Barutca 2014). According to the National Cancer Institute, 235,000 new breast cancer cases are projected in the USA in 2014 with approximately 40,000 deaths. Currently, there are 5 approved drugs for the prevention of breast cancer with over 60 drugs approved for the treatment with many of them used in combination. Again, the need for improved therapeutics is critical for the treatment of breast cancer, and DNA vaccines are potential targets for the development of such novel therapeutics.

Cervical cancer is almost always caused by HPV infection and accounts for approximately 12,000 new cases in 2014 and results in about 4,000 deaths. There are currently 4 treatments approved for the prevention of cervical cancer including Cervarix® (GlaxoSmithKline), a bivalent vaccine containing VLPs of types 16 and 18, and Gardasil® (Merck), a quadrivalent vaccine containing VLPs of types 6, 11, 16, and 18 (Aggarwal 2014). Potentially precancerous dysplastic tissue, also known as cervical intraepithelial neoplasia (CIN), is sometimes managed with a watch and wait approach and depending on the severity can result in surgical intervention. There is currently no non-surgical alternative treatment option. Cervical cancer is commonly treated with a combination of chemotherapy and radiation, including cisplatin, brachytherapy or internal radiation therapy, and external radiation therapy. A targeted therapy, such as bevacizumab, may also be utilized. This area of cancer is greatly lacking in noninvasive therapeutic strategies, and DNA vaccines may provide a much needed solution.

1.2 DNA Vaccines

pDNA is employed in DNA vaccines and gene therapies against many infectious, acquired, and genetic diseases, including HIV-AIDS (Muthumani et al. 2013; Kalams et al. 2013), Hepatitis C (Latimer et al. 2014; Lang et al. 2008), Ebola (Shedlock et al. 2013), Malaria (Ferraro et al. 2013), different types of cancer, enteric pathogens, and influenza (Yan et al. 2014b; Laddy et al. 2007, 2008, 2009). Compared to conventional vaccines, DNA vaccines have many advantages such as high stability, non-infectious, focusing the immune response to only those antigens desired for immunization, the ability to give repeat doses (boost the immune response), and long-term persistence of vaccine-induced protection. It has been shown that a multivalent vaccine can be employed to target multiple antigens or even multiple pathogens simultaneously (Hirao et al. 2011). Furthermore, the simplicity, low cost to produce, and rapid production of DNA vaccines give them an advantage over many conventional vaccines or treatments and should make the technology accessible to developing countries. DNA vaccines have been shown to elicit tumor-protective cytotoxic T lymphocyte (CTL) immunity but to date have not reached their full potential in larger animals or humans.

Cancer is a worldwide leading cause of death, and several malignancies are incurable or not as successfully treated by current therapies as previously discussed. Therefore, new anti-tumor therapies are necessary to improve the outcome for patients with cancer. The induction of cellular immunity directed against tumor-specific antigens is emerging as a potential pathway for novel and effective drug development. DNA vaccines may prove to be a reliable form of cancer immunotherapy based on safety profile, stability, and can be ease of production. Moreover, tumor-specific antigens are expressed for a longer period of time compared to RNA- or protein-based vaccines. The selection of antigens, vector, delivery route, dose, timing, adjuvants, and boosting agents all affect the outcome of vaccination, in particular, the magnitude and quality of immunity elicited (Kutzler and Weiner 2008). Here, we will discuss the development of DNA vaccines and their potential application in treating cancer.

DNA vaccines are also being investigated as cancer treatments in companion animals. Testing anticancer medicine in companion animals such as dogs as an intermediary step of translational research program also provides clinical data for FDA/USDA approval as a veterinary anticancer drug or vaccine. The veterinary community is in need of novel medicine for the prevention and treatment of canine and feline cancers. More importantly, the benefit of testing anticancer vaccines in companion animals is that spontaneous tumors in dogs may provide invaluable information for human trials due to their heterogeneous nature. p62 (SQSTM1) is a key component of autophagic machinery which is also involved in signal transduction and is over-expressed in a variety of human tumors. It was noted that the administration of p62-encoding plasmid acted as a novel, effective broad-spectrum anti-tumor, and anti-metastatic vaccine (Venanzi et al. 2013). The potential effect of a p62 DNA vaccine on mammary tumors of dogs was also examined (Gabai et al. 2014). It was noted that the p62 DNA vaccine administered intramuscularly decreased or stabilized growth of locally advanced lesions and was associated with lymphocyte infiltration and tumor encapsulation via fibrotic reaction.

All these studies show the importance of tapping the potential of DNA vaccines for the development of novel therapeutics that will benefit cancer patients and concurrently provide much needed anticancer medicines for our four-legged friends. In order to produce the greatest benefit that DNA vaccines can deliver, it will be important to also evaluate effective adjuvants that may boost the immune response as well as utilize EP as a delivery method.

1.3 Adjuvants

Adjuvants are becoming critical components of most clinical vaccines and are used to enhance adaptive immune responses to antigen effecting both the quantity and quality of the immune response. Numerous studies are examining the potential of such adjuvants to increase the efficiency of DNA vaccines.

The potency of DNA-based vaccines co-administered with molecular cytokine adjuvants as part of a vaccine cocktail has been demonstrated to boost the adaptive immune response (Villarreal et al. 2013). Currently, there are numerous cytokine adjuvants that are showing potential as DNA vaccine assistants for cancer therapies. Cytokine adjuvants are of particular interest as they have the ability to induce $CD4^+$ and $CD8^+$ T cell responses that are critical for an effective therapeutic immune response. Cytokines such as the interleukin family members IL-12, IL-15, and IL-33 are all under investigation as potential adjuvants for use with DNA vaccines.

Previously, IL-12 DNA was shown to act as a molecular adjuvant when optimized for high level of expression and delivered using in vivo EP. Co-administration with IL-12 DNA resulted in the detection of systemic IL-12 cytokine in the plasma and was paralleled by a rapid increase of IFN-γ (Jalah et al. 2012). Hirao et al. (2008) have shown in non-human primates that the inclusion of IL-12 into a DNA vaccine delivered with EP resulted in the induction of higher, more rapid responses with increases in IL-2, TNF-α, and IFN-γ compared to the group not receiving IL-12 demonstrating that the combination elicits the most favorable outcome. Furthermore, it was found that when IL-12 was combined with a SIV-mac239 DNA vaccine, significantly higher SIV-specific cellular immune responses developed and persisted up to 6 months after the last vaccination (Jalah et al. 2012). A single therapeutic injection of an optimized murine IL-12 DNA plasmid showed significantly more potent control of tumor development in the B16 melanoma cancer model in mice (Jalah et al. 2013) indicating that optimization of the adjuvant can contribute to the success of therapeutic vaccines. Recently, IL-12 DNA was shown to augment the T cell immunity induced by a DNA vaccine in humans (Kalams et al. 2013).

In another example of the beneficial addition of cytokine adjuvants, the therapeutic response of an HPV DNA vaccine was improved with the inclusion of IL-33 (Villarreal et al. 2014). It was noted that the IL-33 immunoadjuvant induced potent anti-tumor immunity and resulted in regression of established tumors in mice. IL-28B was also examined by Morrow et al. for its potential to booster the immune response as an adjuvant in a non-human primate study for DNA vaccination (Morrow et al. 2010). The IL-28B adjuvant continued to boost the immune response three months after the final immunization.

Other adjuvants such as the novel chemokine adjuvant CCL27/CTACK have been examined for the ability to enhance immune responses to an HIV-1 or SIV antigen in mice and rhesus macaques (Kraynyak et al. 2010). Significant IFN-γ secretion and $CD8^+$ T cell proliferation was observed. Furthermore, plasmids encoding the mucosal chemokines CCL27 and CCL28 have been shown to be effective adjuvants in eliciting antigen-specific immunity in vivo and protected from morbidity and mortality associated with a lethal intranasal influenza challenge (Kutzler et al. 2010). The inclusion of molecular adjuvants into a DNA vaccine or immunotherapy can help drive an immune response tailored to the particular pathogen being targeted.

Other adjuvants have been also examined for their potential to aid the immune response of DNA vaccines in cancer. The Toll-like receptors (TLR) which play a crucial role in innate immune responses to infection are under consideration. TLR3 and TLR9 have been shown to be capable of eliciting strong T cell responses and have been shown to help control the growth of established B16 melanoma tumors after immunization (Zaks et al. 2006). A DNA vaccine incorporating TLR adaptor molecule such as the Toll-interleukin-1 receptor domain-containing adaptor-inducing beta interferon resulted in enhanced cellular immune responses and significantly reduced tumor growth compared to DNA vaccine alone (Takeshita et al. 2006). More recently, it has been shown that TLR3 and TLR7 agonists can be used to enhance the immune response to DNA vaccine encoding HPV-16 E7 (Sajadian et al. 2014).

1.4 Electroporation

To date, numerous delivery methods have been investigated to boost efficacy of non-viral gene therapies such as lipid-mediated entry into cells, jet injection, gene gun delivery, and sonoporation. In this review, we will focus on EP whereby a DNA-based vaccine is delivered intradermally or intramuscularly followed by electric pulses (millisecond electrical fields), resulting in temporary pores in the cellular membrane facilitating significant cellular uptake of the vaccine. Although the exact mechanism of cellular macromolecule entry is still under discussion, entry of small molecules such as anticancer therapeutics seems to occur by simple diffusion after the pulse, and larger molecules such as pDNA are thought to enter through a multistep mechanism involving the interaction of the DNA molecule with the destabilized membrane during the pulse and then its passage across the membrane. The cell membrane then reseals and the cellular machinery uses the DNA code to produce the desired antigen. Antigen-presenting cells then engulf the produced antigen and transport them to the lymph nodes where the antibodies or T cells are produced to eliminate the cancerous cells. The delivery method of EP for DNA-based vaccines in the treatment of cancer and its complications has been previously reviewed (Bodles-Brakhop and Draghia-Akli 2008).

Numerous preclinical studies have examined the effectiveness of EP as a delivery method for DNA vaccines. EP appears to have a great impact on immunogenicity and efficacy by increasing antigen delivery up to a 1000-fold over naked DNA delivery alone (reviewed by (Sardesai and Weiner 2011)). Furthermore, there are currently several ongoing clinical studies examining the administration of DNA vaccines with EP (Khan et al. 2014). DNA vaccines administered with EP in a comparison study with an adenovirus-based vaccine revealed significant differences with the DNA vaccine plus EP being able to booster the immune response with each subsequent vaccination, whereas the adenovirus vaccination failed to boost the immune response after the first immunization (Hirao et al. 2010).

The skin, compared to muscle, is an attractive tissue for DNA vaccination in a clinical setting due to the accessibility of the target, the ease of monitoring, tolerability, and most importantly the immunocompetent nature of the dermis (Broderick et al. 2014). Furthermore, it has been shown that EP of the skin with the use of a topical anesthetic cream prior to vaccination does not affect the number or function of the antigen-specific T cells induced (Roos et al. 2009). Recently, a novel dual depth device that has the ability to deliver both intradermal and intramuscular DNA vaccines simultaneously has been proven to be superior to delivery to either tissue alone for induction of antigen-specific antibody and cellular immunity (Lin et al. 2011). The strategy of intratumoral EP of DNA vaccines has also been explored with successful results. Intratumoral EP with tetanus toxin fragment C and IL-12 cDNA induced an IFN-γ-producing T cell response to tumor-associated antigen, heavy inflammatory infiltration, regression of established tumors, and immune memory to protect mice from repeated tumor challenge (Radkevich-Brown et al. 2010).

The effectiveness of the delivery method of EP has been shown to improve anti-tumor immune responses when used in a prime/boost strategy (Buchan et al. 2005). Furthermore, in a head to head comparison of EP with gene gun and conventional intramuscular injection in the ability to generate antigen-specific cytotoxic CD8+ T cell responses as well as anti-tumor immune responses against an HPV-16 E7 expressing tumor cell line using the pNGVL4a-CRT/E7(detox) DNA vaccine, EP was the most effective delivery method (Best et al. 2009). In addition, different procedures of DNA vaccine delivery, namely intradermal injection, gene gun delivery, and intramuscular injection alone or with EP, were compared in a murine transgenic model of mammary carcinoma overexpressing HER2/neu. In this study, intramuscular delivery followed by EP elicited better protection against HER2/neu spontaneous tumor development and induced an immune response (Smorlesi et al. 2006).

Overall, EP has been shown to be an efficient method for enhancing the uptake and expression of DNA vaccine candidates, enabling the use of a lower dose of vaccine with similar or higher efficacy. Optimization of EP will also increase its acceptability as a delivery method by potentially reducing the associated pain with the procedure. The current of intradermal vaccination by EP impacts antigen expression, inflammation, and the induction of both humoral and cellular immunity. It was observed that a lower (0.1 A) current reduced inflammation and improved antigen expression compared with a 0.2 A current and highlights the need for optimization of EP conditions in vivo (Hutnick et al. 2012). Minimally invasive low-voltage EP delivery has been accomplished with no evidence of injection site inflammation or local tissue damage (Broderick et al. 2012; Lin et al. 2012). In general, the delivery of DNA vaccines via either intramuscular, intratumoral, or intradermal EP has been proven to enhance antigen-specific antibody and cellular immunity compared to delivery to tissue alone (Lin et al. 2011).

2 Potential of DNA Vaccines in Cancer—Preclinical Studies

2.1 Melanoma

The delivery of pDNA by in vivo EP has been widely tested in preclinical melanoma models. Intratumoral delivery has been shown to generate a direct anti-tumor effect, whereas delivery to other sites can result in additional therapeutic effects such as anti-angiogenesis, reviewed by Heller and Heller (2010).

It has previously been shown that a combination of therapies can provide significant results. In a mouse model, in vivo EP of plasmids encoding granulocyte–monocyte colony-stimulating factor (GM-CSF) and interleukin-2 (IL2) into B16 mouse melanomas combined with electrochemotherapy resulted in the induction of long-term immunity to recurrence and resistance to challenge (Heller et al. 2000). Furthermore, it has been shown that optimization of a plasmid vaccine delivered by

EP can dramatically improve outcome compared to EP with plasmids encoding the full-length autologous melanocyte antigen tyrosinase-related protein-2 in mice when challenged with B16F10M melanoma cells (Kalat et al. 2002).

The combination of cancer vaccination with angiogenesis inhibition is appealing, due to favorable safety profile of both approaches, as well as possible biological synergies. The administration of pDNA vaccination (encoding gp100, TRP2, and Ii-PADRE) and anti-angiogenesis (pDNAs encoding angiostatin and/or endostatin) in B16F10 murine model was investigated. In an optimized administration protocol, the melanoma vaccination together with intratumoral delivery of pDNAs encoding angiostatin and endostatin resulted in 57 % tumor-free survival over 90 days after challenge (Chan et al. 2009). Furthermore, the intradermal EP with a survivin DNA vaccine has been shown to suppress angiogenesis in vivo and elicit protection against highly aggressive syngeneic B16 melanoma tumor challenge (Lladser et al. 2010).

The HIV-1 accessory protein Vpr (viral protein R) has previously been demonstrated to induce G2 cell cycle arrest as well as in vitro growth inhibition/killing of a number of tumor cells by apoptosis. When established, subcutaneous B16.F10 melanoma tumors were injected intratumorally with plasmid Vpr followed by EP complete tumor regression with long-term survival was noted (McCray et al. 2006). In a follow-up study, refinement of the pVPr plus EP regimen resulted in a higher percentage of complete tumor regression with long-term survival (McCray et al. 2007). It has also been shown that the HIV accessory protein Vpr has anti-proliferation/anticancer properties (Muthumani et al. 2009) and when administered as a plasmid by in vivo EP can result in regression of established B16.F10 melanoma tumors in mice (Muthumani et al. 2010).

The p42.3 gene is involved in cell cycle regulation, tumorigenesis and has significantly high expression levels in cancer cells including melanoma (Mao et al. 2014). When tested as a DNA vaccine in the B16F10 melanoma mouse model by EP, prophylactic and therapeutic effects were observed such as tumor growth inhibition and decrease in tumor weight (Liu et al. 2013).

The ability to treat melanoma with a DNA-based vaccine is gaining ground although there are still obstacles to be overcome. The utilization of canines which offer many similarities to human counterparts has led to a study where the therapeutic efficacy of a human chondroitin sulfate proteoglycan-4 (hCSPG4) DNA-based vaccine has been investigated. Homology between the human and canine forms is 80 % warranting its use. Intramuscular administration followed by EP resulted in significantly longer overall and disease-free survival times in 14 vaccinated dogs as compared with 13 non-vaccinated controls with the development of antibodies against both hCSPG4 and cCSPG4 (Riccardo et al. 2014). These results demonstrate the important potential advances for the veterinary field as well as providing an opportunity for translation into the human clinical setting.

Most recently, the role and significance of myeloid-derived suppressor cells (MDSCs) in the maintenance of the tumor microenvironment has been examined as they have the ability to suppress immune responses and, as such, facilitate tumor growth. A novel synthetic tyrosinase (Tyr) DNA vaccine therapy delivered by EP in both prophylactic and therapeutic models was investigated in conjunction with the role of MDSCs in immune suppression of T cells in an antigen-specific B16 melanoma murine system. A robust and broad immune response was induced as well as a reduction in the number of MDSCs in the tumor microenvironment. Overall, DNA vaccination by EP resulted in a significantly reduced melanoma tumor burden and increased survival in vivo (Yan et al. 2014a).

2.2 Prostate Cancer

The identification and measurement of prostate-specific antigen (PSA) has led to earlier diagnosis of prostate cancer. The knowledge that PSA expression is limited to prostate cells and has been shown to be found at higher expression levels in prostate-specific cancer cells makes it a good candidate for the development of immunotherapies and DNA-based vaccines (Kim et al. 1998). The safety and immunogenicity of a PSA DNA vaccine was evaluated in rhesus macaques. Overall, it was found to result in induction of PSA-specific humoral responses with no adverse effects (Kim et al. 2001b) establishing it as a potential cancer vaccine target. Furthermore, it has been shown that the co-immunization of PSA vaccine with cytokine adjuvants can result in significant enhancement of the PSA-specific antibody responses (Kim et al. 2001a). The intradermal EP of the prostate cancer vaccine encoding PSA has been shown to result in significantly higher gene expression levels and increased levels of PSA-specific T cells compared to DNA vaccine alone, without EP (Roos et al. 2006). Furthermore, the optimization of the intradermal EP delivery of a PSA DNA vaccine has been shown to enhance efficiency (Roos et al. 2008). The intramuscular EP of plasmid PSA has also been shown to be an effective strategy for inducing effective anti-tumor immune responses, tumor reduction, and increased survival (Ahmad et al. 2010).

Prostate stem cell antigen (PSCA) is a cell surface antigen expressed in normal human prostate and it is also over-expressed in prostate cancer correlating with increased tumor stage and increased bone metastases (Reiter et al. 1998). Intramuscular EP of a PSCA plasmid vaccine results in effective anti-tumor immune responses, inhibition of tumor growth, and increased survival while also inhibiting metastases (Ahmad et al. 2009).

Other novel DNA vaccines delivered by EP have also been evaluated. A DNA vaccine encoding the prostate-specific antigen prostatic acid phosphatase (PAP) delivered with EP in mice resulted in strong PAP-specific cellular immune responses and inhibited tumor growth in the transgenic adenocarcinoma of the mouse prostate (TRAMP) mouse model that closely resembles human prostate cancer (Spies et al. 2012). A dual antigen approach has also been investigated as a potential therapeutic strategy toward prostate cancer with the premise that a more comprehensive collection of antigens could improve the effectiveness of the vaccine. Highly optimized

DNA vaccines encoding both PSA and PSMA were evaluated in a mouse model inducing robust antigen-specific immune responses (Ferraro et al. 2011) and warranting further investigation of this novel dual approach.

2.3 Human Papillomavirus Infections and Associated Cancer

DNA vaccination has become an effective strategy for the development of therapeutics against many types of cancer, including cervical carcinoma. Human papillomavirus (HPV) is the leading cause of a broad spectrum of disease, including genital warts, precancerous lesions, cervical, and anal cancer, and is a worldwide public health problem of epidemic proportions. Persistent infection with HPV is the main etiological factor in cervical cancer, the second most common cancer in women worldwide. HPV, particularly HPV type 16, is the primary causative agent of cervical cancer; thus, HPV-associated cervical malignancies might be prevented or treated by the induction of the appropriate specific immune responses in patients (Han and Sin 2013). Moreover, HPV16 accounts for more than 90 % of HPV-related head and neck squamous cell carcinomas (Marur et al. 2010). HPV18 is the most prevalent high-risk HPV after type 16. Therefore, HPV18 antigen development, with the goal of increasing anti-HPV18 cellular immunity, has been shown to result in a strong cellular immune response against HPV18 E6 and E7 antigens in a murine model. Moreover, when applied to rhesus monkeys, this construct is also able to elicit cellular immunity, providing evidence as a candidate for further study in the eventual context of immunotherapy for HPV-associated cancers (Yan et al. 2008).

Viral E6 and E7 oncoproteins are suitable targets for therapeutic vaccination (Gan et al. 2014), and it has been shown that HPV E6 and E7 are promising tumor antigens as they are regulatory proteins that are constitutively expressed in HPV-associated cancer cells (Morrow et al. 2013) and, therefore, were investigated as potential HPV DNA vaccine candidates (Seo et al. 2009). In one approach, E6 and E7 antigens were engineered to generate an optimal HPV DNA vaccine by codon optimization, fusion of E6 and E7, the addition of a tissue plasminogen activator signal sequence, and the addition of CD40 ligand (CD40L) or Fms-like tyrosine kinase-3 ligand (Flt3L). The results indicated that the inclusion of a tpa signal sequence, Flt3L, fusion of E6 and E7, and codon optimization induced strong E6- and E7-specific $CD8^+$ T cell responses that were further enhanced by intramuscular EP leading to complete tumor regression (Seo et al. 2009). The addition of adjuvants to a HPV-16 E7-based DNA vaccine was investigated as a means to improve immunogenicity (Ohlschlager et al. 2009). DNA encoded cytokines (IL-2, IL-12, GM-CSF, and IFN-γ) and the chemokine MIP1-alpha were co-applied either simultaneously or at different time points pre- or post-E7SH vaccination. The timing of adjuvant administration was found to be critical for success in mice, with MIP-1α pretreatment (day 5) in combination with sequence-optimized IFN-γ (day 3) resulting in the more significant tumor regression. In a further study, it was shown that the immunogenicity of the HPV-16 E7SH DNA vaccine was greatly enhanced by the introduction of a highly optimized CpG cassette into the plasmid backbone, as well as by improving DNA delivery using EP technology (Ohlschlager et al. 2011).

Although most effects have been directed against the high-risk subtypes 16 and 18 of HPV, investigation into the so-called lower-risk subtypes 6 and 11 that are also associated with otolaryngologic malignancies, carcinoma of the lung, tonsil, larynx, and low-grade cervical lesions is needed. Optimized DNA vaccines that encode HPV 6 and 11 consensus E6/E7 fusion proteins (p6E6E7 and p11E6E7) were delivered to mice using in vivo EP. p6E6E7 and p11E6E7 proved to be highly immunogenic vaccines that mounted very robust HPV 6 or HPV 11 E6- and E7-specific T cell immune responses (Shin et al. 2012).

2.4 Other Potential Cancer Targets

To date, there is no effective vaccine available for breast cancer patients. Although major advancements have been achieved especially with the advent of HER-2 transgenic mice (Lollini et al. 2013), there is still a lot of work to be done. However, it has been shown that intramuscular EP with DNA plasmids coding for the extracellular and transmembrane domains of the protein product of the Her-2/neu oncogene can result in tumor clearance (Quaglino et al. 2004). Furthermore, it has been shown that a single administration with EP was enough to markedly delay carcinogenesis progression in mice with multiple microscopic invasive carcinomas and keep about 50 % of mice tumor free at one year of age (Curcio et al. 2008).

Moreover, the first administration of a Her2-pDNA vaccine in humans has been reported (Norell et al. 2010). The vaccine, encoding a full-length signaling-deficient version of the oncogene Her2, was administered together with low doses of GM-CSF and IL-2 to patients with metastatic Her2-expressing breast carcinoma who were also treated with trastuzumab in a pilot clinical trial. This pilot clinical trial demonstrates that Her2-pDNA vaccination in conjunction with GM-CSF and IL-2 administration is safe, well-tolerated and can induce long-lasting cellular and humoral immune responses against Her2 in patients with advanced breast cancer.

High levels of human telomerase reverse transcriptase (hTERT) are detected in more than 85 % of solid tumors, while normal cells showed undetectable levels of telomerase expression making it an attractive immunotherapeutic target as a universal cancer vaccine. A DNA-based hTERT vaccine delivered by EP was examined in mice and non-human primates. Robust and broad immune responses were generated in vaccinated mice compared to the control group, and in an HPV16-associated tumor model, vaccination of phTERT with EP slowed tumor growth and improved survival rate in both prophylactic and therapeutic studies. The success of these results suggests that phTERT may have a role as a broad therapeutic cancer vaccine candidate (Yan et al. 2013). Similar immune responses were achieved in non-human primates (Yan et al. 2013). More recently, it has been shown that an intradermal administration of a hTERT vaccine with EP induces an intense specific $CD8^+$ T cell response (Calvet et al. 2014) and has warranted further investigation in a phase 1 clinical trial.

2.5 Clinical Trials

According to the Journal of Gene Medicine, there have been over 2000 clinical trials worldwide investigating gene therapy with 379 trials investigating pDNA (http://www.wiley.com//legacy/wileychi/genmed/clinical/). This is a staggering increase over the last five years (Bodles-Brakhop et al. 2009). The majority of the gene therapy clinical trials address cancers (64.1 %, $n = 1{,}331$). Of these, there are 216 studies that are examining the potential of naked pDNA in the treatment of various cancers. Cancer DNA vaccines administered by EP are shown in Fig. 1.

A vaccine that encodes a domain of fragment C of tetanus toxin to induce $CD4^+$ T cell help, fused to a tumor-derived epitope from prostate-specific membrane antigen (PSMA) for use in HLA-A2(+) patients with recurrent prostate cancer was investigated for safety and tolerability. The immune response in an open label phase I/II two arm dose escalation trial with and without intramuscular EP was also investigated (Low et al. 2009). The results indicated that delivery of the vaccine with EP yielded the highest humoral response that persisted up to 18 months. Reports of an encouraging phase 1 safety, tolerability, and immunogenicity trial for

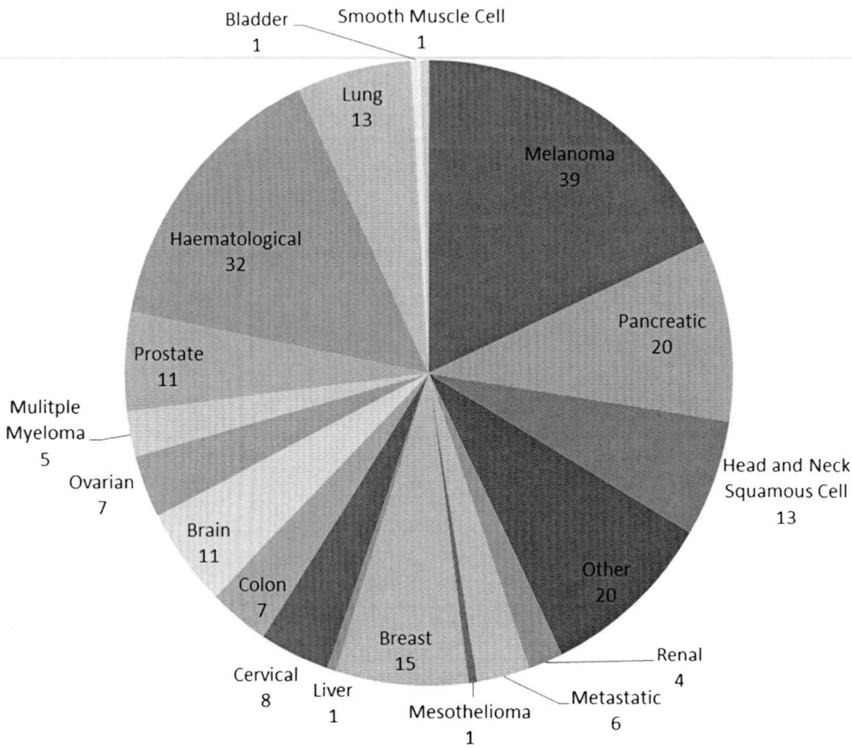

Fig. 1 Clinical trials of naked plasmid DNA for the treatment of cancer by type. The number of clinical trials using naked plasmid DNA for individual cancers is indicated

Table 1 Clinical trials involving DNA vaccines administered with EP for the treatment of cancer

NCT ID	Phase	Status	Sponsor	Condition	Intervention	Objective
NCT00859729	1 & 2	Completed	Uppsala University	Prostate cancer	pVAXrcPSAv53, DERMA VAX™ ID DNA delivery system	Feasibility and safety, immune response, anti-tumor effect
NCT01440816	2	Recruiting	OncoSec Medical Incorporated	Merkel cell carcinoma	IL-12 gene, IT EP-mediated plasmid DNA vaccine therapy	Twofold increase in IL-12 successful outcome, safety, survival, immunological effects
NCT01064375	1 & 2	Unknown	Maria Liljefors	Colorectal cancer	tetwtCEA DNA, DERMA VAX™ (EP device)	Safety and immunogenicity
NCT00685412	1	Completed	Inovio Pharmaceuticals	Human papilloma virus	VGX-3100, DNA plasmid delivered via IM injection + EP using CELLECTRA® device	Safety and tolerability, humoral and cellular immune responses
NCT01634503	1	Completed	Genexine, Inc.	Cervical cancer	GX-188E administered by EP	Safety and immunogenicity
NCT01304524	2	Ongoing	Inovio Pharmaceuticals	Cervical intraepithelial neoplasia 2/3 or 3	VGX-3100, DNA plasmid delivered via IM injection + EP using CELLECTRA® device	Histopathological regression, Virologically-proven clearance
NCT02139267	2	Not yet open	Genexine, Inc.	Cervical cancer	GX-188E, administered IM by EP	Histopathological regression of cervical lesions
NCT00471133	1	Completed	Ichor Medical Systems Incorporated	Melanoma	Xenogeneic tyrosinase DNA vaccine, TriGrid™ delivery system for IM by EP	Safety and feasibility, immunological and anti-tumor response
NCT01334060	2	Suspended	University Hospital Southampton NHS Foundation Trust	Haematological malignancies	p.DOM-WT1-37 DNA vaccine and p. DOM-WT1-126 DNA vaccine, IM by EP	Molecular response, time to disease progression, overall survival

(continued)

Table 1 (continued)

NCT ID	Phase	Status	Sponsor	Condition	Intervention	Objective
NCT02172911	**1 & 2**	**Recruiting**	**Inovio Pharmaceuticals**	**Cervical cancer**	**VGX-3100 and INO-9012 delivered via IM EP with CELLECTRA®-5P**	**Safety and tolerability, immunogenicity**
NCT01493154	1	Terminated	Sidney Kimmel Comprehensive Cancer Center	Head and neck cancer	pNGVL4a-CRT/E7(Detox) DNA vaccine using the IM TriGrid™ delivery system	Safety and immunogenicity
NCT02100085	1	Ongoing	Genexine, Inc.	Cervical intraepithelial neoplasia 3	GX-188E administered by EP, follow up study from NCT01634503	Immune response, lesion and infection status, compared to that of the final visit in phase I study
NCT01188850	1	Completed	Inovio Pharmaceuticals	Human papilloma virus	VGX-3100, delivered via IM injection + EP using CELLECTRA® device	Safety and tolerability, humoral and cellular immune responses
NCT01138410	1 & 2	Recruiting	Scancell Ltd	Malignant melanoma	SCIB1 administered by IM injection using the TDS-IM EP device (Ichor Medical Systems, Inc.)	Safety, tolerability, biological, and clinical effects
NCT01579318	2	Recruiting	OncoSec Medical Incorporated	Cutaneous T cell lymphomas	IT injection of pIL-12 with EP	Response rate, safety, and immunogenicity
NCT02204098	1	Not yet open	Washington University School of Medicine	Breast cancer	Mammaglobin-A DNA vaccine given IM using an integrated EP administration system	Safety and immunogenicity
NCT01502293	2	Recruiting	OncoSec Medical Incorporated	Melanoma	Plasmid interleukin-12, IT with EP	Safety, response rate, overall survival
NCT01664273	1	Terminated	Copenhagen University Hospital at Herlev	Metastatic malignant neoplasm	Plasmid AMEP injected IM and immediately followed by application of electric pulses via a needle electrode inserted into the muscle	Safety, efficacy, pharmokinetics

(continued)

Table 1 (continued)

NCT ID	Phase	Status	Sponsor	Condition	Intervention	Objective
NCT02241369	**1**	**Recruiting**	**Inovio Pharmaceuticals**	**Aerodigestive malignancies (e.g., squamous cell carcinoma)**	**INO-3106 alone or in combination with INO-9012 (DNA plasmid encoding human IL-12) delivered by EP**	**Safety, tolerability, and immunogenicity**
NCT02163057	**1 & 2**	**Recruiting**	**Inovio Pharmaceuticals**	**Head and neck squamous cell cancer**	**VGX-3100 and INO-9012 delivered via IM EP**	**Safety, tolerability, and immunogenicity, anti-tumor effects**
NCT01764009	1 & 2	Ongoing	BioAlliance Pharma SA	Melanoma	Naked DNA coding for protein AMEP delivered by IM EP	Safety and tolerability
NCT01045915	1	Terminated	BioAlliance Pharma SA	Melanoma	Naked DNA coding for protein AMEP delivered by IM EP	Determination of dose-limiting toxicity
NCT00685412	1	Completed	Inovio Pharmaceuticals	Cervical cancer	VGX-3100, DNA plasmid delivered via IM injection + EP using CELLECTRA® device	Safety and tolerability, humoral and cellular immune responses
NCT02301754	1	Recruiting	Invectys	Solid tumors	INVAC-1, a DNA vaccine encoding human telomerase reverse transcriptase (hTERT), delivered ID with EP	Safety, immunogenicity and pharmacodynamics

There are a total of 22 clinical trials worldwide, with 9 of these studies currently open of which 7 are occurring in North America (USA), 1 in Europe, and 1 in East Asia. Three studies, highlighted in bold, are examining the safety, tolerability, and immunogenicity of a DNA vaccine administered with a plasmid adjuvant by EP (search conducted November 2014)

EP electroporation; *ID* intradermal; *IM* intramuscular; *IT* intratumoral a therapeutic HPV16/18 candidate vaccine, VGX-3100, delivered by in vivo EP indicate it is capable of driving a robust immune response to antigens from high-risk HPV serotypes and could contribute to elimination of HPV-infected cells and subsequent regression of the dysplastic process (Bagarazzi et al. 2012).

3 Summary

Overall, the preclinical and clinical studies discussed demonstrate that DNA vaccines administered with an adjuvant by EP could provide a potential alternative to standard therapies. To date, four DNA plasmid products are currently licensed for veterinary applications. This includes two infectious disease vaccines, one for West Nile virus in horses (Ft Dodge Animal Health) and one for infectious haematopoietic necrosis virus in salmon (Novartis). A melanoma cancer vaccine for dogs (Manufacturer: Merial) and a growth hormone releasing factor therapy for pigs (Manufacturer: VGX Animal Health) are also approved. The canine melanoma vaccine (Trade name: Oncept) consists of highly purified pDNA capable of expressing the human tyrosinase protein and is a therapeutic vaccine administered to dogs with stage II or stage III oral melanoma to aid in extending overall survival (Peruzzi et al. 2010). The vaccine was evaluated by the Canadian Centre for Veterinary Biologics of the Canadian Food Inspection Agency for licensing in Canada. The vaccine is given by transdermal administration, targeting intramuscular deposition using the VET JET needle-free transdermal vaccination system (a high-pressure device placed on the skin which deposits injectate transdermally into the muscular tissue) with four doses of vaccine given at two-week intervals, with a booster dose administered every six months for the life of the animal. The results of a double-arm clinical trial revealed immune responses, no adverse effects, and an extended overall survival time compared to historical controls that were treated with a chemotherapy regimen (Gavazza et al. 2013). These results in pet dogs represent exceptional translational models for advancement of cancer research because they reflect the complex heterogeneity also observed in human cancer. Currently, there are three clinical trials that are examining the potential of DNA vaccines administered by EP with an adjuvant as highlighted in Table 1 in bold. These studies and others are paving the way for future clinical studies and will play an important role in advancing DNA vaccines as a significant therapeutic option.

Most recently, it has been shown that a combination therapy of old and new treatment concepts may prove effective and should be considered when the health and well-being of a patient is under consideration. For example, a combination therapy consisting of intratumoral IL-12 gene therapy, human tyrosinase (hTyr) DNA vaccination, and metronomic cyclophosphamide (CPX) was evaluated in a B16-F10 mouse model revealing that each component of this combination treatment contributed a unique immunologic trait with associated clinical benefits

(Denies et al. 2014). As we progress toward developing DNA vaccines for cancer, the inclusion of adjuvants and delivery by EP should be investigated fully in combination approaches with and without existing therapies in an effort to make every effort to provide the best outcome for patients.

References

Abdulla A, Kapoor A (2011) Emerging novel therapies in the treatment of castrate-resistant prostate cancer. Can Urol Assoc J (Journal de l'Association des urologues du Canada) 5 (2):120–133. doi:10.5489/cuaj.10160

Adamo V, Noto L, Franchina T, Chiofalo G, Picciotto M, Toscano G, Caristi N (2012) Emerging targeted therapies for castration-resistant prostate cancer. Front Endocrinol 3:73. doi:10.3389/fendo.2012.00073

Agarwal N, Di Lorenzo G, Sonpavde G, Bellmunt J (2014) New agents for prostate cancer. Ann Oncol Official J Eur Soc Med Oncol/ESMO 25(9):1700–1709. doi:10.1093/annonc/mdu038

Aggarwal P (2014) Cervical cancer: can it be prevented? World J Clin Oncol 5 (4):775–780. doi:10.5306/wjco.v5.i4.775

Ahmad S, Casey G, Sweeney P, Tangney M, O'Sullivan GC (2009) Prostate stem cell antigen DNA vaccination breaks tolerance to self-antigen and inhibits prostate cancer growth. Mol Ther: J Am Soc Gene Ther 17(6):1101–1108. doi:10.1038/mt.2009.66

Ahmad S, Casey G, Sweeney P, Tangney M, O'Sullivan GC (2010) Optimised electroporation mediated DNA vaccination for treatment of prostate cancer. Genet Vaccines Ther 8(1):1. doi:10.1186/1479-0556-8-1

Bagarazzi ML, Yan J, Morrow MP, Shen X, Parker RL, Lee JC, Giffear M, Pankhong P, Khan AS, Broderick KE, Knott C, Lin F, Boyer JD, Draghia-Akli R, White CJ, Kim JJ, Weiner DB, Sardesai NY (2012) Immunotherapy against HPV16/18 generates potent TH1 and cytotoxic cellular immune responses. Sci Transl Med 4(155):155ra138

Best SR, Peng S, Juang CM, Hung CF, Hannaman D, Saunders JR, Wu TC, Pai SI (2009) Administration of HPV DNA vaccine via electroporation elicits the strongest CD8+ T cell immune responses compared to intramuscular injection and intradermal gene gun delivery. Vaccine 27(40):5450–5459. doi:10.1016/j.vaccine.2009.07.005

Bodles-Brakhop AM, Draghia-Akli R (2008) DNA vaccination and gene therapy: optimization and delivery for cancer therapy. Expert Rev Vaccines 7(7):1085–1101

Bodles-Brakhop AM, Heller R, Draghia-Akli R (2009) Electroporation for the delivery of DNA-based vaccines and immunotherapeutics: current clinical developments. Mol Ther 17(4):585–592

Broderick KE, Chan A, Lin F, Shen X, Kichaev G, Khan AS, Aubin J, Zimmermann TS, Sardesai NY (2012) Optimized in vivo transfer of small interfering RNA targeting dermal tissue using in vivo surface electroporation. Mol Ther Nucleic Acids 1:e11. doi:10.1038/mtna.2012.1

Broderick KE, Khan AS, Sardesai NY (2014) DNA vaccination in skin enhanced by electroporation. Methods Mol Biol (Clifton, NJ) 1143:123–130. doi:10.1007/978-1-4939-0410-5_8

Buchan S, Gronevik E, Mathiesen I, King CA, Stevenson FK, Rice J (2005) Electroporation as a "prime/boost" strategy for naked DNA vaccination against a tumor antigen. J Immunol 174 (10):6292–6298

Calvet CY, Thalmensi J, Liard C, Pliquet E, Bestetti T, Huet T, Langlade-Demoyen P, Mir LM (2014) Optimization of a gene electrotransfer procedure for efficient intradermal immunization with an hTERT-based DNA vaccine in mice. Mol Ther Methods Clin Dev 1. doi:10.1038/mtm.2014.45

Chan RC, Gutierrez B, Ichim TE, Lin F (2009) Enhancement of DNA cancer vaccine efficacy by combination with anti-angiogenesis in regression of established subcutaneous B16 melanoma. Oncol Rep 22(5):1197–1203

Curcio C, Khan AS, Amici A, Spadaro M, Quaglino E, Cavallo F, Forni G, Draghia-Akli R (2008) DNA immunization using constant-current electroporation affords long-term protection from autochthonous mammary carcinomas in cancer-prone transgenic mice. Cancer Gene Ther 15 (2):108–114

Denies S, Cicchelero L, Van Audenhove I, Sanders NN (2014) Combination of interleukin-12 gene therapy, metronomic cyclophosphamide and DNA cancer vaccination directs all arms of the immune system towards tumor eradication. J Control Release 187:175–182. doi:10.1016/j.jconrel.2014.05.045

DeSantis CE, Lin CC, Mariotto AB, Siegel RL, Stein KD, Kramer JL, Alteri R, Robbins AS, Jemal A (2014) Cancer treatment and survivorship statistics, 2014. CA: A Cancer J Clin 64 (4):252–271. doi:10.3322/caac.21235

Ferraro B, Cisper NJ, Talbott KT, Philipson-Weiner L, Lucke CE, Khan AS, Sardesai NY, Weiner DB (2011) Co-delivery of PSA and PSMA DNA vaccines with electroporation induces potent immune responses. Hum Vaccine 7:120–127

Ferraro B, Talbott KT, Balakrishnan A, Cisper N, Morrow MP, Hutnick NA, Myles DJ, Shedlock DJ, Obeng-Adjei N, Yan J, Kayatani AK, Richie N, Cabrera W, Shiver R, Khan AS, Brown AS, Yang M, Wille-Reece U, Birkett AJ, Sardesai NY, Weiner DB (2013) Inducing humoral and cellular responses to multiple sporozoite and liver-stage malaria antigens using exogenous plasmid DNA. Infect Immun 81(10):3709–3720. doi:10.1128/iai.00180-13

Flingai S, Czerwonko M, Goodman J, Kudchodkar SB, Muthumani K, Weiner DB (2013) Synthetic DNA vaccines: improved vaccine potency by electroporation and co-delivered genetic adjuvants. Front Immunol 4:354. doi:10.3389/fimmu.2013.00354

Gabai V, Venanzi FM, Bagashova E, Rud O, Mariotti F, Vullo C, Catone G, Sherman MY, Concetti A, Chursov A, Latanova A, Shcherbinina V, Shifrin V, Shneider A (2014) Pilot study of p62 DNA vaccine in dogs with mammary tumors. Oncotarget 5(24):12803–12810

Gan L, Jia R, Zhou L, Guo J, Fan M (2014) Fusion of CTLA-4 with HPV16 E7 and E6 enhanced the potency of therapeutic HPV DNA vaccine. PLoS One 9(9):e108892. doi:10.1371/journal.pone.0108892

Gavazza A, Lubas G, Fridman A, Peruzzi D, Impellizeri JA, Luberto L, Marra E, Roscilli G, Ciliberto G, Aurisicchio L (2013) Safety and efficacy of a genetic vaccine targeting telomerase plus chemotherapy for the therapy of canine B-cell lymphoma. Hum Gene Ther 24(8):728–738. doi:10.1089/hum.2013.112

Han KT, Sin JI (2013) DNA vaccines targeting human papillomavirus-associated diseases: progresses in animal and clinical studies. Clin Exp Vaccine Res 2(2):106–114. doi:10.7774/cevr.2013.2.2.106

Heller L, Pottinger C, Jaroszeski MJ, Gilbert R, Heller R (2000) In vivo electroporation of plasmids encoding GM-CSF or interleukin-2 into existing B16 melanomas combined with electrochemotherapy induces long-term antitumour immunity. Melanoma Res 10(6):577–583

Heller LC, Heller R (2010) Electroporation gene therapy preclinical and clinical trials for melanoma. Curr Gene Ther 10(4):312–317

Hirao L, Wu L, Khan AS, Hokey D, Yan J, Dai A, Betts M, Draghia-Akli R, Weiner DB (2008) Combined effects of IL-12 and electroporation enhances the potency of DNA vaccination in macaques. Vaccine 26(25):3112–3120

Hirao LA, Draghia-Akli R, Prigge JT, Yang M, Satishchandran A, Wu L, Hammarlund E, Khan AS, Babas T, Rhodes L, Silvera P, Slifka M, Sardesai NY, Weiner DB (2011) Multivalent smallpox DNA vaccine delivered by intradermal electroporation drives protective immunity in nonhuman primates against lethal monkeypox challenge. J Infect Dis 203(1):95–102. doi:10.1093/infdis/jiq017

Hirao LA, Wu L, Satishchandran A, Khan AS, Draghia-Akli R, Finnefrock AC, Bett AJ, Betts MR, Casimiro DR, Sardesai NY, Kim JJ, Shiver JW, Weiner DB (2010) Comparative analysis of immune responses induced by vaccination with SIV antigens by recombinant Ad5 vector or plasmid DNA in rhesus macaques. Mol Ther J Am Soc Gene Ther 18(8):1568–1576. doi:10.1038/mt.2010.112

Hutnick NA, Myles DJ, Ferraro B, Lucke C, Lin F, Yan J, Broderick KE, Khan AS, Sardesai NY, Weiner DB (2012) Intradermal DNA vaccination enhanced by low-current electroporation improves antigen expression and induces robust cellular and humoral immune responses. Hum Gene Ther 23(9):943–950. doi:10.1089/hum.2012.055

Jacobs JJ, Snackey C, Geldof AA, Characiejus D, Van Moorselaar RJ, Den Otter W (2014) Inefficacy of therapeutic cancer vaccines and proposed improvements. Casus prostate cancer. Anticancer Res 34(6):2689–2700

Jalah R, Patel V, Kulkarni V, Rosati M, Alicea C, Ganneru B, von Gegerfelt A, Huang W, Guan Y, Broderick KE, Sardesai NY, LaBranche C, Montefiori DC, Pavlakis GN, Felber BK (2012) IL-12 DNA as molecular vaccine adjuvant increases the cytotoxic T cell responses and breadth of humoral immune responses in SIV DNA vaccinated macaques. Hum Vaccines Immunotherapeutics 8(11):1620–1629. doi:10.4161/hv.21407

Jalah R, Rosati M, Ganneru B, Pilkington GR, Valentin A, Kulkarni V, Bergamaschi C, Chowdhury B, Zhang GM, Beach RK, Alicea C, Broderick KE, Sardesai NY, Pavlakis GN, Felber BK (2013) The p40 subunit of interleukin (IL)-12 promotes stabilization and export of the p35 subunit: implications for improved IL-12 cytokine production. J Biol Chem 288 (9):6763–6776. doi:10.1074/jbc.M112.436675

Kalams SA, Parker SD, Elizaga M, Metch B, Edupuganti S, Hural J, De Rosa S, Carter DK, Rybczyk K, Frank I, Fuchs J, Koblin B, Kim DH, Joseph P, Keefer MC, Baden LR, Eldridge J, Boyer J, Sherwat A, Cardinali M, Allen M, Pensiero M, Butler C, Khan AS, Yan J, Sardesai NY, Kublin JG, Weiner DB (2013) Safety and comparative immunogenicity of an HIV-1 DNA vaccine in combination with plasmid interleukin 12 and impact of intramuscular electroporation for delivery. J Infect Dis 208(5):818–829. doi:10.1093/infdis/jit236

Kalat M, Kupcu Z, Schuller S, Zalusky D, Zehetner M, Paster W, Schweighoffer T (2002) In vivo plasmid electroporation induces tumor antigen-specific CD8+ T-cell responses and delays tumor growth in a syngeneic mouse melanoma model. Cancer Res 62(19):5489–5494

Khan AS, Broderick KE, Sardesai NY (2014) Clinical development of intramuscular electroporation: providing a "boost" for DNA vaccines. Methods in molecular biology (Clifton, NJ) 1121:279-289. doi:10.1007/978-1-4614-9632-8_25

Kim JJ, Trivedi NN, Wilson DM, Mahalingam S, Morrison L, Tsai A, Chattergoon MA, Dang K, Patel M, Ahn L, Boyer JD, Chalian AA, Schoemaker H, Kieber-Emmons T, Agadjanyan MA, Weiner DB (1998) Molecular and immunological analysis of genetic prostate specific antigen (PSA) vaccine. Oncogene 17(24):3125–3135. doi:10.1038/sj.onc.1201736

Kim JJ, Yang JS, Dang K, Manson KH, Weiner DB (2001a) Engineering enhancement of immune responses to DNA-based vaccines in a prostate cancer model in rhesus macaques through the use of cytokine gene adjuvants. Clin Cancer Res 7(3 Suppl):882s–889s

Kim JJ, Yang JS, Nottingham LK, Tang W, Dang K, Manson KH, Wyand MS, Wilson DM, Weiner DB (2001b) Induction of immune responses and safety profiles in rhesus macaques immunized with a DNA vaccine expressing human prostate specific antigen. Oncogene 20 (33):4497–4506. doi:10.1038/sj.onc.1204542

Kraynyak KA, Kutzler MA, Cisper NJ, Khan AS, Draghia-Akli R, Sardesal NY, Lewis MG, Yan J, Weiner DB (2010) Systemic immunization with CCL27/CTACK modulates immune responses at mucosal sites in mice and macaques. Vaccine 28(8):1942–1951. doi:10.1016/j.vaccine.2009.10.095

Kutzler MA, Kraynyak KA, Nagle SJ, Parkinson RM, Zharikova D, Chattergoon M, Maguire H, Muthumani K, Ugen K, Weiner DB (2010) Plasmids encoding the mucosal chemokines CCL27 and CCL28 are effective adjuvants in eliciting antigen-specific immunity in vivo. Gene Ther 17(1):72–82. doi:10.1038/gt.2009.112

Kutzler MA, Weiner DB (2008) DNA vaccines: ready for prime time? Nat Rev Genet 9(10):776–788

Laddy DJ, Yan J, Corbitt N, Kobasa D, Kobinger GP, Weiner DB (2007) Immunogenicity of novel consensus-based DNA vaccines against avian influenza. Vaccine 25(16):2984–2989

Laddy DJ, Yan J, Khan AS, Anderson H, Cohn A, Greenhouse J, Lewis M, Manischewitz J, King LR, Golding H, Draghia-Akli R, Weiner DB (2009) Electroporation of synthetic DNA antigens offers protection in non-human primates challenged with highly pathogenic avian influenza. J Virol 83(9):4624–4630

Laddy DJ, Yan J, Kutzler M, Kobasa D, Kobinger GP, Khan AS, Draghia-Akli R, Greenhouse J, Sardesai NY, Weiner DB (2008) Induction of heterosubtypic protection against pathogenic human and avian influenza viruses by synthetic consensus DNA antigens. Vaccine 3(6):e2517. doi:10.1371/journal.pone.0002517

Lang KA, Yan J, Draghia-Akli R, Khan A, Weiner DB (2008) Strong HCV NS3- and NS4A-specific cellular immune responses induced in mice and Rhesus macaques by a novel HCV genotype 1a/1b consensus DNA vaccine. Vaccine 26(49):6225–6231

Latimer B, Toporovski R, Yan J, Pankhong P, Morrow MP, Khan AS, Sardesai NY, Welles SL, Jacobson JM, Weiner DB, Kutzler MA (2014) Strong HCV NS3/4a, NS4b, NS5a, NS5b-specific cellular immune responses induced in Rhesus macaques by a novel HCV genotype 1a/1b consensus DNA vaccine. Hum Vaccines Immunotherapeutics 10(8):2357–2365. doi:10.4161/hv.29590

Lin F, Shen X, Kichaev G, Mendoza JM, Yang M, Armendi P, Yan J, Kobinger GP, Bello A, Khan AS, Broderick KE, Sardesai NY (2012) Optimization of electroporation-enhanced intradermal delivery of DNA vaccine using a minimally invasive surface device. Hum Gene Ther Methods 23(3):157–168. doi:10.1089/hgtb.2011.209

Lin F, Shen X, McCoy JR, Mendoza JM, Yan J, Kemmerrer SV, Khan AS, Weiner DB, Broderick KE, Sardesai NY (2011) A novel prototype device for electroporation-enhanced DNA vaccine delivery simultaneously to both skin and muscle. Vaccine 29(39):6771–6780. doi:10.1016/j.vaccine.2010.12.057

Liu H, Geng S, Feng C, Xie X, Wu B, Chen X, Zou Q, Wang S, Cui J, Xing R, Li W, Lu Y, Wang B (2013) A DNA vaccine targeting p42.3 induces protective antitumor immunity via eliciting cytotoxic CD8+T lymphocytes in a murine melanoma model. Hum Vaccines Immunotherapeutics 9(10):2196–2202. doi:10.4161/hv.25013

Lladser A, Ljungberg K, Tufvesson H, Tazzari M, Roos AK, Quest AF, Kiessling R (2010) Intradermal DNA electroporation induces survivin-specific CTLs, suppresses angiogenesis and confers protection against mouse melanoma. Cancer Immunol Immunother CII 59(1):81–92. doi:10.1007/s00262-009-0725-4

Lollini PL, Cavallo F, De Giovanni C, Nanni P (2013) Preclinical vaccines against mammary carcinoma. Expert Rev Vaccines 12(12):1449–1463. doi:10.1586/14760584.2013.845530

Low L, Mander A, McCann K, Dearnaley D, Tjelle T, Mathiesen I, Stevenson F, Ottensmeier CH (2009) DNA vaccination with electroporation induces increased antibody responses in patients with prostate cancer. Hum Gene Ther 20(11):1269–1278

Mao L, Sun W, Li W, Cui J, Zhang J, Xing R, Lu Y (2014) Cell cycle-dependent expression of p42.3 promotes mitotic progression in malignant transformed cells. Mol Carcinogenesis 53(5):337–348. doi:10.1002/mc.21982

Marur S, D'Souza G, Westra WH, Forastiere AA (2010) HPV-associated head and neck cancer: a virus-related cancer epidemic. Lancet Oncol 11(8):781–789. doi:10.1016/s1470-2045(10)70017-6

McCray AN, Ugen KE, Heller R (2007) Enhancement of anti-melanoma activity of a plasmid expressing HIV-1 Vpr delivered through in vivo electroporation. Cancer Biol Ther 6(8):1269–1275

McCray AN, Ugen KE, Muthumani K, Kim JJ, Weiner DB, Heller R (2006) Complete regression of established subcutaneous B16 murine melanoma tumors after delivery of an HIV-1 Vpr-expressing plasmid by in vivo electroporation. Mol Ther 14(5):647–655

Morrow MP, Yan J, Pankhong P, Ferraro B, Lewis MG, Khan AS, Sardesai NY, Weiner DB (2010) Unique Th1/Th2 phenotypes induced during priming and memory phases by use of interleukin-12 (IL-12) or IL-28B vaccine adjuvants in rhesus macaques. Clin Vaccine Immunol CVI 17(10):1493–1499. doi:10.1128/cvi.00181-10

Morrow MP, Yan J, Sardesai NY (2013) Human papillomavirus therapeutic vaccines: targeting viral antigens as immunotherapy for precancerous disease and cancer. Expert Rev Vaccines 12 (3):271–283. doi:10.1586/erv.13.23

Muthumani K, Lambert VM, Kawalekar O, Heller R, Kim JJ, Weiner DB, Ugen KE (2010) Anticancer activity of the HIV accessory molecule viral protein R (Vpr): Delivery as a DNA expression plasmid or biologically active peptides. Vaccine 28(8):2005–2010. doi:10.1016/j.vaccine.2009.10.060

Muthumani K, Lambert VM, Shanmugam M, Thieu KP, Choo AY, Chung JC, Satishchandran A, Kim JJ, Weiner DB, Ugen KE (2009) Anti-tumor activity mediated by protein and peptide transduction of HIV viral protein R (Vpr). Cancer Biol Ther 8(2):180–187

Muthumani K, Wise MC, Broderick KE, Hutnick N, Goodman J, Flingai S, Yan J, Bian CB, Mendoza J, Tingey C, Wilson C, Wojtak K, Sardesai NY, Weiner DB (2013) HIV-1 Env DNA vaccine plus protein boost delivered by EP expands B- and T-cell responses and neutralizing phenotype in vivo. PLoS One 8(12):e84234. doi:10.1371/journal.pone.0084234

Norell H, Poschke I, Charo J, Wei WZ, Erskine C, Piechocki MP, Knutson KL, Bergh J, Lidbrink E, Kiessling R (2010) Vaccination with a plasmid DNA encoding HER-2/neu together with low doses of GM-CSF and IL-2 in patients with metastatic breast carcinoma: a pilot clinical trial. J Transl Med 8:53. doi:10.1186/1479-5876-8-53

Ohlschlager P, Quetting M, Alvarez G, Durst M, Gissmann L, Kaufmann AM (2009) Enhancement of immunogenicity of a therapeutic cervical cancer DNA-based vaccine by co-application of sequence-optimized genetic adjuvants. Int J Cancer 125(1):189–198

Ohlschlager P, Spies E, Alvarez G, Quetting M, Groettrup M (2011) The combination of TLR-9 adjuvantation and electroporation-mediated delivery enhances in vivo antitumor responses after vaccination with HPV-16 E7 encoding DNA. Int J Cancer J Int du Cancer 128(2):473–481. doi:10.1002/ijc.25344

Peruzzi D, Gavazza A, Mesiti G, Lubas G, Scarselli E, Conforti A, Bendtsen C, Ciliberto G, La Monica N, Aurisicchio L (2010) A vaccine targeting telomerase enhances survival of dogs affected by B-cell lymphoma. Mol Ther J Am Soc Gene Ther 18(8):1559–1567. doi:10.1038/mt.2010.104

Quaglino E, Iezzi M, Mastini C, Amici A, Pericle F, Di CE, Pupa SM, De GC, Spadaro M, Curcio C, Lollini PL, Musiani P, Forni G, Cavallo F (2004) Electroporated DNA vaccine clears away multifocal mammary carcinomas in her-2/neu transgenic mice. Cancer Res 64(8):2858–2864

Radkevich-Brown O, Piechocki MP, Back JB, Weise AM, Pilon-Thomas S, Wei WZ (2010) Intratumoral DNA electroporation induces anti-tumor immunity and tumor regression. Cancer Immunol Immunother CII 59(3):409–417. doi:10.1007/s00262-009-0760-1

Reiter RE, Gu Z, Watabe T, Thomas G, Szigeti K, Davis E, Wahl M, Nisitani S, Yamashiro J, Le Beau MM, Loda M, Witte ON (1998) Prostate stem cell antigen: a cell surface marker overexpressed in prostate cancer. Proc Natl Acad Sci USA 95(4):1735–1740

Riccardo F, Iussich S, Maniscalco L, Lorda Mayayo S, La Rosa G, Arigoni M, De Maria R, Gattino F, Lanzardo S, Lardone E, Martano M, Morello E, Prestigio S, Fiore A, Quaglino E, Zabarino S, Ferrone S, Buracco P, Cavallo F (2014) CSPG4-specific immunity and survival prolongation in dogs with oral malignant melanoma immunized with human CSPG4 DNA. Clin Cancer Res Official J Am Assoc Cancer Res 20(14):3753–3762. doi:10.1158/1078-0432.ccr-13-3042

Roos AK, Eriksson F, Walters DC, Pisa P, King AD (2009) Optimization of skin electroporation in mice to increase tolerability of DNA vaccine delivery to patients. Mol Ther 17(9):1637–1642

Roos AK, King A, Pisa P (2008) DNA vaccination for prostate cancer. In: Li S (ed) Methods in molecular biology. Electroporation protocols. Preclinical and clinical gene medicine, vol 423. Humana Press, Totowa, New Jersey, 07512, pp 463–472

Roos AK, Moreno S, Leder C, Pavlenko M, King A, Pisa P (2006) Enhancement of cellular immune response to a prostate cancer DNA vaccine by intradermal electroporation. Mol Ther 13(2):320–327

Sajadian A, Tabarraei A, Soleimanjahi H, Fotouhi F, Gorji A, Ghaemi A (2014) Comparing the effect of Toll-like receptor agonist adjuvants on the efficiency of a DNA vaccine. Arch Virol 159(8):1951–1960. doi:10.1007/s00705-014-2024-4

Saranga-Perry V, Ambe C, Zager JS, Kudchadkar RR (2014) Recent developments in the medical and surgical treatment of melanoma. CA Cancer J Clin 64(3):171–185. doi:10.3322/caac.21224

Sardesai NY, Weiner DB (2011) Electroporation delivery of DNA vaccines: prospects for success. Curr Opin Immunol 23(3):421–429

Seo SH, Jin HT, Park SH, Youn JI, Sung YC (2009) Optimal induction of HPV DNA vaccine-induced CD8+ T cell responses and therapeutic antitumor effect by antigen engineering and electroporation. Vaccine 27(42):5906–5912. doi:10.1016/j.vaccine.2009.07.033

Shedlock DJ, Aviles J, Talbott KT, Wong G, Wu SJ, Villarreal DO, Myles DJ, Croyle MA, Yan J, Kobinger GP, Weiner DB (2013) Induction of broad cytotoxic T cells by protective DNA vaccination against Marburg and Ebola. Mol Ther J Am Soc Gene Ther 21(7):1432–1444. doi:10.1038/mt.2013.61

Shin TH, Pankhong P, Yan J, Khan AS, Sardesai NY, Weiner DB (2012) Induction of robust cellular immunity against HPV6 and HPV11 in mice by DNA vaccine encoding for E6/E7 antigen. Hum Vaccines Immunotherapeutics 8(4):470–478. doi:10.4161/hv.19180

Smorlesi A, Papalini F, Amici A, Orlando F, Pierpaoli S, Mancini C, Provinciali M (2006) Evaluation of different plasmid DNA delivery systems for immunization against HER2/neu in a transgenic murine model of mammary carcinoma. Vaccine 24(11):1766–1775

Spies E, Reichardt W, Alvarez G, Groettrup M, Ohlschlager P (2012) An artificial PAP gene breaks self-tolerance and promotes tumor regression in the TRAMP model for prostate carcinoma. Mol Ther J Am Soc Gene Ther 20(3):555–564. doi:10.1038/mt.2011.241

Takeshita F, Tanaka T, Matsuda T, Tozuka M, Kobiyama K, Saha S, Matsui K, Ishii KJ, Coban C, Akira S, Ishii N, Suzuki K, Klinman DM, Okuda K, Sasaki S (2006) Toll-like receptor adaptor molecules enhance DNA-raised adaptive immune responses against influenza and tumors through activation of innate immunity. J Virol 80(13):6218–6224. doi:10.1128/jvi.00121-06

Venanzi F, Shifrin V, Sherman M, Gabai V, Kiselev O, Komissarov A, Grudinin M, Shartukova M, Romanovskaya-Romanko EA, Kudryavets Y, Bezdenezhnykh N, Lykhova O, Semesyuk N, Concetti A, Tsyb A, Filimonova M, Makarchuk V, Yakubovsky R, Chursov A, Shcherbinina V, Shneider A (2013) Broad-spectrum anti-tumor and anti-metastatic DNA vaccine based on p62-encoding vector. Oncotarget 4(10):1829–1835

Villarreal DO, Talbott KT, Choo DK, Shedlock DJ, Weiner DB (2013) Synthetic DNA vaccine strategies against persistent viral infections. Expert Rev Vaccines 12(5):537–554. doi:10.1586/erv.13.33

Villarreal DO, Wise MC, Walters JN, Reuschel EL, Choi MJ, Obeng-Adjei N, Yan J, Morrow MP, Weiner DB (2014) Alarmin IL-33 acts as an immunoadjuvant to enhance antigen-specific tumor immunity. Cancer Res 74(6):1789–1800. doi:10.1158/0008-5472.can-13-2729

Wolff JA, Malone RW, Williams P, Chong W, Acsadi G, Jani A, Felgner PL (1990) Direct gene transfer into mouse muscle in vivo. Science 247(4949 Pt 1):1465–1468

Yan J, Harris K, Khan AS, Draghia-Akli R, Sewell DA, Weiner DB (2008) Cellular immunity induced by a novel HPV18 DNA vaccine encoding an E6/E7 fusion consensus protein in mice and rhesus macaques. Vaccine 26(40):5210–5215

Yan J, Pankhong P, Shin TH, Obeng-Adjei N, Morrow MP, Walters JN, Khan AS, Sardesai NY, Weiner DB (2013) Highly optimized DNA vaccine targeting human telomerase reverse transcriptase stimulates potent antitumor immunity. Cancer Immunol Res 1(3):179–189. doi:10.1158/2326-6066.cir-13-0001

Yan J, Tingey C, Lyde R, Gorham TC, Choo DK, Muthumani A, Myles D, Weiner LP, Kraynyak KA, Reuschel EL, Finkel TH, Kim JJ, Sardesai NY, Ugen KE, Muthumani K, Weiner DB (2014a) Novel and enhanced anti-melanoma DNA vaccine targeting the tyrosinase protein inhibits myeloid-derived suppressor cells and tumor growth in a syngeneic prophylactic and therapeutic murine model. Cancer Gene Ther. doi:10.1038/cgt.2014.56

Yan J, Villarreal DO, Racine T, Chu JS, Walters JN, Morrow MP, Khan AS, Sardesai NY, Kim JJ, Kobinger GP, Weiner DB (2014b) Protective immunity to H7N9 influenza viruses elicited by synthetic DNA vaccine. Vaccine 32(24):2833–2842. doi:10.1016/j.vaccine.2014.02.038
Yersal O, Barutca S (2014) Biological subtypes of breast cancer: prognostic and therapeutic implications. World J Clin Oncol 5(3):412–424. doi:10.5306/wjco.v5.i3.412
Zaks K, Jordan M, Guth A, Sellins K, Kedl R, Izzo A, Bosio C, Dow S (2006) Efficient immunization and cross-priming by vaccine adjuvants containing TLR3 or TLR9 agonists complexed to cationic liposomes. J Immunol (Baltimore, Md: 1950) 176 (12):7335–7345

Targeted Immunotherapy Designed to Treat MUC1-Expressing Solid Tumour

Bruce Acres, Gisele Lacoste and Jean-Marc Limacher

Abstract Several approaches to antigen-specific immunotherapy of cancer antigen-specific immunotherapy of cancer have been tested clinically. In this chapter, we will describe studies done with the antigen MUC1. Tested MUC1 therapeutic vaccines include the following: monoclonal antibodies (MAbs) specific for MUC1; synthetic and recombinant polypeptides from the protein sequence of MUC1; dendritic cells carrying MUC1; RNA and DNA vaccinations; and recombinant viruses carrying the MUC1 DNA sequence. Chemotherapy of cancer aims to be toxic to the cancer cells with manageable side effects to the patient. In contrast, antigen-specific immunotherapy of cancer aims to treat the patient, such that the patient is then able to control and eventually eliminate their cancer cells. It is therefore important to know the immune status of each cancer patient prior to therapy.

Contents

G. Lacoste (✉) · J.-M. Limacher
Department of Medical Affairs, Transgene SA, 400 Blvd Gonthier d'Andernach, Parc d'Innovation CS80166, 67405 Illkirch-Graffenstaden Cedex, France
e-mail: lacoste@transgene.fr

B. Acres
Bruce Acres Consulting, Strasbourg, France

Current Topics in Microbiology and Immunology (2017) 405:79–97
DOI 10.1007/82_2015_429

Published Online: 22 February 2015

1 Introduction

1.1 Historical Background

The ferocity of a full-blown immune reaction to some pathogens and, most dramatically, in organ graft rejection has tempted immunologists for generations, to hope that the destructive power of this force could be focused onto cancer cells. The realization of that dream had a slow start, due to the sequential revelations of the many complexities of the immune system. Now, armed with much better knowledge of the vast array of accelerators and brakes used by the immune system, some progress is being made in the treatment of cancer with immunotherapy (Weber 2014).

The application of immune stimulation to cancer treatment was first attempted over a century ago. Most often with sarcomas, some early success was observed when William Coley injected patients with a concoction of bacterial extracts, Coley's toxins (Coley 1893, 1906). The reaction to the toxins and their eventual success in the elimination of some tumours has been attributed to a strong cytokine reaction to bacterial products.

A more antigen-specific approach was also tried in the early 1900s. Patients were injected with their own tumour cells or extracts, or tumour cells of the same type from other patients (Coca and Lebredo 1912; Coca 1909). Again, some successes were noted, but growth of new tumours was also observed.

During the following decades, the miracle of penicillin led many to believe that any disease could be treated with small chemical molecules. This was in addition to the magic of radiotherapy and advances in surgery. Therefore, these new treatments soon overshadowed any attempts to coax the immune system to eliminate cancer cells.

Fifty years later, interest in immunology was reawakened by the seminal work of Medawar (Billingham et al. 1953) and Burnet (1960), who showed some of the complexities of the immune response in the demonstration that the immune system could be rendered tolerant to some antigens and that the specific immune response was the result of cellular clonal expansion. Therefore, evidence was starting to accumulate to show that the immune response could be manipulated. Over the same period of time, the 1950s, it was demonstrated that the rodent immune system had ability to react and destroy autologous tumour cells (Foley 1953; Prehn and Main 1957; Baldwin 1955). Inbred stains of mice were available, along with continuous tumour cell lines from various mouse strains. The antigens responsible for this recognition were initially called TSTA for tumour-specific transplantation antigens, but are now called tumour-associated antigens or TAAs. Work soon followed to identify some of these antigens from rodent (Harris et al. 1973; De Plaen et al. 1988) and human (Eichmuller et al. 2001) tumour cells.

During the next decade, immunology began to elucidate various immune control mechanisms such as IgG feedback, high-dose and low-dose tolerance, and T suppressor (and contra-suppressor) cells.

In 1975, a major leap forward occurred in the laboratory of Kohler and Milstein: the discovery that antibody-producing murine plasma cells could be fused to murine plasmacytoma cells to create a 'hybridoma'. These hybrid cells could be cloned, grown to large quantities (Kohler and Milstein 1975) and produce almost limitless quantities of antibodies with a single specificity. This was also a turning point with the discovery and purification of many antigenic molecules including TAA. One such antigen, MUC1, was initially thought to be a collection of distinct molecules associated with several different tumour types. Several tumour-specific antibodies were derived in several different laboratories, using different tumour cells as the immunizing antigen. Each laboratory had a different name for their antibody and a different name for their TAA (Keydar et al. 1989; Sekine et al. 1985; Kim et al. 1988; Burchell et al. 1984; Stacker et al. 1989; Lan et al. 1987).

1.2 MUC1

Once the genes for the corresponding proteins were cloned, several of these were shown to be the same MUC1 tumour-associated antigen. This TAA was subsequently shown to be abnormally expressed on a variety of cancer cells, predominantly epithelial tumours (Jonckheere and Van Seuningen 2010). MUC1 is so commonly over-expressed in a tumour-associated form (see below) that it has been estimated to be a potential target of immune therapy for about 80 % of all cancer cases (Kimura and Finn 2013). It has also been shown to be expressed on several normal tissues (Peat et al. 1992) albeit in a different glycoform.

MUC1-specific monoclonal antibodies (MAbs) are able to distinguish healthy MUC1 from cancer-associated MUC1 (Burchell et al. 1984; Sekine et al. 1985; Keydar et al. 1989; Lan et al. 1987; Kim et al. 1988; Stacker et al. 1989). The reason for this was demonstrated in the laboratory of Joyce Taylor-Papadimitriou, who, in an elegant series of experiments, showed that antibodies generated to the human milk fat protein, mucin-1, chemically stripped of its carbohydrate side chains, could react specifically to cancer-associated MUC1 glycoprotein (Burchell et al. 1987; Burchell and Taylor-Papadimitriou 1993). This suggested that cancer-associated MUC1 is non- or at least under-glycosylated with respect to the normal MUC1 glycoprotein.

It was eventually shown that cancer-associated MUC1 has about as many glycosylated sites on the protein core as normal MUC1, but that the carbohydrate side chains are much shorter and terminated with a sialyl group (see Fig. 1). The reason for this was shown to be a cancer-associated perturbation in the relative expression of the numerous glycosyl transferase enzymes responsible for the assembly of the carbohydrate side chains on the MUC1 protein (Dalziel et al. 2001; Picco et al. 2010).

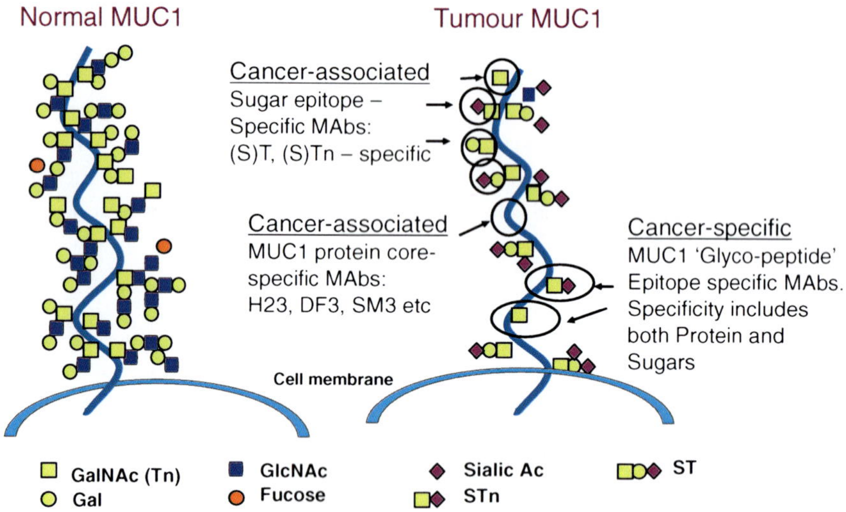

Fig. 1 The MUC1 protein on cancer cells is modified and expresses several types of novel, cancer-associated antigenic epitopes (Re-published, with permission, from Acres and Limacher (2005))

Many pre-clinical and laboratory experiments in mice and rats have provided a wealth information on the potential for MUC1-based vaccines combined with sophisticated vaccinations strategies for the treatment of cancer. These have been reviewed by Tang and Apostolopoulos (2008) and Roulois et al. (2013). This review will focus on a description of the biology of MUC1 and MUC1-based vaccines that have been tested in clinical studies.

2 Biology of MUC1

The molecular biology and biochemistry of MUC1 have been nicely reviewed recently by Nath and Mukherjee (2014). Briefly, MUC1 is a long, rigid protein which towers above the glycocalyx at the cell surface. It is comprised of an intracellular, C-terminal segment, rich in conserved tyrosines; a single-pass trans-membrane region and a large extracellular region comprised mainly of a tandemly repeated 20 amino acid segment, the variable number tandem repeats (VNTR), which can be repeated from 20 to 120 times. In healthy epithelial tissues, MUC1 expression is restricted to the luminal side of epithelial cells lining secretory ducts. It acts as a lubricant for material passing though the duct, but also protects the epithelial cells from the same contents and from bacteria. In contrast, on tumour cells, MUC1 expression is over-expressed, is hypo-glycosylated and is not restricted to any particular cell surface.

Studies have shown that MUC1 contributes to the transcriptional regulation of genes associated with not only immune regulation and inflammation, but also drug resistance, apoptosis, proliferation, angiogenesis, metastases and tumour cell invasion (Nath and Mukherjee 2014). Thus, MUC1 is not only an important target antigen for cancer immunotherapy due to its over-expression and cancer-associated modifications, but MUC1 is a very important target antigen since the reduction of MUC1 expression by immune selection of MUC1-negative variants would have a serious negative impact of the ability of the tumour cells to replicate, invade and metastasize.

3 MUC1 Immunology

3.1 Antibody Responses

Some patients with MUC1-expressing tumours do spontaneously show signs of an antibody response to MUC1, which seems associated with better prognosis (von Mensdorff-Pouilly et al. 2000) without overt signs of autoimmunity. These antibodies were identified using an ELISA with synthetic, non-glycosylated MUC1 VNTR peptides. Early vaccine studies with MUC1 showed that blood samples taken from patients prior to MUC1 immunotherapy did sometimes have a demonstrable level of antibodies to MUC1. Patients who had no anti-MUC1 prior to immunotherapy did not develop antibodies to MUC1 following vaccination, as determined using the same ELISA as described above (Scholl et al. 2003). It has been shown, using human MUC1 transgenic mice, that antibodies to human MUC1 (hMUC1) do not cause any signs of autoimmunity, even when the mice are infused with MUC1-specific antiserum (Tempero et al. 1999).

Immune tolerance to MUC1, at the level of antibodies, appears to be well established as demonstrated in transgenic mice (Rowse et al. 1998; Acres et al. 2000) when using an ELISA in which synthetic non-glycosylated VNTR peptide was used. Interestingly, evidence of a T cell response was observed in MUC1-vaccinated hMUC1 transgenic mice. In another hMUC1 transgenic mouse system, an anti-MUC1 antibody and T cell response could be generated using a complex and very powerful immune stimulation: mouse tumour cells fused with autologous dendritic cells (Gong et al. 1998) or specific glycopeptides (Sorensen et al. 2006).

There is now an accumulation of data showing the complexity of the antibody response to MUC1 by cancer patients and the role of MUC1 glycosylation. Sorensen et al. (2006) showed that some cancer patients do have a detectable antibody response to glycoforms of MUC1. What is even more interesting is that when they used MUC1 VNTR glyco–peptide arrays to assess serum for patients in a vaccine study, they were able to show that patients had no antibody response to MUC1 glycopeptides prior to vaccination. However, once vaccinated with a VNTR peptide glycosylated with the Tn antigen (see Fig. 1), patients generated IgG antibody response to that peptide and peptides with similar glycosylation, but not to unglycosylated MUC1 (Wandall et al. 2010) or unrelated glycoforms.

3.2 MUC1 Glycosylation

Figure 1 demonstrates the glycosylation of MUC1. 'Normal' or 'healthy' MUC1 is decorated with long, complex and branched glycosyl side chains, which are often terminated with a fucose residue. In this conformation, the protein core is covered and not accessible to antibodies specific for protein core epitopes (Burchell and Taylor-Papadimitriou 1993). In contrast, the cancer-associated MUC1 presents several novel epitopes to the immune system:

1. Cancer-associated sugar epitopes, the so-called T and T antigens along with their sialylated counterparts: Sialyl-T and Sialyl Tn;
2. Cancer-associated protein core epitopes, which are exposed by the shorter, truncated carbohydrate side chains and are recognized by MAbs such as SM3 (Burchell et al. 1984) and H23 (Keydar et al. 1989); and
3. Cancer-associated epitopes which are the combination of the protein core and short sugar side chains, as recognized by the antibodies DF3 (Sekine et al. 1985) 2D9 and 5E5 (Tarp et al. 2007).

Some MAbs specific for tumour antigens have now found their way into the clinic and, since the turn of the millennium, have achieved notable successes, such as Herceptin for breast cancer (Brenner and Adams 1999) and rituximab for human B cell malignancies (Maloney 2012). These are now commercially available treatments. The application of anti-MUC1 MAbs to cancer patient treatment has also been tested clinically (Table 1). The lack of dramatic success may well be due to the release of a soluble form of MUC1 from the cancer cell, the CA15.3 tumour marker, such that it acts as a decoy for antibody molecules. Even if there was no soluble MUC1 released, the cell bound form is such a long molecule that antibodies attached to it could well be too far from the cell surface to have any significant impact.

3.3 T Cell Responses to MUC1

T cell responses to MUC1 have been reviewed in detail by Roulois et al. (2013). It is noteworthy that the first-reported human T cell response to MUC1, described in detail, was very unusual in that the T cells were not specific to the combination of MUC1 peptide sequences within the target cell surface major histocompatibility complex (MHC) I (Barnd et al. 1989). Rather, they are MHC unrestricted and were shown to be specifically blocked by the antibody to MUC1 protein core, SM3. This special type of T cell generated some scepticism since it could not be found in any murine responses to MUC1 or other tumour antigens. Nevertheless, independent laboratories have also described this cell population in humans (Noto et al. 1997; Takahashi et al. 1994). There has been some speculation that this could be a sub-population of NKT cells (Wajchman et al. 2004). Whatever their exact lineage,

Table 1 A summary of MUC1-based immunotherapeutics (Re-published, with permission, from Limacher and Acres (2014))

Type of product	Agent	Stage of development	Disease setting	Main results	References
Monoclonal MUC1-specific antibodies	MAb-AR20.5 (Brevarex®)	Phase I	Adenocarcinomas	Antibody response	De Bono et al. (2004, 354)
	AS1402	Phase I	Breast cancer, metastatic	Correct tolerance	Pegram et al. (2009, 356)
		Randomized Phase II	Breast cancer, metastatic, with letrozole	No improvement	Ibrahim et al. (2011, 357)
Radiolabeled MUC1-specific antibodies	C595-^{67}Cu	Phase I	Bladder cancer	Tumour uptake	Hughes et al. (2001, 359)
	C595-^{111}In	Phase I	Bladder cancer	Tumour uptake	Hughes et al. (2001, 359)
	NCRC48-^{111}In	Phase I	Bladder cancer	tumoral uptake	Kunkler et al. (1995, 362)
MUC1 VNTR peptides vaccines	MUC1-MFP (mannan fusion protein)	Phase I	Adenocarcinomas	Antibody and T cell immune response	Karanikas et al. (2001, 366)
		Randomized Phase III	Breast cancer	Decreased recurrence rate	Apostolopoulos et al. (2006, 371)
	L-BLP25 (Stimuvax®)	Randomized Phase II	Non-small-cell lung cancer, advanced	Improved overall survival in stage III patients	Butts et al. (2005, 372, 2011, 374)
		Phase III	Non-small-cell lung cancer, non-resectable stage III	Improved survival in patients who received concurrent chemoradiothaerpy	Butts et al. (2014, 375)
	MUC1-KLH	Phase I	Breast cancer, high risk	Antibody response	Gilewski et al. (2000, 376)

(continued)

Table 1 (continued)

Type of product	Agent	Stage of development	Disease setting	Main results	References
Vaccines based on poxviruses encoding MUC1 DNA sequence	PANVAC (CV 301)	Randomized Phase II	Colorectal, cancer after surgical resection of metastases (treated with vaccine + DC)	Improved overall survival	Morse et al. (2013, 377)
		Phase III	Pancreatic cancer, advanced, after failure of gemcitabine	No improvement of survival	Therion Biologics press release (2006)
		Randomized Phase II	Breast cancer, metastatic, combination with chemotherapy	Improved progression-free survival	Heery et al. (35th CTRC-AACR San Antonio Breast Cancer Symposium)
	TG4010	Phase II	Kidney cancer, metastatic	Favourable overall survival	Oudard et al. 2011, 88)
		Randomized Phase II	Prostate cancer, PSA failure	Improvement in PSA-doubling time	Dreicer et al. (2009, 378)
		Randomized Phase II	Lung cancer, advanced, combination with chemotherapy	Improved response rate	Ramlau et al. (2008, 90)
		Randomized Phase II	Lung cancer, advanced, combination with chemotherapy	Improved 6-month PFS and response rate, TrPAL biomarker	Quoix et al. (2011, 379)
MUC1 mRNA vaccines	In vitro-transcribed naked RNA	Phase I/II	Kidney cancer, metastatic	Stabilizations/response	Rittig et al. (2011, 380)
Adoptive cell therapy	MUC1-stimulated PBMCs	Phase I/II	Breast cancer, advanced	Change tumour burden	Wright et al. (2009, 381)
		Phase I	Ovarian cancer	One complete clinical response	Dobrzanski et al. (2009, 382), Corbiere et al. (2011)
		Phase I/II	Pancreatic cancer	Long-term survival	Lepisto et al. (2008, 383)
	MUC1-MFP-pulsed DCs	Phase I	Adenocarcinomas	Cellular immune response, two long stabilizations	Loveland et al. (2006, 385)
	Dendritic cells and CTL transfer	Phase I	Pancreatic cancer	Clinical response	Kondo et al. (2008, 408)

these cells could be very important in the patient's immune response to MUC1 expressing tumour cells, since so many tumour cells express low or no MHC I molecules. Whether these cells are activated and/or amplified by MUC1 vaccines is not yet known.

MHC I-restricted MUC1 epitopes for more 'traditional' cytotoxic T lymphocytes (CTL) have also been identified (Apostolopoulos et al. 1997; Barnea et al. 2002; Brossart et al. 1999; Dreicer et al. 2009; Heukamp et al. 2001; Roulois et al. 2011). The majority of these epitopes lie outside of the VNTR section of the MUC1 sequence. Therefore, the MUC1-based therapeutic vaccines, which include only the VNTR segment or peptides from that segment, are unlikely to stimulate such a CTL response. In addition, there are some cancer-associated forms of MUC1 devoid of the VNTR (Baruch et al. 1997; Roulois et al. 2013).

Like most non-melanoma TAA, immune monitoring of patient CTL responses to MUC1 has been a challenge. Responses, measured using lymphocytes from peripheral blood of patients, appear to be weak and transient. Measurable CTL specific for MUC1 are not rare in these patients, but do not seem to be systematically activated or amplified by vaccination. Measurable CTL are detectable in circulation of about 20–30 % of patients prior to MUC1 vaccination. Existing T cell immunity to MUC1 has been detected in blood samples from both healthy individuals and breast cancer patients, again with no overt signs of autoimmunity. Pre-existing T cell immunity to MUC1 has been associated with better response to MUC1-based immunotherapy in metastatic renal cell carcinoma and late-stage lung cancer patients (Oudard et al. 2011; Ramlau et al. 2008). The appearance of MUC1-specific CTL, nor its disappearance, was associated with better clinical outcome (Quoix et al. 2011). Nevertheless, there was an association between having a MUC1 CTL response anytime on the study, whether before or during therapy, and clinical improvement (Oudard et al. 2011; Ramlau et al. 2008). In a study with minimal remaining disease following therapy (prostate cancer therapy patients following radiation or surgery for their cancer, who have rising PSA with no apparent disease), a de novo CTL response to MUC1 during MUC1 vaccine immunotherapy was loosely associated with clinical improvement (Dreicer et al. 2009). These observations question the approach of assessing the MUC1-specific CTL response in the periphery, while the key events of this immune process happen in tissues, either lymphatic or tumour.

Monitoring patient CTL responses has become more complex with recent evidence to indicate that CTL may react to glycosylated peptides as well as to naked peptides as previously thought. It has been immunological dogma to believe that polypeptides are associated with MHC I complex without glycosylation. However, it now appears that glycopeptides can be presented to CTL in the cleft of MHC I (Ninkovic et al. 2009; Haurum et al. 1999)

In normal cells, emerging data suggest that the extensive glycosylation could prevent the MUC1 from being processed by the proteasome and thus, MUC1 peptides would not be presented with MHC class I molecules on the cell surface (Hiltbold et al. 2000; Hanisch et al. 2003; Ninkovic et al. 2009). MUC1 expressed by tumour cells is hypoglycosylated so would be more easily processed by antigen-presenting cells. This could be one potential reason why normal cells are not vulnerable to T cells targeting MUC1 epitopes.

Nevertheless, this does complicate monitoring of patient CTL responses during a clinical study due to the numbers of possible glycosylations of each MUC1 peptide epitope. This will require more patient blood per sample and more resources since glycopeptides are very expensive to produce, or new assays to detect T cell responses to a wider variety of MUC1 antigenic epitopes will be required.

CD4+ T cells, while not direct effector T cells, are nonetheless important for the development of both CTL and antibody responses. The state of glycosylation may also affect presentation to CD4+ T 'helper' cells in the context of MHC II (Vlad et al. 2002). CD4+ T cells produce a variety of cytokines which can indirectly affect the growth of tumours by, for example, restricting blood flow to the tumour mass. The traditional method for measuring CD4+ T cell activity is by lymphocyte proliferation, although ELISpot or intracellular cytokine measurement after stimulation with long peptides can also indicate CD4+ reactivity. In clinical studies, MUC1-specific CD4+ activity has been detected in lymphocytes from patient peripheral blood samples; however, no correlation with clinical activity has been described (Oudard et al. 2011; Ramlau et al. 2008).

4 MUC1 Therapeutic Vaccines in the Clinic

MUC1-based immunotherapies in clinical studies are summarized in Table 1. The application of MUC1-specific MAbs has been described above. There are two MUC-based therapeutic vaccines in clinical development, which comprise long, non-glycosylated polypeptides from the VNTR sequence from MUC1 and are most likely to elicit antibody responses. These are mannan fusion protein, MFP (Apostolopoulos et al. 2006), and Stimuvax® (Powell and Chow 2008; Wu et al. 2011).

McKenzie et al. made the important observation (Apostolopoulos et al. 1995) that coupling the carbohydrate mannan to their MUC1 VNTR-GST (glutathione-S-transferase) fusion protein affected the MUC1 VNTR-specific immune response. There are mannose receptors on dendritic (DC) cells. When mannan was coupled to the fusion protein under oxidized conditions, it induced a cytotoxic T lymphocyte (CTL) response in mice, while coupling under reducing conditions, a less effective antibody response was generated. In contrast, MFP produced under oxidizing conditions produced antibody rather than CTL in humans (Apostolopoulos et al. 1998). A small Phase III study testing MFP in breast cancer was undertaken. Over 8 years later, it was observed that rate of recurrence of breast cancer in the MFP-treated patients was significantly lower than in the non-vaccinated patient group (Apostolopoulos et al. 2006). This was an interesting observation, even though initial, protocol defined, end points were not achieved. Stimuvax® (L-BLP25 or Tecemotide) is a therapeutic vaccine based on 25-mer peptides including the pattern repeated in MUC1 VNTR which are incorporated in a liposome formulation. In a Phase II trial, 171 non-small-cell lung cancer (NSCLS) patients received subcutaneous vaccinations of L-BLP25 weekly for 8 weeks, followed by maintenance vaccinations at 6-week intervals plus best supportive care (BSC) or BSC alone. Median survival in patients receiving L-BLP25 plus BSC compared to those receiving BSC alone was 17.2 months versus 13.0 months, respectively. In the subset of patients with stage IIIb loco-regional disease, median survival time was 30.6 versus 13.3 month (Butts et al. 2011). A Phase III trial in unresectable stage III NSCLC patients was conducted (START). It did not reach its primary end point of overall survival, but a large pre-specified subgroup of 806 patients who received concurrent chemoradiotherapy demonstrated a significantly longer survival for the patients who received Stimuvax®: 30.8 versus 20.6 months (Butts et al. 2014). Based on these results, a second Phase III was launched (START2) but unfortunately prematurely terminated for strategic reasons.

As described above, most potential CTL epitopes on the MUC1 molecule lie outside of the VNTR. It is therefore of interest to incorporate the entire MUC1 molecule into therapeutic vaccines. Two such vaccines are described in Table 1, both of which utilize poxviruses as vectors for the MUC1 gene sequence. Poxviruses are useful because large DNA sequences can be inserted, and they are safe and reasonably easy to produce and very immunogenic. In both the PANVAC and TG4010 therapeutic vaccines, additional sequences for immune-stimulating molecules are co-expressed.

PANVAC is based on two poxviruses, vaccinia and fowlpox, engineered to express two tumour antigens, CEA and MUC1, plus a complex series of co-stimulatory molecules, all of which have been administered either together with the cytokine GM-CSF or as infected dendritic cells, in a Phase II study at the NIH. Some clinical benefit was observed.

TG4010, which by comparison, is simpler, since it uses one poxvirus: the non-propagative modified virus of Ankara (MVA), which incorporates MUC1 and the immune stimulatory cytokine IL2. TG4010 has been tested in Phase II studies in breast, kidney, prostate and lung cancers. Now, two controlled Phase IIb studies in late-stage NSCLS have been completed.

MUC1 epitope peptides have been characterized by cell binding assay and iTopia® and have been used to test T cell response by patients treated with TG4010. ELISpot was used to test T cells from lung, prostate and kidney cancer patients who have been treated with TG4010. Many of these epitope peptides have now been incorporated into tetramers (Quoix et al. 2011). At least, some MUC1-specific T cells using most peptides were observed. The strongest and most frequently detected CTL were identified using the HLA-B7 epitopes, with both ELISpot and tetramers. Neither of the HLA-B7 epitopes tested are from the tandem repeat of MUC1. HLA-A2, the most frequent HLA type in Caucasians, has received a lot of attention when looking for TAA epitopes. MUC1 peptides that bind to HLA-A2 have been identified (Heukamp et al. 2001; Barnea et al. 2002; Brossart et al. 1999; Apostolopoulos et al. 1997; Ramlau et al. 2008) and were included in the analyses of immune responses by lymphocytes from T4010-treated patients. CTL detected with these A2 peptides, either in ELISpot or using tetramers, were less frequent as with the B7 peptides.

In both PANVAC and TG4010, the MUC1 antigen is co-expressed with additional signals to provide a local stimulation to a cellular immune response. In PANVAC, these signals are in the form of the co-stimulatory molecules B7.1 (CD80), ICAM-1 (CD54) and LFA-2 (CD58). The vaccine is often given together with another positive immune signal in the form of GM-CSF. TG4010 also provides the positive immune signal IL-2 in addition to the MUC1 antigen. Including these positive immune stimulatory signals is like pressing a bit harder on the accelerator of the immune system. It is felt that this is required since the immune system of late-stage cancer patients is often described as 'tired' or 'anergic' such that additional immune systems can provide a secondary boost to the local immune response. From this perspective, the viral vectors themselves are seen by immune system as a danger system, further contributing to co-signalling messages during antigen presentation by dendritic cells to lymphocytes.

Another concept, which holds great potential, is to inhibit the immune inhibitors. Using the same analogy as above, it is like removing, or at least weakening, the brakes on the immune system. This is done by applying antibodies which inhibit negative immune signals such as PD-1 (Herbst et al. 2014; Hamid et al. 2013; Tumeh et al. 2014) or CTLA-4 (Robert et al. 2014; Ribas et al. 2012). This may require more caution since it removes some elements of control, which may be required to guide the immune response through its many dips and turns and avoid collateral damage such as autoimmunity.

A similar approach, removing growth controls altogether from the amplification of immune effector cells, is the in vitro amplification and activation of a patient's own tumour infiltrating or other tumour-specific T cells. These cells develop without any of the in vivo checks and balances exerted on immune development in vivo. They are grown to large numbers in vitro and then injected back into patients. A recent editorial in Nature Biotechnology (2013) advises caution for the treatment of cancer with in vitro-activated, tumour antigen-specific T cells. In theory, the T cells are exquisitely specific for tumour antigens. Nevertheless, severe toxicity can be associated with these treatments.

It has been estimated that decades can elapse between, for instance, the first lung cancer cell division and eventual diagnosis of lung cancer. During that time, the cancer and the immune system develop a relationship which is both dynamic and patient specific. At the time of diagnosis, some patients have evidence of a dominant inflammatory response with abnormally high blood levels of inflammation-related proteins and cytokines such as CRP, sCD54, IL-6, IL-10 and CSF-1. Inflammation is usually associated with poor clinical response to treatments such as chemotherapy or immunotherapy. Other patients do not show any particular signs of inflammation, but have a measurable immune response to tumour antigens, cellular and/or antibody, both of which have been associated with better response to therapy (Ramlau et al. 2008; von Mensdorff-Pouilly et al. 2000; Oudard et al. 2011). Some patients have abnormally high levels of cells with activated natural killer and/or natural killer T cell phenotype (CD16+ CD56+ CD69+) at the time of diagnosis (Quoix et al. 2011). These cells have come to be called TrPAL for triple-positive activated lymphocytes. Abnormally, high levels of these cells in lung cancer patients, prior to therapy, are associated with poor response to TG4010 in combination with chemotherapy. No such association is seen in response to chemotherapy alone.

The correlation between lower levels of TrPAL cells and better response to TG4010 therapy has now been further supported in a second Phase IIb study in stage IV lung cancer patients (Quoix et al. 2014).

Therefore, the status of the patient's immune system should be considered when deciding whether to treat with some immunotherapeutics. In addition to the TrPAL biomarker, other soluble signs of immune imbalance were also associated with poorer or better response to TG 4010, namely sCD-54, IL-10 or CSF-1 (Quoix et al. 2011).

Chemotherapy is designed to be toxic for the disease with hopes for usually manageable side effects to the patient. In contrast, vaccine immunotherapy treats the patient with the intention that the patient's own immune system will then treat the cancer. Thus, it is imperative that the patient's immune system is still adequately and correctly reactive.

The fine specificity of the 'therapeutic' T cells following an immunotherapeutic vaccination is an interesting question. One could question whether the immune response to the vaccine is responsible for observed clinical responses. Alternatively, the response to the vaccine may sufficiently disturb the established anergy, which allows the immune system to react and to find the most effective therapeutic antigen specificity. Such antigen spreading has been observed in melanoma (Corbiere et al. 2011).

5 Conclusion

Lung cancer is the leading cause of cancer-related mortality in both men and women. Most new cases of lung cancer are NSCLC, and about 60 % of cases are diagnosed as unresectable or advanced. In patients with unresectable, localized, NSCLC chemotherapy combined with radiation is a viable option. For patients with advanced or metastatic NSCLC, there are fewer treatment options. Chemotherapy has demonstrated some improvement in survival, but the treatment of these patients remains unsatisfactory. More effective therapies need to be found. Most targeted therapies for NSCLC are based on either small inhibitory molecules or MAbs which interfere with tumour growth, angiogenesis or both (Auberger et al. 2006). Vaccine-based therapeutic immunotherapy is designed to induce or amplify an immune response directed against the population of tumour cells (O'Mahony et al. 2005). Due to its over-expression on many cancer cells and in cancer-specific forms, MUC1 is a potential target for immunotherapy of many cancers (Cheever et al. 2009). Recent data indicate that there is a true potential for the treatment of late-stage lung cancer patients, as well as many other MUC1+ cancers, with therapeutic vaccines such as TG4010.

References

Editorial (2013) Do no harm. Nat Biotechnol 31(5):365. doi: 10.310.1038/nbt.2587

Acres B, Apostolopoulos V, Balloul JM, Wreschner D, Xing PX, Ali-Hadji D, Bizouarne N, Kieny MP, McKenzie IF (2000) MUC1-specific immune responses in human MUC1 transgenic mice immunized with various human MUC1 vaccines. Cancer Immunol Immunother 48(10):588–594

Acres B, Limacher JM (2005) MUC1 as a target antigen for cancer immunotherapy. Expert Rev Vaccines 4(4): 493–502

Apostolopoulos V, Karanikas V, Haurum JS, McKenzie IF (1997) Induction of HLA-A2-restricted CTLs to the mucin 1 human breast cancer antigen. J Immunol 159(11):5211–5218

Apostolopoulos V, Osinski C, McKenzie IF (1998) MUC1 cross-reactive Gal alpha(1,3)Gal antibodies in humans switch immune responses from cellular to humoral. Nat Med 4(3):315–320

Apostolopoulos V, Pietersz GA, Tsibanis A, Tsikkinis A, Drakaki H, Loveland BE, Piddlesden SJ, Plebanski M, Pouniotis DS, Alexis MN, McKenzie IF, Vassilaros S (2006) Pilot phase III immunotherapy study in early-stage breast cancer patients using oxidized mannan-MUC1 [ISRCTN71711835]. Breast Cancer Res 8(3):R27

Apostolopoulos V, Pietersz GA, Xing PX, Lees CJ, Michael M, Bishop J, McKenzie IF (1995) The immunogenicity of MUC1 peptides and fusion protein. Cancer Lett 90(1):21–26

Auberger J, Loeffler-Ragg J, Wurzer W, Hilbe W (2006) Targeted therapies in non-small cell lung cancer: proven concepts and unfulfilled promises. Curr Cancer Drug Targets 6(4):271–294

Baldwin RW (1955) Immunity to methylcholanthrene-induced tumours in inbred rats following atrophy and regression of the implanted tumours. Br J Cancer 9(4):652–657

Barnd DL, Lan MS, Metzgar RS, Finn OJ (1989) Specific, major histocompatibility complex-unrestricted recognition of tumor-associated mucins by human cytotoxic T cells. Proc Natl Acad Sci U S A 86(18):7159–7163

Barnea E, Beer I, Patoka R, Ziv T, Kessler O, Tzehoval E, Eisenbach L, Zavazava N, Admon A (2002) Analysis of endogenous peptides bound by soluble MHC class I molecules: a novel approach for identifying tumor-specific antigens. Eur J Immunol 32(1):213–222

Baruch A, Hartmann M, Zrihan-Licht S, Greenstein S, Burstein M, Keydar I, Weiss M, Smorodinsky N, Wreschner DH (1997) Preferential expression of novel MUC1 tumor antigen isoforms in human epithelial tumors and their tumor-potentiating function. Int J Cancer 71 (5):741–749

Billingham RE, Brent L, Medawar PB (1953) Actively acquired tolerance of foreign cells. Nature 172(4379):603–606

de Bono JS, Rha SY, Stephenson J, Schultes BC, Monroe P, Eckhardt GS, Hammond LA, Whiteside TL, Nicodemus CF, Cermak JM, Rowinsky EK, Tolcher AW (2004) Phase I trial of a murine antibody to Muc1 in patients with metastatic cancer: evidence for the activation of humoral and cellular antitumor immunity. Ann Oncol 15(12):1825–1833

Brenner TL, Adams VR (1999) First MAb approved for treatment of metastatic breast cancer. J Am Pharm Assoc (Wash) 39(2):236–238

Brossart P, Heinrich KS, Stuhler G, Behnke L, Reichardt VL, Stevanovic S, Muhm A, Rammensee HG, Kanz L, Brugger W (1999) Identification of HLA-A2-restricted T-cell epitopes derived from the MUC1 tumor antigen for broadly applicable vaccine therapies. Blood 93(12): 4309–4317

Burchell J, Gendler S, Taylor-Papadimitriou J, Girling A, Lewis A, Millis R, Lamport D (1987) Development and characterization of breast cancer reactive monoclonal antibodies directed to the core protein of the human milk mucin. Cancer Res 47(20):5476–5482

Burchell J, Taylor-Papadimitriou J (1993) Effect of modification of carbohydrate side chains on the reactivity of antibodies with core-protein epitopes of the MUC1 gene product. Epithelial Cell Biol 2(4):155–162

Burchell J, Wang D, Taylor-Papadimitriou J (1984) Detection of the tumour-associated antigens recognized by the monoclonal antibodies HMFG-1 and 2 in serum from patients with breast cancer. Int J Cancer 34(6):763–768

Burnet FM (1960) Theories of immunity. Perspect Biol Med 3:447–458

Butts C, Maksymiuk A, Goss G, Soulières D, Marshall E, Cormier Y, Ellis PM, Price A, Sawhney R, Beier F, Falk M, Murray N (2011) Updated survival analysis in patients with stage IIIB or IV non-small-cell lung cancer receiving BLP25 liposome vaccine (L-BLP25): phase IIB randomized, multicenter, open-label trial. J Cancer Res Clin Oncol 137(9):1337–1342

Butts C, Murray N, Maksymiuk A, Goss G, Marshall E, Soulières D, Cormier Y, Ellis P, Price A, Sawhney R, Davis M, Mansi J, Smith C, Vergidis D, Ellis P, MacNeil M, Palmer M (2005) Randomized phase IIb trial of BLP25 liposome vaccine in stage IIIB and IV non-small-cell lung cancer. J Clin Oncol 23(27):6674–6681

Butts C, Socinski MA, Mitchell PL, Thatcher N, Havel L, Krzakowski M, Nawrocki S, Ciuleanu TE, Bosquee L, Trigo JM, Spira A, Tremblay L, Nyman J, Ramlau R, Wickart-Johansson G, Ellis P, Gladkov O, Pereira JR, Eberhardt WE, Helwig C, Schroder A, Shepherd FA, Team S.t (2014) Tecemotide (L-BLP25) versus placebo after chemoradiotherapy for stage III non-small-cell lung cancer (START): a randomised, double-blind, phase 3 trial. Lancet Oncol 15(1): 59–68

Cheever MA, Allison JP, Ferris AS, Finn OJ, Hastings BM, Hecht TT, Mellman I, Prindiville SA, Viner JL, Weiner LM, Matrisian LM (2009) The prioritization of cancer antigens: a national cancer institute pilot project for the acceleration of translational research. Clin Cancer Res 15 (17):5323–5337

Coca AF, Lebredo MG (1912) A report of the results of the vaccination therapy as applied in 79 cases of Human Cancer. Z Immunitatsforschung und Exp 13:543–585

Coca AF (1909) The specific treatment of carcinoma. Philippine J Sci 4(6):391–402

Coley WB (1893) The treatment of malignant tumors by repeated inoculations of erysipelas: with a report of ten original cases. Am J Med Sci 105(5):487–511

Coley WB (1906) Late results of the treatment of inoperable sarcoma by the mixed toxins of erysipelas and bacillus prodigiosus. Am J Med Sci 131(3):377–430

Corbiere V, Chapiro J, Stroobant V, Ma W, Lurquin C, Lethe B, van Baren N, Van den Eynde BJ, Boon T, Coulie PG (2011) Antigen spreading contributes to MAGE vaccination-induced regression of melanoma metastases. Cancer Res 71(4):1253–1262

Dalziel M, Whitehouse C, McFarlane I, Brockhausen I, Gschmeissner S, Schwientek T, Clausen H, Burchell JM, Taylor-Papadimitriou J (2001) The relative activities of the C2GnT1 and ST3Gal-I glycosyltransferases determine O-glycan structure and expression of a tumor-associated epitope on MUC1. J Biol Chem 276(14):11007–11015

De Plaen E, Lurquin C, Van Pel A, Mariame B, Szikora JP, Wolfel T, Sibille C, Chomez P, Boon T (1988) Immunogenic (tum-) variants of mouse tumor P815: cloning of the gene of tum-antigen P91A and identification of the tum-mutation. Proc Natl Acad Sci U S A 85(7): 2274–2278

Dobrzanski MJ, Rewers-Felkins KA, Quinlin IS, Samad KA, Phillips CA, Robinson W, Dobrzanski DJ, Wright SE (2009) Autologous Muc1-specific Th1 effector cell immunotherapy induces differential levels of systemic TReg cell subpopulations that result in increased ovarian cancer patient survival. Clin Immunol 133(3):333–352

Dreicer R, Stadler WM, Ahmann FR, Whiteside T, Bizouarne N, Acres B, Limacher JM, Squiban P, Pantuck A (2009) MVA-MUC1-IL2 vaccine immunotherapy (TG4010) improves PSA doubling time in patients with prostate cancer with biochemical failure. Invest New Drugs 27 (4):379–386

Eichmuller S, Usener D, Dummer R, Stein A, Thiel D, Schadendorf D (2001) Serological detection of cutaneous T-cell lymphoma-associated antigens. Proc Natl Acad Sci U S A 98 (2):629–634

Foley EJ (1953) Attempts to induce immunity against mammary adenocarcinoma in inbred mice. Cancer Res 13(8):578–580

Gilewski T, Adluri S, Ragupathi G, Zhang S, Yao TJ, Panageas K, Moynahan M, Houghton A, Norton L, Livingston PO (2000) Vaccination of high-risk breast cancer patients with mucin-1 (Muc1) keyhole limpet hemocyanin conjugate plus QS-21. Clin Cancer Res 6:1693–1701

Gong J, Chen D, Kashiwaba M, Li Y, Chen L, Takeuchi H, Qu H, Rowse GJ, Gendler SJ, Kufe D (1998) Reversal of tolerance to human MUC1 antigen in MUC1 transgenic mice immunized with fusions of dendritic and carcinoma cells. Proc Natl Acad Sci U S A 95(11):6279–6283

Hamid O, Robert C, Daud A, Hodi FS, Hwu WJ, Kefford R, Wolchok JD, Hersey P, Joseph RW, Weber JS, Dronca R, Gangadhar TC, Patnaik A, Zarour H, Joshua AM, Gergich K, Elassaiss-Schaap J, Algazi A, Mateus C, Boasberg P, Tumeh PC, Chmielowski B, Ebbinghaus SW, Li XN, Kang SP, Ribas A (2013) Safety and tumor responses with lambrolizumab (anti-PD-1) in melanoma. N Engl J Med 369(2):134–144

Hanisch FG, Schwientek T, Von Bergwelt-Baildon MS, Schultze JL, Finn O (2003) O-Linked glycans control glycoprotein processing by antigen-presenting cells: a biochemical approach to the molecular aspects of MUC1 processing by dendritic cells. Eur J Immunol 33(12): 3242–3254

Harris JR, Price MR, Baldwin RW (1973) The purification of membrane-associated tumour antigens by preparative polyacrylamide gel electrophoresis. Biochim Biophys Acta 311 (4):600–614

Haurum JS, Hoier IB, Arsequell G, Neisig A, Valencia G, Zeuthen J, Neefjes J, Elliott T (1999) Presentation of cytosolic glycosylated peptides by human class I major histocompatibility complex molecules in vivo. J Exp Med 190(1):145–150

Herbst RS, Soria JC, Kowanetz M, Fine GD, Hamid O, Gordon MS, Sosman JA, McDermott DF, Powderly JD, Gettinger SN, Kohrt HE, Horn L, Lawrence DP, Rost S, Leabman M, Xiao Y, Mokatrin A, Koeppen H, Hegde PS, Mellman I, Chen DS, Hodi FS (2014) Predictive correlates of response to the anti-PD-L1 antibody MPDL3280A in cancer patients. Nature 515 (7528):563–567

Heukamp LC, van der Burg SH, Drijfhout JW, Melief CJ, Taylor-Papadimitriou J, Offringa R (2001) Identification of three non-VNTR MUC1-derived HLA-A*0201-restricted T-cell epitopes that induce protective anti-tumor immunity in HLA-A2/K(b)-transgenic mice. Int J Cancer 91(3):385–392

Hiltbold EM, Vlad AM, Ciborowski P, Watkins SC, Finn OJ (2000) The mechanism of unresponsiveness to circulating tumor antigen MUC1 is a block in intracellular sorting and processing by dendritic cells. J Immunol 165(7):3730–3741

Hughes OD, Perkins AC, Frier M, Wastie ML, Denton G, Price MR, Denley H, Bishop MC (2001) Imaging for staging bladder cancer: a clinical study of intravenous 111 Indium-labelled anti-Muc1 mucin monoclonal antibody c595. BJU Int 87(1):39–46

Ibrahim NK, Yariz KO, Bondarenko I, Manikhas A, Semiglazov V, Alyasova A, Komisarenko V, Shparyk Y, Murray JL, Jones D, Senderovich S, Chau A, Erlandsson F, Acton G, Pegram M (2011) Randomized phase II trial of letrozole plus anti-muc1 antibody as1402 in hormone receptor-positive locally advanced or metastatic breast cancer. Clin Cancer Res 17(21): 6822–6830

Jonckheere N, Van Seuningen I (2010) The membrane-bound mucins: From cell signalling to transcriptional regulation and expression in epithelial cancers. Biochimie 92(1):1–11

Karanikas V, Thynne G, Mitchell P, Ong CS, Gunawardana D, Blum R, Pearson J, Lodding J, Pietersz G, Broadbent R, Tait B, McKenzie IF (2001) Mannan mucin-1 peptide immunization: Influence of cyclophosphamide and the route of injection. J Immunother 24(2):172–183

Keydar I, Chou CS, Hareuveni M, Tsarfaty I, Sahar E, Selzer G, Chaitchik S, Hizi A (1989) Production and characterization of monoclonal antibodies identifying breast tumor-associated antigens. Proc Natl Acad Sci U S A 86(4):1362–1366

Kim YD, Robinson DY, Tomita JT (1988) Monoclonal antibody PR92 with restricted specificity for tumor-associated antigen of prostate and breast carcinoma. Cancer Res 48(16):4543–4548

Kimura T, Finn OJ (2013) MUC1 immunotherapy is here to stay. Expert Opin Biol Ther 13(1): 35–49

Kohler G, Milstein C (1975) Continuous cultures of fused cells secreting antibody of predefined specificity. Nature 256(5517):495–497
Kondo H, Hazama S, Kawaoka T, Yoshino S, Yoshida S, Tokuno K, Takashima M, Ueno T, Hinoda Y, Oka M (2008) Adoptive immunotherapy for pancreatic cancer using MUC1 peptide-pulsed dendritic cells and activated T lymphocytes. Anticancer Res 28(1B):379–387
Kunkler RB, Bishop MC, Green DJ, Pimm MV, Price MR, Frier M (1995) Targeting of bladder cancer with monoclonal antibody NCRC48–a possible approach for intravesical therapy. Br J Urol 76(1):81–86
Lan MS, Khorrami A, Kaufman B, Metzgar RS (1987) Molecular characterization of a mucin-type antigen associated with human pancreatic cancer. The DU-PAN-2 antigen. J Biol Chem 262 (26):12863–12870
Lepisto AJ, Moser AJ, Zeh H, Lee K, Bartlett D, McKolanis JR, Geller BA, Schmotzer A, Potter DP, Whiteside T, Finn OJ, Ramanathan RK (2008) A phase I/II study of a Muc1 peptide pulsed autologous dendritic cell vaccine as adjuvant therapy in patients with resected pancreatic and biliary tumors. Cancer Ther 6(B):955–964
Limacher JM, Acres B (2014) MUC1 as a therapeutic target in cancer. In: 'Mucins and Cancer' Future Medicine, pp 125–137
Loveland BE, Zhao A, White S, Gan H, Hamilton K, Xing PX, Pietersz GA, Apostolopoulos V, Vaughan H, Karanikas V, Kyriakou P, McKenzie IF, Mitchell PL (2006) Mannan-MUC1-pulsed dendritic cell immunotherapy: a phase I trial in patients with adenocarcinoma. Clin Cancer Res 12(3 Pt 1):869–877
Maloney DG (2012) Anti-CD20 antibody therapy for B-cell lymphomas. N Engl J Med 366 (21):2008–2016
Morse MA, Niedzwiecki D, Marshall JL, Garrett C, Chang DZ, Aklilu M, Crocenzi TS, Cole DJ, Dessureault S, Hobeika AC, Osada T, Onaitis M, Clary BM, Hsu D, Devi GR, Bulusu A, Annechiarico RP, Chadaram V, Clay TM, Lyerly HK (2013) A randomized phase II study of immunization with dendritic cells modified with poxvectors encoding cea and muc1 compared with the same poxvectors plus GM-CSF for resected metastatic colorectal cancer. Ann Surg 7:7
Nath S, Mukherjee P (2014) MUC1: a multifaceted oncoprotein with a key role in cancer progression. Trends Mol Med 20(6):332–342
Ninkovic T, Kinarsky L, Engelmann K, Pisarev V, Sherman S, Finn OJ, Hanisch FG (2009) Identification of O-glycosylated decapeptides within the MUC1 repeat domain as potential MHC class I (A2) binding epitopes. Mol Immunol 47(1):131–140
Noto H, Takahashi T, Makiguchi Y, Hayashi T, Hinoda Y, Imai K (1997) Cytotoxic T lymphocytes derived from bone marrow mononuclear cells of multiple myeloma patients recognize an underglycosylated form of MUC1 mucin. Int Immunol 9(5):791–798
O'Mahony D, Kummar S, Gutierrez ME (2005) Non-small-cell lung cancer vaccine therapy: a concise review. J Clin Oncol 23(35):9022–9028
Oudard S, Rixe O, Beuselinck B, Linassier C, Banu E, Machiels JP, Baudard M, Ringeisen F, Velu T, Lefrere-Belda MA, Limacher JM, Fridman WH, Azizi M, Acres B, Tartour E (2011) A phase II study of the cancer vaccine TG4010 alone and in combination with cytokines in patients with metastatic renal clear-cell carcinoma: clinical and immunological findings. Cancer Immunol Immunother 60(2):261–271
Peat N, Gendler SJ, Lalani N, Duhig T, Taylor-Papadimitriou J (1992) Tissue-specific expression of a human polymorphic epithelial mucin (MUC1) in transgenic mice. Cancer Res 52(7): 1954–1960
Pegram MD, Borges VF, Ibrahim N, Fuloria J, Shapiro C, Perez S, Wang K, Schaedli Stark F, Courtenay Luck N (2009) Phase I dose escalation pharmacokinetic assessment of intravenous humanized anti-Muc1 antibody as1402 in patients with advanced breast cancer. Breast Cancer Res 11(5):R73
Picco G, Julien S, Brockhausen I, Beatson R, Antonopoulos A, Haslam S, Mandel U, Dell A, Pinder S, Taylor-Papadimitriou J, Burchell J (2010) Over-expression of ST3Gal-I promotes mammary tumorigenesis. Glycobiology 20(10):1241–1250

Powell E, Chow LQ (2008) BLP-25 liposomal vaccine: a promising potential therapy in non-small-cell lung cancer. Expert Rev Respir Med 2(1):37–45

Prehn RT, Main JM (1957) Immunity to methylcholanthrene-induced sarcomas. J Natl Cancer Inst 18(6):769–778

Quoix E, Losonczy G, Forget F, Chouaid C, Papai Z, Gervais R, Ottensmeier C, Szczesna A, Kazarnowicz A, Felip E, Debieuvre D, Madroszyk A, Lacoste G, Tavernaro A, Bastien B, Palanche T, Limacher J-M (2014) TIME, a phase 2b/3 study evaluating TG4010 in combination with first line therapy advanced non small cell lung cancer (NSCLC). Phase 2b results. In: 39th ESMO congress, Madrid 2014—European Society for Medical Oncology esmocongress.org. Abstract 5152

Quoix E, Ramlau R, Westeel V, Papai Z, Madroszyk A, Riviere A, Koralewski P, Breton JL, Stoelben E, Braun D, Debieuvre D, Lena H, Buyse M, Chenard MP, Acres B, Lacoste G, Bastien B, Tavernaro A, Bizouarne N, Bonnefoy JY, Limacher JM (2011) Therapeutic vaccination with TG4010 and first-line chemotherapy in advanced non-small-cell lung cancer: a controlled phase 2B trial. Lancet Oncol 12(12):1125–1133

Ramlau R, Quoix E, Rolski J, Pless M, Lena H, Levy E, Krzakowski M, Hess D, Tartour E, Chenard MP, Limacher JM, Bizouarne N, Acres B, Halluard C, Velu T (2008) A phase II study of Tg4010 (Mva-Muc1-Il2) in association with chemotherapy in patients with stage III/IV non-small cell lung cancer. J Thorac Oncol 3(7):735–744

Rittig SM, Haentschel M, Weimer KJ, Heine A, Muller MR, Brugger W, Horger MS, Maksimovic O, Stenzl A, Hoerr I, Rammensee HG, Holderried TA, Kanz L, Pascolo S, Brossart P (2011) Intradermal vaccinations with RNA coding for taa generate CD8+ and CD4+ immune responses and induce clinical benefit in vaccinated patients. Mol Ther 19(5):990–999

Ribas A, Chesney JA, Gordon MS, Abernethy AP, Logan TF, Lawson DH, Chmielowksi B, Glaspy JA, Lewis K, Huang B, Wang E, Hsyu PH, Gomez-Navarro J, Gerhardt D, Marshall MA, Gonzalez R (2012) Safety profile and pharmacokinetic analyses of the anti-CTLA4 antibody tremelimumab administered as a one hour infusion. J Trans Med 10:236

Robert L, Harview C, Emerson R, Wang X, Mok S, Homet B, Comin-Anduix B, Koya RC, Robins H, Tumeh PC, Ribas A (2014) Distinct immunological mechanisms of CTLA-4 and PD-1 blockade revealed by analyzing TCR usage in blood lymphocytes. Oncoimmunology 3: e29244

Roulois D, Gregoire M, Fonteneau JF (2013) MUC1-specific cytotoxic T lymphocytes in cancer therapy: induction and challenge. Biomed Res Int 2013:871936

Roulois D, Vignard V, Gueugnon F, Labarriere N, Gregoire M, Fonteneau JF (2011) Recognition of pleural mesothelioma by mucin-1(950-958)/human leukocyte antigen A*0201-specific CD8 + T-cells. Eur Respir J 38(5):1117–1126

Rowse GJ, Tempero RM, VanLith ML, Hollingsworth MA, Gendler SJ (1998) Tolerance and immunity to MUC1 in a human MUC1 transgenic murine model. Cancer Res 58(2):315–321

Scholl S, Squiban P, Bizouarne N, Baudin M, Acres B, Von Mensdorff-Pouilly S, Shearer M, Beuzeboc P, Van Belle S, Uzielly B, Pouillart P, Taylor-Papadimitriou J, Miles D (2003) Metastatic breast tumour regression following treatment by a gene-modified vaccinia virus expressing MUC1 and IL-2. J Biomed Biotechnol 2003(3):194–201

Sekine H, Hayes DF, Ohno T, Keefe KA, Schaetzl E, Bast RC, Knapp R, Kufe DW (1985) Circulating DF3 and CA125 antigen levels in serum from patients with epithelial ovarian carcinoma. J Clin Oncol 3(10):1355–1363

Sorensen AL, Reis CA, Tarp MA, Mandel U, Ramachandran K, Sankaranarayanan V, Schwientek T, Graham R, Taylor-Papadimitriou J, Hollingsworth MA, Burchell J, Clausen H (2006) Chemoenzymatically synthesized multimeric Tn/STn MUC1 glycopeptides elicit cancer-specific anti-MUC1 antibody responses and override tolerance. Glycobiology 16(2):96–107

Stacker SA, Tjandra JJ, Xing PX, Walker ID, Thompson CH, McKenzie IF (1989) Purification and biochemical characterisation of a novel breast carcinoma associated mucin-like glycoprotein defined by antibody 3E1.2. Br J Cancer 59(4):544–553

Takahashi T, Makiguchi Y, Hinoda Y, Kakiuchi H, Nakagawa N, Imai K, Yachi A (1994) Expression of MUC1 on myeloma cells and induction of HLA-unrestricted CTL against MUC1 from a multiple myeloma patient. J Immunol 153(5):2102–2109

Tang CK, Apostolopoulos V (2008) Strategies used for MUC1 immunotherapy: preclinical studies. Expert Rev Vaccines 7(7):951–962

Tarp MA, Sorensen AL, Mandel U, Paulsen H, Burchell J, Taylor-Papadimitriou J, Clausen H (2007) Identification of a novel cancer-specific immunodominant glycopeptide epitope in the MUC1 tandem repeat. Glycobiology 17(2):197–209

Tempero RM, Rowse GJ, Gendler SJ, Hollingsworth MA (1999) Passively transferred anti-MUC1 antibodies cause neither autoimmune disorders nor immunity against transplanted tumors in MUC1 transgenic mice. Int J Cancer 80(4):595–599

Therion Biologics press release (2006) http://www.prnewswire.com/news-releases/therion-reports-results-of-phase-3-panvac-vf-trial-and-announces-plansfor-company-sale-56997582.html

Tumeh PC, Harview CL, Yearley JH, Shintaku IP, Taylor EJ, Robert L, Chmielowski B, Spasic M, Henry G, Ciobanu V, West AN, Carmona M, Kivork C, Seja E, Cherry G, Gutierrez AJ, Grogan TR, Mateus C, Tomasic G, Glaspy JA, Emerson RO, Robins H, Pierce RH, Elashoff DA, Robert C, Ribas A (2014) PD-1 blockade induces responses by inhibiting adaptive immune resistance. Nature 515(7528):568–571

Vlad AM, Muller S, Cudic M, Paulsen H, Otvos L Jr, Hanisch FG, Finn OJ (2002) Complex carbohydrates are not removed during processing of glycoproteins by dendritic cells: processing of tumor antigen MUC1 glycopeptides for presentation to major histocompatibility complex class II-restricted T cells. J Exp Med 196(11):1435–1446

von Mensdorff-Pouilly S, Verstraeten AA, Kenemans P, Snijdewint FG, Kok A, Van Kamp GJ, Paul MA, Van Diest PJ, Meijer S, Hilgers J (2000) Survival in early breast cancer patients is favorably influenced by a natural humoral immune response to polymorphic epithelial mucin. J Clin Oncol 18(3):574–583

Wajchman HJ, Pierce CW, Varma VA, Issa MM, Petros J, Dombrowski KE (2004) Ex vivo expansion of CD8+ CD56+ and CD8+ CD56− natural killer T cells specific for MUC1 mucin. Cancer Res 64(3):1171–1180

Wandall HH, Blixt O, Tarp MA, Pedersen JW, Bennett EP, Mandel U, Ragupathi G, Livingston PO, Hollingsworth MA, Taylor-Papadimitriou J, Burchell J, Clausen H (2010) Cancer biomarkers defined by autoantibody signatures to aberrant O-glycopeptide epitopes. Cancer Res 70(4):1306–1313

Weber JS (2014) Immuno-oncology comes of age-introduction. Semin Oncol 41(5): S1–2. doi: 10.1053/j.seminoncol.2014.1009.1002. (Epub 2014 Sep 1056)

Wright SE, Rewers-Felkins KA, Quinlin IS, Phillips CA, Townsend M, Philip R, Zorsky P, Klug P, Dai L, Hussain M, Thomas AA, Sundaramurthy C (2009) Tumor burden influences cytotoxic T cell development in metastatic breast cancer patients-a phase I/II study. Immunol Invest 38(8):820–838

Wu YL, Park K, Soo RA, Sun Y, Tyroller K, Wages D, Ely G, Yang JC, Mok T (2011) INSPIRE: a phase III study of the BLP25 liposome vaccine (L-BLP25) in Asian patients with unresectable stage III non-small cell lung cancer. BMC Cancer 11:430

Chimeric DNA Vaccines: An Effective Way to Overcome Immune Tolerance

Federica Riccardo, Elisabetta Bolli, Marco Macagno, Maddalena Arigoni, Federica Cavallo and Elena Quaglino

Abstract The fact that cancer immunotherapy is considered to be a safe and successful weapon for use in combination with surgery, radiation, and chemotherapy treatments means that it has recently been chosen as Breakthrough of the Year 2013 by Science editors. Anticancer vaccines have been extensively tested, in this field, both in preclinical cancer models and in the clinic. However, tumor-associated antigens (TAAs) are often self-tolerated molecules and cancer patients suffer from strong immunosuppressive effects, meaning that the triggering of an effective anti-tumor immune response is difficult. One possible means to overcome immunological tolerance to self-TAAs is of course the use of vaccines that code for xenogeneic proteins. However, a low-affinity antibody response against the self-homologous protein expressed by cancer cells is generally induced by xenovaccination. This issue becomes extremely limiting when working with tumors in which the contribution of the humoral rather than the cellular immune response is required if tumor growth is to be hampered. A possible way to avoid this problem is to use hybrid vaccines which code for chimeric proteins that include both homologous and xenogeneic moieties. In fact, a superior protective anti-tumor immune response against $ErbB2^{+}$ transplantable and autochthonous mammary tumors was observed over plasmids that coded for the fully rat or fully human proteins when hybrid plasmids that coded for chimeric rat/human ErbB2 protein were tested in ErbB2 transgenic mice. In principle, these findings may become the basis for a new rational means of designing effective vaccines against TAAs.

F. Riccardo · E. Bolli · M. Macagno · M. Arigoni · F. Cavallo · E. Quaglino (✉)
Department of Molecular Biotechnology and Health Sciences,
Molecular Biotechnology Center, University of Torino, via Nizza 52,
10126 Torino, Italy
e-mail: elena.quaglino@unito.it

Current Topics in Microbiology and Immunology (2017) 405:99–122
DOI 10.1007/82_2014_426

Published Online: 08 October 2014

Contents

1 Introduction

Its specificity and long-term memory furnishes the immune system with great potential for specifically eliminating tumor cells without harming normal cells and for preventing cancer recurrence. Considerable effort has therefore been invested in discovering molecular biomarkers associated with each specific cancer and in designing effective vaccines for their targeting, all with the final aim of boosting or restoring the ability of patients' immune system to fight cancer. Thus, cancer vaccines have the potential to become a therapeutic treatment which is used synergistically in combination with traditional therapies. Recent decades have seen several types of anticancer vaccines successfully designed, manufactured, and preclinically tested, with this final aim in mind. However, only few have been proven to be effective in inducing a measurable immune response when used in clinical trials and overall clinical benefit has been so far limited. Indeed, only a single anticancer vaccine (Provenge®, or APC8015) has so far been approved by the Food and Drug Administration (FDA) (Kantoff et al. 2010).

One problem, in terms of clinical setting, is that cancer vaccine studies are generally carried out in end-stage cancer patients with high tumor burden and impaired immune capacity. Studies are, therefore, now moving toward patients with minimal disease, thereby preventing recurrence and metastasis (Frelin et al. 2010). Other factors that may account for this failure concern the choice of target antigens, vaccine formulation, and overcoming tolerance. We herein discuss these limitations and propose the use of chimeric DNA vaccines against oncoantigens as a possible solution.

2 Choice of Successful Vaccination Targets

2.1 Oncoantigens

The starting point in the development of an effective anti-tumor vaccine is identifying an appropriate target antigen. Several reports have demonstrated that cancer control through active immunotherapy is an attainable goal only when the vaccine targets a tumor-associated antigen (TAA) that displays a high level of expression in cancer cells but low levels in healthy cells, holds a potent oncogenic role, and is not prone to escape from immune recognition. TAAs with these features are defined as oncoantigens (Lollini et al. 2006).

Oncoantigens can be secreted or expressed by both cancer and non-neoplastic cells that form the tumor microenvironment (Iezzi et al. 2011). They can be classified into three classes according to their function and cellular localization. Class I oncoantigens (receptors, adhesion molecules, etc.) are expressed on the cell surface, class II (growth factors, angiogenic factors, etc.) are present in the tumor microenvironment, while class III (non-receptor tyrosine kinases, transcription factors, cell cycle molecules) are intracellular proteins.

The benefits of using oncoantigens as targets for effective immunotherapy rest on several pillars. Firstly, they are not susceptible to cancer immunoediting (Dunn et al. 2004) as they play a key role in tumor growth and survival and, furthermore, their loss impairs or blocks tumor progression. Inevitably, tumor cells are less likely to down-regulate this protein and, even if oncoantigen-loss variants occur, they will cause impaired tumorigenic potential and negative selection (Friedman et al. 2005). Secondly, their low expression level on normal cells makes the risk of inducing an autoimmunity reaction following oncoantigen vaccination almost negligible. Thirdly, they can be targeted by different immune mechanisms according to their diverse functions and localizations. Class I oncoantigens are considered to be the best targets for effective anticancer immunotherapeutic strategies (Iezzi et al. 2012) as they are susceptible to the attack of both T cell and antibodies at the same time.

2.2 ErbB2 as a Prototype Oncoantigen

Of all the TAAs identified as possible targets for cancer immunotherapy so far, ErbB2 has the makings of an "ideal" oncoantigen as it is expressed at low levels by few healthy cells in adult life, and its overexpression and dysregulation occur in several types of cancer, including invasive breast cancers, colorectal cancers, ovarian cancers, pancreatic cancers, and prostate cancers. These aberrations are associated with poor prognosis because of greater tumor aggressiveness and an increased risk of recurrence (Spears et al. 2012). Moreover, its localization on the tumor cell surface makes ErbB2 a target for both cell-mediated and antibody-mediated immunity. As a consequence, the development of innovative therapeutic options that specifically target ErbB2 has become one of the most outstanding achievements in clinical oncology.

Since the intrinsic kinase activity of the ErbB2 receptor is essential for many of its oncogenic functions, several small-molecule tyrosine kinase inhibitors (TKI) have been tested (Albanell and Gascon 2005) and approved by the FDA. These include Gefitinib (Iressa®) and Erlotinib (Tarceva®) (Rukazenkov et al. 2009), which have been approved for the treatment of patients with $ErbB2^{+}$ advanced or metastatic non small cell lung cancer (NSCLC) and Lapatinib (Tyverb®) for the treatment of $ErbB2^{+}$ breast cancer patients. Unfortunately, ErbB2 inhibitors often fail to elicit a clinical response, even when tumors express high levels of the activated receptor. Several explanations are possible for this and include insufficient target inhibition due to poor drug penetration of the tumor, or alternatively, it is possible that some tumors are intrinsically resistant to TKI or can acquire different mechanisms of resistance to therapeutic inhibitors (Wykosky et al. 2011).

The field of passive immunotherapy has seen the successful clinical testing of monoclonal antibodies (mAbs) that target ErbB2 and, thus, the FDA approval of Trastuzumab and Pertuzumab. The first has become standard of care treatment for women with ErbB2-overexpressing metastatic breast cancer. Its clinical efficacy is clear, both when used as a single agent (Vogel et al. 2002) and when used in combination with a variety of chemotherapy agents (Cortes and Roche 2012). Pertuzumab has recently shown promising results when used against metastatic breast cancer, leading to the exploration of a combination of targeted therapies in the adjuvant setting (Baselga et al. 2012). Although the clinical results observed in Trastuzumab and Pertuzumab therapy have been encouraging, the high rate of cardiac side effects (Shak 1999) and the evidence of the short-lived therapeutic action of mAbs, associated with the relapse of most treated patients, suggests that tumors intrinsically possess or acquire mechanisms for escape (Anido et al. 2006; Castiglioni et al. 2006). All these limitations highlight the need to develop other strategies to provide a wider immunotherapeutic armamentarium against $ErbB2^{+}$ tumors.

Active therapies, such as cancer vaccines, offer a number of advantages over passive therapies, including the induction of a specific long-lasting immunological memory against the antigen and of a wider vaccine-elicited immune response that may be able to overcome tumor resistance mechanisms (Eschenburg et al. 2010). In reality, while the ability of several anti-ErbB2 vaccine formulations to induce a specific humoral and cellular response has been demonstrated in cancer patients (Kutzler and Weiner 2008; Norell et al. 2010), along with their safety, their therapeutic clinical benefits remain questionable. Several hypotheses have been put forward to explain these results, and besides the deleterious impact on the immune system caused by treatments such as chemotherapy and radiotherapy prior to vaccination, the difficulty in breaking the immune tolerance against the self-ErbB2 antigen would appear to play a key role in hampering an effective anti-tumor immune response.

2.3 Oncoantigens are Self-tolerated Molecules

The priceless opportunity provided by anti-tumor vaccination relies on its ability to specifically amplify a patient's own immune response against definite oncoantigens in order to induce long-lasting memory against cancer cells (Eschenburg et al. 2010). However, one of the most important challenges is found in the intrinsic nature of oncoantigens: most of them are self-tolerated proteins, overexpressed by cancer cells but non-mutated and therefore showing various degrees of tolerogenicity (Even-Desrumeaux et al. 2011). Even if the overexpression of self-oncoantigens exceeded the threshold for T cell activation and break immune tolerance, they may show low immunogenicity potential (Zinkernagel and Hengartner 2001). Tolerogenicity causes reactive high-avidity T cells to be deleted or transformed into natural Foxp3^{+} regulatory T cells (Treg), a T cell subset with immunosuppressive properties that limits the magnitude of effector T cell responses (Josefowicz et al. 2012; Stritesky et al. 2012). As consequence of central tolerance, low-frequency tumor-specific T cell precursors are present and display a suboptimal TCR affinity or an immunosuppressive phenotype. Potentially self-reactive, low-avidity T cells that evade from central tolerance mechanisms are controlled in the periphery by steady-state antigen-presenting cells, which present tumor antigens to T cells in the presence of coinhibitory receptors (e.g., programmed cell death ligands, PD-L1 and PD-L2) or in the absence of costimulatory signals (e.g., CD40 and CD86), rendering T cells almost unresponsive (anergic or exhausted) or Foxp3^{+} (inducible Treg). Both natural Treg and inducible Treg further suppress self-reactive T cells by antigen-specific and non-specific mechanisms that involve the expression of inhibitory molecules, such as cytotoxic T lymphocyte antigen (CTLA)-4, and the secretion of anti-inflammatory cytokines, such as TGF-β and IL-10, which suppress dendritic cell (DC)-mediated induction and effector T cell function (Sakaguchi et al. 2001; Yagi et al. 2004). These dysfunctions in T cell response against tumors may all contribute to the failure of the anticancer vaccines that have been evaluated in human clinical trials (Kutzler and Weiner 2008).

The real challenge for anti-tumor vaccines is, therefore, to overcome all these types of T cell dysfunctions, inducing the activation of non-tolerized, non-exhausted, and self-cross-reactive low-affinity T cell clones (Jacob et al. 2006).

2.4 Tumors Limit Vaccine-Induced Immune Response

Besides the difficulty in inducing an effective anti-tumor immune response against self-tolerated molecules, recent data demonstrate that tumors can also escape from immune destruction via dominant negative regulatory pathways that impart a state of peripheral T cell tolerance against TAAs. These inhibitory pathways can take the form of cytokines, suppressive cell populations (e.g., Treg, myeloid-derived suppressor cells, (MDSC) and tumor-associated macrophages) (Takenaka et al. 2013;

Pollard 2004; Kim et al. 2006), amino acid-catabolizing enzymes (e.g., indoleamine-2, 3-dioxygenase, and arginase), and the ligation of inhibitory receptors on activated T cells (e.g., CTLA-4 and PD-1) (Pentcheva-Hoang et al. 2009). Indeed, increased Treg frequencies in the blood, draining lymph nodes, and tumor tissues of cancer patients have been described and associated with impaired immune response against cancer (Liyanage et al. 2002). For this reason, Treg depletion in cancer immunotherapy may be a useful adjuvant strategy. The targeting of the CD25 Treg surface marker with specific mAb has been shown to be effective in enhancing vaccine-induced anti-tumor activity in various preclinical models (Ludwig-Portugall et al. 2009; LaCelle and Jensen 2009; Goforth et al. 2009; Viehl et al. 2006; Casares et al. 2003; Quezada et al. 2008). Moreover, the use of US FDA-approved humanized mAb against CD25 (Daclizumab) in a peptide vaccination trial of breast cancer patients was shown to be effective in inducing an anti-peptide immune response (Rech et al. 2012). However, the autoimmune reactions potentially associated with the administration of anti-CD25 mAb and the risk of inhibiting the tumor-specific cytotoxic T cells that transiently express this molecule after activation are critical issues for its application in human patients. Therefore, alternative strategies with which to potentiate vaccine-induced immune responses and improve tumor control have to be developed (Stewart and Smyth 2011). One possible method is combining anti-tumor vaccines with the use of antibodies that block or suppress inhibitory receptors on activated T cells (Sarnaik et al. 2011; Yuan et al. 2011). Improved advanced metastatic melanoma patient survival has recently been described in a phase III clinical trial which combined a gp-100 peptide vaccine with CTLA-4 blockade using the fully human antagonistic anti-CTLA-4 mAb, Ipilimumab (Gajewski 2010; Hodi et al. 2010). However, it is worth noting that severe adverse events occurred in around 15 % of patients treated with Ipilimumab, most of which were immune-related, and included seven patient deaths.

In conclusion, even if the combined use of mAbs blocking checkpoint inhibitors together with anticancer vaccines is a potentially powerful strategy, safer drugs have to be developed.

3 Chimeric DNA Vaccines

3.1 Xenogeneic Vaccines

One way to overcome the major limitations of a successful anticancer vaccine, namely the host immune tolerance to self-oncoantigens and the tumor-induced immunesuppression, is to use xenogeneic proteins or peptides from a different species, which is significantly homologous with the self-ortholog, as immunogens. This strategy has been widely studied, and several papers have demonstrated its potential (Jacob et al. 2006; Kianizad et al. 2007; Soong et al. 2013; Yuan et al. 2009).

Many oncoantigens are phylogenetically conserved to various degrees of similarity; however, they are recognized by the immune systems as "non-self-antigens" as they are not identical in their sequences. Therefore, a vaccine coding for a xenogeneic oncoantigen can circumvent immune tolerance and may acquire the proper immunogenic and anti-tumor potential.

Although the xenogeneic vaccination mechanism of action has not been completely elucidated, it is believed that subtle differences between epitopes of the orthologue and the native protein are responsible for eliciting T and B cell responses against the xenoantigen that may cross-react with the native target. From the mechanistic point of view, the foreign epitopes of an orthologue protein which is used as vaccine may lead to the formation of heteroclitic epitopes (Dyall et al. 1998; Kianizad et al. 2007) that possess an enhanced ability to bind to MHC glycoproteins and effectively prime both $CD8^+$ and $CD4^+$ T cells which are able to cross-react against the original non-mutated peptide. The release of helper cytokines by activated $CD4^+$ T cells may rescue bystander anergic T and B lymphocytes (Jensen and Kapp 1986) and lead to the activation of DCs (Smith et al. 2004). Moreover, the interaction between B cells, reacting with self-epitopes, and their cognate-activated $CD4^+$ T cells provides proper signals to B cells and triggers the production of high-affinity antibodies which may potentially cross-react with the self-protein (Zhang et al. 2001; Sobel et al. 1994).

The efficacy of this strategy has been extensively demonstrated in several murine models of cancer both in prophylactic and therapeutic settings (Cavallo et al. 2014). Moreover, xenovaccination has recently been shown to hamper cancer growth and to improve survival in veterinary cancer patients, mainly in dogs affected by spontaneous disease (Riccardo et al. 2014; Alexander et al. 2006; Kamstock et al. 2007; Yu et al. 2011). These positive results obtained in veterinary trials led to the approval by the United States Department of Agriculture (USDA) of the first xenogeneic DNA vaccine against tyrosinase, ONCEPT (Merial), for the treatment of oral malignant melanomas (Grosenbaugh et al. 2011) in 2010. Although the therapeutic efficacy of ONCEPT has been recently questioned (Ottnod et al. 2013), its licensing has renewed enthusiasm for heterologous DNA vaccination as an alternative and potentially effective immunotherapeutic strategy. Finally, the safety and immunogenicity of xenovaccination against human tumor antigens have also been demonstrated in several phase I/II human clinical trials (Fong et al. 2001; Wolchok et al. 2007; Yuan et al. 2009, 2013; Ginsberg et al. 2010; Eriksson et al. 2013), thus facilitating the opening up of new perspectives in the management of cancer.

3.2 *An Easy and Versatile Means of Oncoantigen Delivery: DNA*

Many different oncoantigen sources have been tested for use as vaccines in preclinical models and in clinical studies (Berzofsky et al. 2004). These include whole tumor cells, tumor lysates, purified tumor antigens (protein- or peptide-containing vaccines), recombinant viruses, and nucleic acids (DNA and mRNA) that encode for the oncoantigen of choice. Even if proof of principle of the potential efficacy of all these strategies has been demonstrated, specific pitfalls have to be taken into consideration when developing a successful anti-tumor vaccination strategy.

The use of autologous whole tumor cells or tumor cell lysates as the source of tumor antigens for vaccination (Kircheis et al. 2000; Kayaga et al. 1999) faces a number of logistical challenges which come in the form of the preparation of patient-specific therapies and high production costs. Thus, researcher interest has shifted toward molecularly defined synthetic vaccines which are more suitable for large-scale pharmaceutical manufacturing processes (Mocellin et al. 2009). However one of the major issues with peptide-based vaccination is the fact that individual peptides will only be useful in patients who possess appropriate HLA molecules capable of presenting that peptide. However, encouraging data from two trials in patients with advanced renal carcinoma suggest that targeting multiple tumor-associated HLA-restricted peptides elicits specific vaccine-induced immune responses associated with clinical benefit (Walter et al. 2012).

A more hopeful scenario seemed to be presented by DC-based anticancer vaccines. The best example can be traced to 2010, when sipuleucel-T (also known as Provenge), a DC-enriched autologous cell preparation which is expanded ex vivo in the presence of a prostate acid phosphatase/granulocyte macrophage colony-stimulating factor (PAP/GM-CSF) fusion protein, was approved by the US FDA for use in patients with asymptomatic or minimally symptomatic metastatic castration-refractory prostate cancer (Cheever and Higano 2011). Overall, experience with DC has shown that these cells can be safely administrated with no, or only mild, side effects. The induction of an immune response against the target antigens has been demonstrated, but the actual clinical benefits for patients with cancer have so far been marginal (Sabado and Bhardwaj 2013).

Advances in recombinant techniques have provided the opportunity to introduce oncoantigens, or simply epitopes (if needed, along with costimulatory molecules and cytokines), into viral vectors. Indeed, a number of trials for the treatment of cancer which use recombinant viruses, i.e., adenovirus, vaccinia, and the avipox virus, that express oncoantigens have been reported or are in progress (Odunsi et al. 2012; Madan et al. 2012; Marshall et al. 2000). However, the use of these vectors in clinical cancer immunotherapy brings with it some important limitations which can be traced to the potential dangers associated with live virus use and the presence of preexisting anti-vector immune responses and a high prevalence of anti-viral neutralizing antibodies in patients.

The high versatility, ease of production, and low cost of manufacturing combined with the high stability and easy scalability of DNA plasmids may provide an important base from which to further develop this approach into the effective cancer therapies of the twenty-first century (Fioretti et al. 2010). A DNA vaccine is composed of a plasmid DNA, which includes the entire or partial coding region of the TAA of interest under the control of a mammalian promoter, a transcription termination signal, and a prokaryotic antibiotic resistance gene (Glenting and Wessels 2005). Sometimes, instead of the partial or entire TAA sequence, a string of epitopes which is specifically selected as a highly immunogenic sequence of the TAA can be used as immunogens (Aurisicchio et al. 2014). The plasmid DNA vaccine mode of action appears to be twofold. On the one hand, DNA plasmids appear to act as a pathogen-associated molecular pattern which is able to stimulate the innate immune system (Klinman et al. 1997). On the other hand, DNA plasmids directly transfect resident cells that start producing the vaccine-encoded antigen.

Several DNA vaccines against TAAs have been successfully tested in preclinical models of different cancers. In parallel, human trials performed with DNA vaccines, which target some of the best-known tumor antigens, have shown clinical evidence of strong immunogenicity and preliminary evidence of clinical activity (Chudley et al. 2012; Thomas and Kwak 2012; Eriksson et al. 2013; Diaz et al. 2013; Ginsberg et al. 2010; Norell et al. 2010).

Of the several means of delivering a naked plasmid in vivo, sophisticated electroporators have recently rendered intramuscular plasmid electroporation, one of the most effective methods for securing safe, efficient DNA immunization both in animals and humans (Aurisicchio et al. 2013; Low et al. 2009). The induction of local inflammation at the injection site and the production of a pro-immunogenic microenvironment results in effective antigen cross-presentation which has been indicated as the principal route by which DNA vaccines elicit a potent antibody and cytotoxic response (Cavallo et al. 2006; Heath et al. 2004; Shedlock and Weiner 2000; Rice et al. 2008; Liu et al. 2008).

However, rather limited overall efficacy in inducing effective anti-tumor protection has so far been demonstrated (Stevenson et al. 2010; Kutzler and Weiner 2008) and no DNA vaccines have been licensed for human use to date. Preclinical studies have revealed that one reason for failure is the insufficient induction of the $CD4^+$ T cell help engagement provided by DNA vaccine coding for the oncoantigen alone (Janssen et al. 2003). Besides the use of xenogeneic sequence of the oncoantigen, several other strategies have been developed and tested. Among them, the coinjection of the vaccine with a $CD4^+$ T cell inducing peptide such as the Pan HLA-DR epitope (PADRE) peptide or the use of long peptides, which have the advantage of both potentially activating T cell help and also being preferentially processed by DCs (Melief and van der Burg 2008). A more recent approach is represented by the use of DNA vaccines coding for fusion proteins between the oncoantigen and tetanus toxin or plant viral coat proteins (Stevenson et al. 2011). This strategy has been demonstrated to be highly effective when tested in mice, and although not yet in clinical trials, it has considerable potential.

Nevertheless, it is important to mention that DNA vaccination is the youngest of the vaccination strategies for cancer immunotherapy and, thus, has probably not yet lived up to its potential. Moreover, if one takes into account the fact that a timeline of more than a century was needed for the development of antibodies into effective cancer drugs, DNA vaccines may yet be considered to be on fast track development.

3.3 Hybrid Plasmids Coding for Chimeric Antigens

Thanks to the capability of xenoantigens to induce a potent cross-reactive T cell immune response against self-tolerated TAAs, xenovaccination using DNA has been demonstrated to effectively halt tumor growth in several preclinical mouse model of cancer (Cavallo et al. 2014). However, it must be noted that an antibody-mediated contribution may be fundamental in hampering tumor growth rather than just T cell immunity, depending upon the oncoantigen used and the disease model. Indeed, as discussed above, the role of $CD8^+$ T cells is prominent in the case of oncoantigens with intracellular localization (class III oncoantigens), while the contribution of $CD4^+$ T cells and antibodies might be determinant in the case of oncoantigens expressed on the cell membrane (class I oncoantigens). Several studies have demonstrated that self-reactive antibodies are better induced by autologous rather than xenogeneic vaccination, reflecting the exquisite specificity for the cognate antigen of antibodies induced by DNA vaccines (Jacob et al. 2006, 2010; Quaglino et al. 2010). Therefore, one of the major issues concerning xenogeneic vaccination is the low-affinity antibody response generally induced against the self-homolog protein, thus limiting the anticancer efficacy of the vaccine.

One possible means by which to induce a combined potent cross-reactive T cell and antibody response is to use hybrid plasmids which code for chimeric proteins that include both xenogeneic and homologous oncoantigen domains. The potential efficacy of these plasmids relies on the presence of the homologous sequence which ensures the specificity of the immune response and the presence of the xenogeneic determinants which are instrumental in circumventing immune tolerance. In particular, the chimeric protein produced by transfected cells can be uptaken by DCs and also be recognized and internalized by B cells. In this way, peptides from both the xenogeneic and homologous domains of the internalized chimeric protein are presented by DCs and B cells through MHC class I (MHC I) and class II (MHC II) glycoproteins. The presentation of xenogeneic peptides by DCs is instrumental for the effective priming and the expansion of both $CD8^+$ and $CD4^+$ T cells which are specific for xenogeneic moieties and potentially cross-reactive against the homologous one. The interaction between the expanded $CD4^+$ T cells with B cells, which recognize the xenogeneic domain of the chimeric protein, leads to the differentiation of plasma cells which produce antibodies which are specifically against the xenogeneic domain of the vaccine. By contrast, the interaction of expanded $CD4^+$ T cells with B cells which recognize the homologous domain leads to the production of antibodies which are specific for the self-tolerated homologous domain of the protein, by differentiated plasma cells (Fig. 1). The slight differences in the amino acid sequence and in the tertiary structure of the chimeric protein, encoded by the hybrid plasmids, may result in the exposition of subdominant and/or new conformational epitopes, triggering an even more efficient humoral immune response than that induced by the xenogeneic and homologous vaccines.

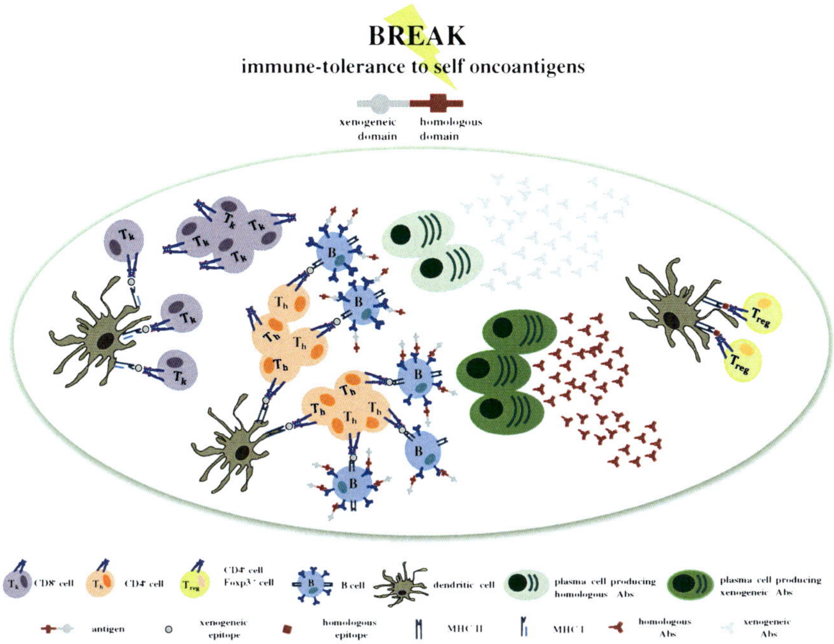

Fig. 1 Schematic representation of the mechanisms leading to the induction of potent cross-reactive T cell and antibody responses using chimeric proteins which combine xenogeneic and homologous domains of the self-oncoantigen. The chimeric protein used as vaccine is taken up by DCs and recognized by B cells that internalize it and present peptides through MHC II. The presentation of xenogeneic peptides (*white circles*) by DCs is instrumental for the effective priming and the expansion of both CD8$^+$ and CD4$^+$ T cells. The interaction between the expanded CD4$^+$ T cells with B cells, which recognize the xenogeneic domain of the chimeric protein, leads to the differentiation of plasma cells which produce antibodies which are specifically against the xenogeneic domain of the vaccine (xenogeneic-Abs). By contrast, the interaction of expanded CD4$^+$ T cells with B cells which recognize the homologous domain (*red squares*) leads to the production of antibodies which are specific for the self-tolerated homologous domain of the protein (homologous-Abs), by differentiated plasma cells. The presentation of peptides which derive from the homologous domain of the vaccine by DCs, through MHC II, leads to the expansion of Tregs

In principle, the strategy of combining heterologous with self-antigens can be applied to any TAA and could provide an initial starting point for the development of an effective anti-tumor vaccine to be used in clinic.

3.4 *Significant Mouse Models for the Study of ErbB2$^+$ Breast Cancer*

The evaluation of the power of hybrid DNA vaccines, which code for chimeric proteins, unquestionably requires the availability of appropriate animal models. Since immune tolerance to TAAs in cancer patients poses a major obstacle to the mounting of an effective anti-tumor immune response, the development of genetically engineered mice which carry an oncoantigen as a transgene offers an unprecedented opportunity to evaluate vaccine efficacy. The early expression of the oncoantigen in the thymus of transgenic mice causes immune tolerance that may be analogous to that observed in cancer patients.

In view of the causal correlation between ErbB2 receptor overexpression and mammary carcinogenesis, several laboratories have assessed the tumorigenic potential of ErbB2 in the mammary epithelium of transgenic mice, over the last 20 years (Quaglino et al. 2008). Indeed, several strains of ErbB2-transgenic mice which overexpress the rat or human ErbB2 ortholog and which spontaneously develop mammary tumors have been generated. They mimic crucial features of the human nature of breast cancer, such as slow progression, the natural occurrence of invasion and metastasis, and the presence of a long-lasting interaction between the evolving tumor and the host immune system (Cavallo et al. 2006).

One of the first and more commonly used genetically engineered mouse models in immunological studies is transgenic for an activated form of the rat ErbB2 protein under the transcriptional control of the mouse mammary tumor virus promoter long terminal repeats (MMTV-LTR promoter). The single-point mutation at position 664 in the transmembrane domain of the rat ErbB2 receptor, involving the replacement of valine with glutamic acid, results in the formation of homo- and heterodimers that spontaneously transduce the proliferative signals that are responsible for the transformation of mammary epithelial cells (Boggio et al. 1998). Rat ErbB2 transgenic mice acquire a central tolerance to rat ErbB2 as its early expression in the thymus causes a central deletion of T cell clones that react with high affinity to dominant rat ErbB2 peptides (Rolla et al. 2006; Ambrosino et al. 2006). All rat ErbB2 transgenic females are genetically predestinated to develop mammary tumors at 100 % penetrance. Carcinogenesis is completed over the course of 5 months, and spontaneous lung metastases become evident during the late stages of tumor progression. Notably, mammary carcinogenesis in ErbB2 transgenic mice displays consistent, stepwise, and directly age-related progression that mimics several features of human breast carcinoma (Quaglino et al. 2008). Moreover, the progressive expansion of both Treg cells (Ambrosino et al. 2006) and MDSC (Melani et al. 2003) can be measured in function of tumor progression and both further hamper the induction of an effective immune response. Similar observations have been made in human cancer patients.

Although rat ErbB2 transgenic mice provide an interesting and useful model, the 10% difference in amino acid sequence between rat and human ErbB2 receptors may be of critical importance for the accurate evaluation and translation of immunotherapeutic strategies against ErbB2 in patients. This concept led to the generation of human ErbB2 transgenic mouse models. Indeed, several strains have been generated, including those in which the human ErbB2 transgene is under the transcriptional control of the whey acidic protein (Piechocki et al. 2003), or of the MMTV-LTR promoter (Finkle et al. 2004). Both these mouse models are fully tolerant to human ErbB2 (Piechocki et al. 2003); however, only MMTV-LTR-

ErbB2 transgenic mice develop spontaneous asynchronous mammary tumors, although with long latency and incomplete penetrance.

The availability of these transgenic mice is of crucial importance to the pre-clinical evaluation of the efficacy of ErbB2 DNA vaccines and their potential benefits. However, they are all subject to major limitations as conventional transgenic mice do not model the sporadic nature of human cancer. Indeed, while the initiating mutation that drives cancer development in humans occurs in a single cell surrounded by a genetically wild-type microenvironment, early and widespread oncogene overexpression in the mammary epithelium does not follow the same expression pattern in ErbB2 transgenic mice giving rise to multifocal and scattered neoplastic lesions all over the mammary glands. Therefore, the efficacy of the anti-ErbB2 vaccines tested so far may be somehow underestimated and the generation of an ErbB2 conditional mouse model in which the oncogene is expressed in a tissue-specific and time-controlled manner could be instrumental to more faithfully gaining insight into the treatment of breast cancer in the future.

3.5 ErbB2 Chimeric DNA Vaccines

As previously described, the ErbB2 oncoantigen can be considered a peculiar archetype of self-tolerated TAA and one of the "ideal" targets to be used as a proof of concept for the effectiveness of hybrid plasmids. Existing immunological tolerance against ErbB2 may, indeed, represent a barrier to the effective vaccination of $ErbB2^+$ cancer patients; however, extreme sensitivity to the antibody-mediated immunity of most $ErbB2^+$ tumors (Wong and Lee 2012) points to DNA vaccination with ErbB2 hybrid plasmids as an appealing strategy for anti-tumor immunotherapy.

Actually, a DNA vaccination strategy using a plasmid which codes for the full-length human ErbB2 protein in conjunction with GM-CSF and IL-2 in patients with advanced breast cancer has been proven to be safe, well tolerated, and effective in inducing long-lasting cellular and humoral immune responses against the oncoantigen. However, measurable therapeutic clinical benefits have not been observed, most probably because of the chemo- and radiotherapy-induced immunosuppression of the patients and of the use of a homologous antigen, which is powerless to effectively circumvent immune tolerance, as a vaccine (Norell et al. 2010).

Considering the potential and the limits of xenogeneic vaccines, a significant amount of effort has been invested in producing hybrid plasmids that code for chimeric ErbB2 proteins which are partly derived from xenogeneic and partly from homologous sequences, with the final aim of inducing both a specific cellular and humoral response. The high amino acid homology (84.5 %) between rat and human extracellular (EC) and transmembrane (TM) domains of the ErbB2 protein has spurred us to generate two different plasmids which code for chimeric rat/human and human/rat EC-TM domains of the ErbB2 protein (named RHuT and HuRT plasmids, respectively) (Quaglino et al. 2010). While the chimeric plasmid RHuT encodes for a protein in which the 410 NH_2-terminal residues are from the rat ErbB2 domain and the remaining residues are from the human ErbB2 domain, almost symmetrically, HuRT encodes a protein in which 390 NH_2-terminal residues are from the human domain and the remainder from the rat domain. The availability of both rat and human ErbB2 transgenic mice has proven to be of crucial importance to the preclinical evaluation of the potential benefit of using hybrid RHuT and HuRT plasmids as compared to those which code for fully rat (RRT) or fully human (HuHuT) EC-TM ErbB2 domains.

When RRT and the HuHuT plasmids were used as autologous vaccines in rat and human ErbB2 transgenic mice, respectively, they induced high levels of antibodies with consummate specificity to the ErbB2 ortholog, used as an immunogen, but the T cell response was almost nil, as expected. However, a delay in cancer progression was observed, thanks to the pivotal role that antibodies play in the inhibition of ErbB2$^+$ tumors (Quaglino et al. 2010; Jacob et al. 2010). By contrast, when the RRT and the HuHuT plasmids were used as xenovaccines in human and rat ErbB2 transgenic mice, respectively, the humoral and cellular immune response induced were poorly cross-reactive against the self-oncoantigen expressed by the neoplastic cells (Iezzi et al. 2012) and thus completely ineffective in hampering the growth of transplantable or autochthonous ErbB2 tumors (Quaglino et al. 2010; Jacob et al. 2010), suggesting that xenogeneic vaccination may not be the strategy of choice in this model of cancer.

The use of hybrid RHuT and HuRT plasmids was found to be superior both to the fully autologous and to the fully xenogeneic vaccines in inducing a protective anti-tumor immune response against ErbB2$^+$ transplantable and autochthonous tumors, highlighting the importance of hybrid plasmids as effective anti-tumor vaccines.

The generation of a robust B and T cell response to the ErbB2 self-antigen together with a measurable anti-tumor effect in ErbB2 transgenic, tolerant mice (Quaglino et al. 2010, 2011), provided proof of concept of the power of combining target antigen heterologous and self-sequences for effective anti-tumor DNA vaccination. However, the rational design of chimeric DNA vaccines has to be carried out in order to potentially broaden this strategy to any TAA.

3.6 How to Design an Effective Hybrid Plasmid

Although the basic concepts behind the potential advantages of using hybrid instead of xenogeneic or homologous plasmids are clear, setting up the strategy for the design of an effective vaccine which codes for the oncoantigen of interest is less obvious and more complicated.

Seeing as the final goal of the hybrid plasmid strategy is the translation of chimeric vaccine into clinical practice, part of the antigen sequence must be derived from the human sequence. As far as the choice of species from which to derive the xenogeneic sequence used as the vaccine determinant is concerned, no defined indications are readily available. In principle, this heterologous sequence has to be different enough from that of the self-tolerated antigen in order to provide the heteroclitic peptides which are necessary to overcome T cell tolerance (Kianizad et al. 2007). However, it must, at the same time, be sufficiently similar to guarantee an effective cross-reactive immune response (Jacob et al. 2010). In general, a good degree of homology with the self-homologous oncoantigen can range from 85 to 95% (Cavallo et al. 2014). Practically, the choice of the xenogeneic part, from the several options available, can be dictated by the preclinical model that will be used to evaluate the efficacy of the chimeric vaccine. An example of this is provided by our chimeric human/rat ErbB2 vaccines described above. Moreover, other important issues to take into consideration in the generation of effective vaccines are both the location of the autologous and the xenogeneic domains in the chimeric protein and the ability of the hybrid plasmid to give rise to a protein which presents a structural conformation which is similar to the homologous one. Finally, it has been suggested that vaccine-encoded specific homologous sequences may actually activate the Treg population, thus limiting vaccine-induced anti-tumor immune response (Jacob et al. 2010). Therefore, when designing a hybrid plasmid for a given oncoantigen, self-regions involved in Treg expansion should be defined and replaced with the corresponding xenogeneic sequences. Based on all previous considerations, the design of hybrid vaccines which target oncoantigens should be theoretically performed once the critical regions for immune activation in the self and in the heterologous antigens have been clearly defined.

As far as our oncoantigen of choice, the ErbB2 receptor, and the two different hybrid plasmids generated which combine rat and human ErbB2 sequences are concerned, the rationale behind our design was formed around the availability of a consistent model of breast cancer in which the development of autochthonous mammary tumors is dictated by the expression of a rat ErbB2 transgene. In these mice, the rat ErbB2 is a fully tolerated self-protein. Moreover, rat ErbB2 has a high degree of homology with the human counterpart. To assess the weight of the position of the xenogeneic determinants, we compared the immunogenicity of two hybrid plasmids which differ from one another simply in the location of the rat and human domains in the coded chimeric protein.

Superior immunogenicity and anti-tumor efficacy over fully homologous or fully xenogeneic vaccines was demonstrated by both hybrid plasmids. This suggests, first of all, that the slight differences in the amino acid sequence between the human and rat EC-TM domains of the ErbB2 receptor are enough to circumvent self-tolerance (Quaglino et al. 2010, 2011). Moreover, the anti-tumor efficacy of the RHuT plasmid was found to be superior to HuRT when tested in ErbB2-transgenic and tolerant mice, suggesting that, in this preclinical model, the optimal immune response is elicited when the NH_2-terminal portion of the chimeric protein and the corresponding portion on the targeted ErbB2 orthologue are identical. The availability of mice which are transgenic and tolerant for the human ErbB2 protein allowed us to further confirm this result; HuRT was more immunogenic than RHuT, in this context (Quaglino et al. 2010, 2011). Moreover, it has been demonstrated that there is a Treg activation epitope in the human ErbB2 protein, embedded in the amino acid sequence ranging from amino acid 501 to 687 (Jacob et al. 2010). The replacement of this Treg-activating sequence with the corresponding rat sequence in the HuRT plasmid may explain its superior efficacy over the fully human ErbB2 vaccine.

This finding was also evident when the ability of ErbB2 hybrid plasmids to activate the suppressive effects of the tumor-induced Tregs, derived from ErbB2$^+$ cancer patients, was compared with that of fully human ErbB2 plasmid (Occhipinti et al. 2014). Indeed, while cancer patient DCs which had been transfected with the fully human HuHuT plasmid promoted the suppressive activity of autologous Tregs, those transfected with chimeric RHuT and HuRT plasmids were found to be ineffective at Treg activation. Therefore, these human surrogate experiments have provided proof of concept that chimeric rat/human ErbB2 DNA plasmids are useful in overcoming tumor-induced T cell dysfunction in ErbB2$^+$ cancer patients.

4 Conclusions

It is when oncology meets immunology that cancer immunotherapy becomes a reality. Strengthening a patient's own immune response against cancer cells is one of the most challenging and exciting concepts in active cancer immunotherapy. Thanks to striking progress in both the understanding of anti-tumor immune response and the characterization of several TAAs, a more rational design and more sophisticated strategies for anti-tumor vaccination have been possible. In this evolving scenario, selecting the best tumor target and the most appropriate vaccine administration route are of paramount importance. Only when vaccines are directed against oncoantigens can effective tumor control be achieved. DNA vaccines are an attractive and potentially effective tool for oncoantigen-specific cancer immunotherapy, and electroporation is one of the most sophisticated and promising strategies of the different delivery approaches tested so far.

However, despite successful studies in murine models, the anti-tumor efficacy of DNA vaccination in human clinical trials has been modest, reflecting the difficulty found in translating the plethora of convincing preclinical and early clinical results to an effective treatment for patients. Existing immunological tolerance against self-oncoantigens and tumor-suppressive mechanisms and the consequent difficulty in inducing an effective anti-tumor immune response may dramatically impact the success of cancer vaccination. Moreover, several studies have reported that despite the robust induction of specific antibodies, a paradoxical expansion of Tregs, of immunosuppressive phenotypes, is associated with vaccines that code for self-sequences.

Vaccination with a xenogeneic protein or peptide has been labeled as an effective means by which to overcome both central and peripheral immunological tolerance to self-proteins. The effective triggering of T cells can be induced, thanks to the generation of the so-called heteroclitic epitope. However, only low-affinity and poor cross-reactive humoral immune responses have been measured, because of the exquisite specificity of antibodies.

The ability of hybrid plasmids, which combine xenogeneic and homologous domains of the oncoantigen, to harness the power of xenogeneic vaccination to circumvent immune tolerance without losing the specificity of the immune response elicited by autologous vaccines may be a useful addition to the immunotherapeutic armamentarium for the fight against cancer. A demonstration of the power of this strategy is offered by the superior immunogenicity and anti-tumor efficacy elicited by the two rat/human (RHuT and HuRT) hybrid plasmids as compared to that of their fully rat (RRT) or fully human (HuHuT) counterparts in an ErbB2-tolerant context. Taken together, our preclinical data offer a proof of concept for the power of ErbB2 chimeric vaccines in cancer immunotherapy and have laid the foundation for the approval of a phase I clinical trial in patients with ErbB2^{+} carcinomas (EudraCT Number: 2011-001104-34).

Acknowledgments The authors thank Dr. Dale Lawson for his revision and editing of the article. This work was supported by grants from the Italian Association for Cancer Research (IG 11675), University of Torino, the Compagnia di San Paolo (Progetti di Ricerca Ateneo/CSP), and Fondazione Ricerca Molinette Onlus.

References

Albanell J, Gascon P (2005) Small molecules with EGFR-TK inhibitor activity. Curr Drug Targets 6(3):259–274

Alexander AN, Huelsmeyer MK, Mitzey A, Dubielzig RR, Kurzman ID, Macewen EG, Vail DM (2006) Development of an allogeneic whole-cell tumor vaccine expressing xenogeneic gp100 and its implementation in a phase II clinical trial in canine patients with malignant melanoma. Cancer Immunol Immunother 55(4):433–442. doi:10.1007/s00262-005-0025-6

Ambrosino E, Spadaro M, Iezzi M, Curcio C, Forni G, Musiani P, Wei WZ, Cavallo F (2006) Immunosurveillance of Erbb2 carcinogenesis in transgenic mice is concealed by a dominant regulatory T-cell self-tolerance. Cancer Res 66(15):7734–7740. doi:10.1158/0008-5472.CAN-06-1432 66/15/7734 [pii]

Anido J, Scaltriti M, Bech Serra JJ, Santiago Josefat B, Todo FR, Baselga J, Arribas J (2006) Biosynthesis of tumorigenic HER2 C-terminal fragments by alternative initiation of translation. EMBO J 25(13):3234–3244. doi:10.1038/sj.emboj.7601191 7601191 [pii]

Aurisicchio L, Mancini R, Ciliberto G (2013) Cancer vaccination by electro-gene-transfer. Expert Rev Vaccines 12(10):1127–1137. doi:10.1586/14760584.2013.836903

Aurisicchio L, Fridman A, Bagchi A, Scarselli E, La Monica N, Ciliberto G (2014) A novel minigene scaffold for therapeutic cancer vaccines. Oncoimmunology 3(1):e27529. doi:10.4161/onci.27529 2013ONCOIMM0318R [pii]

Baselga J, Cortes J, Kim SB, Im SA, Hegg R, Im YH, Roman L, Pedrini JL, Pienkowski T, Knott A, Clark E, Benyunes MC, Ross G, Swain SM (2012) Pertuzumab plus trastuzumab plus docetaxel for metastatic breast cancer. N Engl J Med 366(2):109–119. doi:10.1056/NEJMoa1113216

Berzofsky JA, Terabe M, Oh S, Belyakov IM, Ahlers JD, Janik JE, Morris JC (2004) Progress on new vaccine strategies for the immunotherapy and prevention of cancer. J Clin Invest 113(11):1515–1525. doi:10.1172/JCI21926

Boggio K, Nicoletti G, Di Carlo E, Cavallo F, Landuzzi L, Melani C, Giovarelli M, Rossi I, Nanni P, De Giovanni C, Bouchard P, Wolf S, Modesti A, Musiani P, Lollini PL, Colombo MP, Forni G (1998) Interleukin 12-mediated prevention of spontaneous mammary adenocarcinomas in two lines of Her-2/neu transgenic mice. J Exp Med 188(3):589–596

Casares N, Arribillaga L, Sarobe P, Dotor J, de Cerio ALD, Melero I, Prieto J, Borras-Cuesta F, Lasarte JJ (2003) CD4+/CD25+ regulatory cells inhibit activation of tumor-primed CD4+ T cells with IFN-gamma-dependent antiangiogenic activity, as well as long-lasting tumor immunity elicited by peptide vaccination. J Immunol 171(11):5931–5939

Castiglioni F, Tagliabue E, Campiglio M, Pupa SM, Balsari A, Menard S (2006) Role of exon-16-deleted HER2 in breast carcinomas. Endocr Relat Cancer 13(1):221–232. doi:10.1677/erc.1.01047 13/1/221 [pii]

Cavallo F, Offringa R, van der Burg SH, Forni G, Melief CJ (2006) Vaccination for treatment and prevention of cancer in animal models. Adv Immunol 90:175–213. doi:10.1016/S0065-2776(06)90005-4 S0065-2776(06)90005-4 [pii]

Cavallo F, Aurisicchio L, Mancini R, Ciliberto G (2014) Xenogene vaccination in the therapy of cancer. Expert Opin Biol Ther 1–16. doi:10.1517/14712598.2014.927433

Cheever MA, Higano CS (2011) PROVENGE (Sipuleucel-T) in prostate cancer: the first FDA-approved therapeutic cancer vaccine. Clin Cancer Res 17(11):3520–3526. doi:10.1158/1078-0432.CCR-10-3126 1078-0432.CCR-10-3126 [pii]

Chudley L, McCann K, Mander A, Tjelle T, Campos-Perez J, Godeseth R, Creak A, Dobbyn J, Johnson B, Bass P, Heath C, Kerr P, Mathiesen I, Dearnaley D, Stevenson F, Ottensmeier C (2012) DNA fusion-gene vaccination in patients with prostate cancer induces high-frequency CD8(+) T-cell responses and increases PSA doubling time. Cancer Immunol Immunother 61(11):2161–2170. doi:10.1007/s00262-012-1270-0

Cortes J, Roche H (2012) Docetaxel combined with targeted therapies in metastatic breast cancer. Cancer Treat Rev 38(5):387–396. doi:10.1016/j.ctrv.2011.08.001 S0305-7372(11)00176-9 [pii]

Diaz CM, Chiappori A, Aurisicchio L, Bagchi A, Clark J, Dubey S, Fridman A, Fabregas JC, Marshall J, Scarselli E, La Monica N, Ciliberto G, Montero AJ (2013) Phase 1 studies of the safety and immunogenicity of electroporated HER2/CEA DNA vaccine followed by adenoviral boost immunization in patients with solid tumors. J Transl Med 11:62. doi:10.1186/1479-5876-11-62 1479-5876-11-62 [pii]

Dunn GP, Old LJ, Schreiber RD (2004) The three Es of cancer immunoediting. Annu Rev Immunol 22:329–360. doi:10.1146/annurev.immunol.22.012703.104803

Dyall R, Bowne WB, Weber LW, LeMaoult J, Szabo P, Moroi Y, Piskun G, Lewis JJ, Houghton AN, Nikolic-Zugic J (1998) Heteroclitic immunization induces tumor immunity. J Exp Med 188(9):1553–1561

Eriksson F, Totterman T, Maltais AK, Pisa P, Yachnin J (2013) DNA vaccine coding for the rhesus prostate specific antigen delivered by intradermal electroporation in patients with relapsed prostate cancer. Vaccine 31(37):3843–3848. doi:10.1016/j.vaccine.2013.06.063 S0264-410X(13)00855-4 [pii]

Eschenburg G, Stermann A, Preissner R, Meyer HA, Lode HN (2010) DNA vaccination: using the patient's immune system to overcome cancer. Clin Dev Immunol 2010:169484. doi:10.1155/2010/169484

Even-Desrumeaux K, Baty D, Chames P (2011) State of the art in tumor antigen and biomarker discovery. Cancers (Basel) 3(2):2554–2596. doi:10.3390/cancers3022554 cancers3022554 [pii]

Finkle D, Quan ZR, Asghari V, Kloss J, Ghaboosi N, Mai E, Wong WL, Hollingshead P, Schwall R, Koeppen H, Erickson S (2004) HER2-targeted therapy reduces incidence and progression of midlife mammary tumors in female murine mammary tumor virus huHER2-transgenic mice. Clin Cancer Res 10(7):2499–2511

Fioretti D, Iurescia S, Fazio VM, Rinaldi M (2010) DNA vaccines: developing new strategies against cancer. J Biomed Biotechnol 2010:174378. doi:10.1155/2010/174378

Fong L, Brockstedt D, Benike C, Breen JK, Strang G, Ruegg CL, Engleman EG (2001) Dendritic cell-based xenoantigen vaccination for prostate cancer immunotherapy. J Immunol 167 (12):7150–7156

Frelin L, Brass A, Ahlen G, Brenndorfer ED, Chen M, Sallberg M (2010) Electroporation: a promising method for the nonviral delivery of DNA vaccines in humans? Drug News Perspect 23(10):647–653. doi:10.1358/dnp.2010.23.10.1513492 1513492 [pii]

Friedman LM, Rinon A, Schechter B, Lyass L, Lavi S, Bacus SS, Sela M, Yarden Y (2005) Synergistic down-regulation of receptor tyrosine kinases by combinations of mAbs: implications for cancer immunotherapy. Proc Natl Acad Sci USA 102(6):1915–1920. doi:10.1073/pnas.0409610102 0409610102 [pii]

Gajewski TF (2010) Improved melanoma survival at last! Ipilimumab and a paradigm shift for immunotherapy. Pigment Cell Melanoma Res 23(5):580–581. doi:10.1111/j.1755-148X.2010.00737.xPCR737 PCR737 [pii]

Ginsberg BA, Gallardo HF, Rasalan TS, Adamow M, Mu Z, Tandon S, Bewkes BB, Roman RA, Chapman PB, Schwartz GK, Carvajal RD, Panageas KS, Terzulli SL, Houghton AN, Yuan JD, Wolchok JD (2010) Immunologic response to xenogeneic gp100 DNA in melanoma patients: comparison of particle-mediated epidermal delivery with intramuscular injection. Clin Cancer Res 16(15):4057–4065. doi:10.1158/1078-0432.CCR-10-1093 1078-0432.CCR-10-1093 [pii]

Glenting J, Wessels S (2005) Ensuring safety of DNA vaccines. Microb Cell Fact 4:26. doi:10.1186/1475-2859-4-26 1475-2859-4-26 [pii]

Goforth R, Salem AK, Zhu X, Miles S, Zhang XQ, Lee JH, Sandler AD (2009) Immune stimulatory antigen loaded particles combined with depletion of regulatory T-cells induce potent tumor specific immunity in a mouse model of melanoma. Cancer Immunol Immunother 58(4):517–530. doi:10.1007/s00262-008-0574-6

Grosenbaugh DA, Leard AT, Bergman PJ, Klein MK, Meleo K, Susaneck S, Hess PR, Jankowski MK, Jones PD, Leibman NF, Johnson MH, Kurzman ID, Wolchok JD (2011) Safety and efficacy of a xenogeneic DNA vaccine encoding for human tyrosinase as adjunctive treatment for oral malignant melanoma in dogs following surgical excision of the primary tumor. Am J Vet Res 72(12):1631–1638. doi:10.2460/ajvr.72.12.1631

Heath WR, Belz GT, Behrens GM, Smith CM, Forehan SP, Parish IA, Davey GM, Wilson NS, Carbone FR, Villadangos JA (2004) Cross-presentation, dendritic cell subsets, and the generation of immunity to cellular antigens. Immunol Rev 199:9–26. doi:10.1111/j.0105-2896.2004.00142.x IMR142 [pii]

Hodi FS, O'Day SJ, McDermott DF, Weber RW, Sosman JA, Haanen JB, Gonzalez R, Robert C, Schadendorf D, Hassel JC, Akerley W, van den Eertwegh AJ, Lutzky J, Lorigan P, Vaubel JM, Linette GP, Hogg D, Ottensmeier CH, Lebbe C, Peschel C, Quirt I, Clark JI, Wolchok JD, Weber JS, Tian J, Yellin MJ, Nichol GM, Hoos A, Urba WJ (2010) Improved survival with ipilimumab in patients with metastatic melanoma. N Engl J Med 363(8):711–723. doi:10.1056/NEJMoa1003466 NEJMoa1003466 [pii]

Iezzi M, Quaglino E, Cappello P, Toto V, Sabatini F, Curcio C, Garotta G, Musiani P, Cavallo F (2011) HCG hastens both the development of mammary carcinoma and the metastatization of HCG/LH and ERBB-2 receptor-positive cells in mice. Int J Immunopathol Pharmacol 24 (3):621–630 8 [pii]

Iezzi M, Quaglino E, Amici A, Lollini PL, Forni G, Cavallo F (2012) DNA vaccination against oncoantigens: A promise. Oncoimmunology 1(3):316–325. doi:10.4161/onci.19127 2011ONCOIMM0110 [pii]

Jacob J, Radkevich O, Forni G, Zielinski J, Shim D, Jones RF, Wei WZ (2006) Activity of DNA vaccines encoding self or heterologous Her-2/neu in Her-2 or neu transgenic mice. Cell Immunol 240(2):96–106. doi:10.1016/j.cellimm.2006.07.002 S0008-8749(06)00119-5 [pii]

Jacob JB, Quaglino E, Radkevich-Brown O, Jones RF, Piechocki MP, Reyes JD, Weise A, Amici A, Wei WZ (2010) Combining human and rat sequences in her-2 DNA vaccines blunts immune tolerance and drives antitumor immunity. Cancer Res 70(1):119–128. doi:10.1158/0008-5472.CAN-09-2554 0008-5472.CAN-09-2554 [pii]

Janssen EM, Lemmens EE, Wolfe T, Christen U, von Herrath MG, Schoenberger SP (2003) CD4+ T cells are required for secondary expansion and memory in CD8+ T lymphocytes. Nature 421 (6925):852–856. doi:10.1038/nature01441 nature01441 [pii]

Jensen PE, Kapp JA (1986) Bystander help in primary immune responses in vivo. J Exp Med 164 (3):841–854

Josefowicz SZ, Lu LF, Rudensky AY (2012) Regulatory T cells: mechanisms of differentiation and function. Annu Rev Immunol 30:531–564. doi:10.1146/annurev.immunol.25.022106.141623

Kamstock D, Elmslie R, Thamm D, Dow S (2007) Evaluation of a xenogeneic VEGF vaccine in dogs with soft tissue sarcoma. Cancer Immunol Immunother 56(8):1299–1309. doi:10.1007/s00262-007-0282-7

Kantoff PW, Higano CS, Shore ND, Berger ER, Small EJ, Penson DF, Redfern CH, Ferrari AC, Dreicer R, Sims RB, Xu Y, Frohlich MW, Schellhammer PF (2010) Sipuleucel-T immunotherapy for castration-resistant prostate cancer. N Engl J Med 363(5):411–422. doi:10.1056/NEJMoa1001294

Kayaga J, Souberbielle BE, Sheikh N, Morrow WJ, Scott-Taylor T, Vile R, Chong H, Dalgleish AG (1999) Anti-tumour activity against B16-F10 melanoma with a GM-CSF secreting allogeneic tumour cell vaccine. Gene Ther 6(8):1475–1481. doi:10.1038/sj.gt.3300961

Kianizad K, Marshall LA, Grinshtein N, Bernard D, Margl R, Cheng S, Beermann F, Wan Y, Bramson J (2007) Elevated frequencies of self-reactive CD8+ T cells following immunization with a xenoantigen are due to the presence of a heteroclitic CD4+ T-cell helper epitope. Cancer Res 67(13):6459–6467. doi:10.1158/0008-5472.CAN-06-4336 67/13/6459 [pii]

Kim R, Emi M, Tanabe K, Arihiro K (2006) Tumor-driven evolution of immunosuppressive networks during malignant progression. Cancer Res 66(11):5527–5536. doi:10.1158/0008-5472.CAN-05-4128 66/11/5527 [pii]

Kircheis R, Kupcu Z, Wallner G, Rossler V, Schweighoffer T, Wagner E (2000) Interleukin-2 gene-modified allogeneic melanoma cell vaccines can induce cross-protection against syngeneic tumors in mice. Cancer Gene Ther 7(6):870–878. doi:10.1038/sj.cgt.7700183

Klinman DM, Yamshchikov G, Ishigatsubo Y (1997) Contribution of CpG motifs to the immunogenicity of DNA vaccines. J Immunol 158(8):3635–3639

Kutzler MA, Weiner DB (2008) DNA vaccines: ready for prime time? Nat Rev Genet 9 (10):776–788. doi:10.1038/nrg2432 nrg2432 [pii]

LaCelle MG, Jensen SM, Fox BA (2009) Partial CD4 depletion reduces regulatory T cells induced by multiple vaccinations and restores therapeutic efficacy. Clin Cancer Res 15(22):6881–6890. doi:10.1158/1078-0432.CCR-09-1113 1078-0432.CCR-09-1113 [pii]

Liu J, Kjeken R, Mathiesen I, Barouch DH (2008) Recruitment of antigen-presenting cells to the site of inoculation and augmentation of human immunodeficiency virus type 1 DNA vaccine immunogenicity by in vivo electroporation. J Virol 82(11):5643–5649. doi:10.1128/JVI.02564-07JVI.02564-07 JVI.02564-07 [pii]

Liyanage UK, Moore TT, Joo HG, Tanaka Y, Herrmann V, Doherty G, Drebin JA, Strasberg SM, Eberlein TJ, Goedegebuure PS, Linehan DC (2002) Prevalence of regulatory T cells is increased in peripheral blood and tumor microenvironment of patients with pancreas or breast adenocarcinoma. J Immunol 169(5):2756–2761

Lollini PL, Cavallo F, Nanni P, Forni G (2006) Vaccines for tumour prevention. Nat Rev Cancer 6 (3):204–216. doi:10.1038/nrc1815 nrc1815 [pii]

Low L, Mander A, McCann K, Dearnaley D, Tjelle T, Mathiesen I, Stevenson F, Ottensmeier CH (2009) DNA vaccination with electroporation induces increased antibody responses in patients with prostate cancer. Hum Gene Ther 20(11):1269–1278. doi:10.1089/hum.2009.067

Ludwig-Portugall I, Hamilton-Williams EE, Gotot J, Kurts C (2009) CD25+ T(reg) specifically suppress auto-Ab generation against pancreatic tissue autoantigens. Eur J Immunol 39 (1):225–233. doi:10.1002/eji.200838699

Madan RA, Mohebtash M, Arlen PM, Vergati M, Rauckhorst M, Steinberg SM, Tsang KY, Poole DJ, Parnes HL, Wright JJ, Dahut WL, Schlom J, Gulley JL (2012) Ipilimumab and a poxviral vaccine targeting prostate-specific antigen in metastatic castration-resistant prostate cancer: a phase I dose-escalation trial. Lancet Oncol 13(5):501–508. doi:10.1016/S1470-2045(12)70006-2 S1470-2045(12)70006-2 [pii]

Marshall JL, Hoyer RJ, Toomey MA, Faraguna K, Chang P, Richmond E, Pedicano JE, Gehan E, Peck RA, Arlen P, Tsang KY, Schlom J (2000) Phase I study in advanced cancer patients of a diversified prime-and-boost vaccination protocol using recombinant vaccinia virus and recombinant nonreplicating avipox virus to elicit anti-carcinoembryonic antigen immune responses. J Clin Oncol 18(23):3964–3973

Melani C, Chiodoni C, Forni G, Colombo MP (2003) Myeloid cell expansion elicited by the progression of spontaneous mammary carcinomas in c-erbB-2 transgenic BALB/c mice suppresses immune reactivity. Blood 102(6):2138–2145. doi:10.1182/blood-2003-01-0190-01-0190 2003-01-0190 [pii]

Melief CJ, van der Burg SH (2008) Immunotherapy of established (pre)malignant disease by synthetic long peptide vaccines. Nat Rev Cancer 8(5):351–360. doi:10.1038/nrc2373 nrc2373 [pii]

Mocellin S, Pilati P, Nitti D (2009) Peptide-based anticancer vaccines: recent advances and future perspectives. Curr Med Chem 16(36):4779–4796. doi:10.2174/092986709789909648 CMC-AbsEpub-086 [pii]

Norell H, Poschke I, Charo J, Wei WZ, Erskine C, Piechocki MP, Knutson KL, Bergh J, Lidbrink E, Kiessling R (2010) Vaccination with a plasmid DNA encoding HER-2/neu together with low doses of GM-CSF and IL-2 in patients with metastatic breast carcinoma: a pilot clinical trial. J Transl Med 8:53. doi:10.1186/1479-5876-8-53 1479-5876-8-53 [pii]

Occhipinti S, Sponton L, Rolla S, Caorsi C, Novarino A, Donadio M, Bustreo S, Satolli MA, Pecchioni C, Marchini C, Amici A, Cavallo F, Cappello P, Pierobon D, Novelli F, Giovarelli M (2014) Chimeric Rat/Human HER2 efficiently circumvents HER2 tolerance in cancer patients. Clin Cancer Res 20(11):2910–2921. doi:10.1158/1078-0432.CCR-13-2663 1078-0432.CCR-13-2663 [pii]

Odunsi K, Matsuzaki J, Karbach J, Neumann A, Mhawech-Fauceglia P, Miller A, Beck A, Morrison CD, Ritter G, Godoy H, Lele S, duPont N, Edwards R, Shrikant P, Old LJ, Gnjatic S, Jager E (2012) Efficacy of vaccination with recombinant vaccinia and fowlpox vectors expressing NY-ESO-1 antigen in ovarian cancer and melanoma patients. Proc Natl Acad Sci USA 109(15):5797–5802. doi:10.1073/pnas.1117208109 1117208109 [pii]

Ottnod JM, Smedley RC, Walshaw R, Hauptman JG, Kiupel M, Obradovich JE (2013) A retrospective analysis of the efficacy of Oncept vaccine for the adjunct treatment of canine oral malignant melanoma. Vet Comp Oncol 11(3):219–229. doi:10.1111/vco.12057

Pentcheva-Hoang T, Corse E, Allison JP (2009) Negative regulators of T-cell activation: potential targets for therapeutic intervention in cancer, autoimmune disease, and persistent infections. Immunol Rev 229(1):67–87. doi:10.1111/j.1600-065X.2009.00763.x IMR763 [pii]

Piechocki MP, Ho YS, Pilon S, Wei WZ (2003) Human ErbB-2 (Her-2) transgenic mice: a model system for testing Her-2 based vaccines. J Immunol 171(11):5787–5794

Pollard JW (2004) Tumour-educated macrophages promote tumour progression and metastasis. Nat Rev Cancer 4(1):71–78. doi:10.1038/nrc1256 nrc1256 [pii]

Quaglino E, Mastini C, Forni G, Cavallo F (2008) ErbB2 transgenic mice: a tool for investigation of the immune prevention and treatment of mammary carcinomas. Curr Protoc Immunol Chapter 20:Unit 20 29 21–20 29–10. doi:10.1002/0471142735.im2009s82

Quaglino E, Mastini C, Amici A, Marchini C, Iezzi M, Lanzardo S, De Giovanni C, Montani M, Lollini PL, Masucci G, Forni G, Cavallo F (2010) A better immune reaction to Erbb-2 tumors is elicited in mice by DNA vaccines encoding rat/human chimeric proteins. Cancer Res 70(7):2604–2612. doi:10.1158/0008-5472.CAN-09-2548 0008-5472.CAN-09-2548 [pii]

Quaglino E, Riccardo F, Macagno M, Bandini S, Cojoca R, Ercole E, Amici A, Cavallo F (2011) Chimeric DNA Vaccines against ErbB2+ Carcinomas: from mice to humans. Cancers (Basel) 3(3):3225–3241. doi:10.3390/cancers3033225 cancers3033225 [pii]

Quezada SA, Peggs KS, Simpson TR, Shen Y, Littman DR, Allison JP (2008) Limited tumor infiltration by activated T effector cells restricts the therapeutic activity of regulatory T cell depletion against established melanoma. J Exp Med 205(9):2125–2138. doi:10.1084/jem.20080099 jem.20080099 [pii]

Rech AJ, Mick R, Martin S, Recio A, Aqui NA, Powell DJ, Jr., Colligon TA, Trosko JA, Leinbach LI, Pletcher CH, Tweed CK, DeMichele A, Fox KR, Domchek SM, Riley JL, Vonderheide RH (2012) CD25 blockade depletes and selectively reprograms regulatory T cells in concert with immunotherapy in cancer patients. Sci Transl Med 4(134):134ra162. doi:10.1126/scitranslmed.3003330 4/134/134ra62 [pii]

Riccardo F, Iussich S, Maniscalco L, Lorda-Mayayo S, La Rosa G, Arigoni M, De Maria R, Gattino F, Lanzardo S, Lardone E, Martano M, Morello E, Prestigio S, Fiore A, Quaglino E, Zabarino S, Ferrone S, Buracco P, Cavallo F (2014) CSPG4-specific immunity and survival prolongation in dogs with oral malignant melanoma immunized with human CSPG4 DNA. Clin Cancer Res. doi:clincanres.3042.2013 [pii] 1078-0432.CCR-13-3042 [pii] 10.1158/1078-0432.CCR-13-3042

Rice J, Ottensmeier CH, Stevenson FK (2008) DNA vaccines: precision tools for activating effective immunity against cancer. Nat Rev Cancer 8(2):108–120. doi:10.1038/nrc2326

Rolla S, Nicolo C, Malinarich S, Orsini M, Forni G, Cavallo F, Ria F (2006) Distinct and non-overlapping T cell receptor repertoires expanded by DNA vaccination in wild-type and HER-2 transgenic BALB/c mice. J Immunol 177(11):7626–7633 177/11/7626 [pii]

Rukazenkov Y, Speake G, Marshall G, Anderton J, Davies BR, Wilkinson RW, Mark Hickinson D, Swaisland A (2009) Epidermal growth factor receptor tyrosine kinase inhibitors: similar but different? Anticancer Drugs 20(10):856–866. doi:10.1097/CAD.0b013e32833034e1

Sabado RL, Bhardwaj N (2013) Dendritic cell immunotherapy. Ann NY Acad Sci 1284:31–45. doi:10.1111/nyas.12125

Sakaguchi S, Takahashi T, Yamazaki S, Kuniyasu Y, Itoh M, Sakaguchi N, Shimizu J (2001) Immunologic self tolerance maintained by T-cell-mediated control of self-reactive T cells: implications for autoimmunity and tumor immunity. Microbes Infect 3(11):911–918. doi:10.1016/S1286-4579(01)01452-6

Sarnaik AA, Yu B, Yu D, Morelli D, Hall M, Bogle D, Yan L, Targan S, Solomon J, Nichol G, Yellin M, Weber JS (2011) Extended dose ipilimumab with a peptide vaccine: immune correlates associated with clinical benefit in patients with resected high-risk stage IIIc/IV melanoma. Clin Cancer Res 17(4):896–906. doi:10.1158/1078-0432.CCR-10-2463 1078-0432.CCR-10-2463 [pii]

Shak S (1999) Overview of the trastuzumab (Herceptin) anti-HER2 monoclonal antibody clinical program in HER2-overexpressing metastatic breast cancer. Herceptin Multinational Investigator Study Group. Semin Oncol 26(4 Suppl 12):71–77

Shedlock DJ, Weiner DB (2000) DNA vaccination: antigen presentation and the induction of immunity. J Leukoc Biol 68(6):793–806

Smith CM, Wilson NS, Waithman J, Villadangos JA, Carbone FR, Heath WR, Belz GT (2004) Cognate CD4(+) T cell licensing of dendritic cells in CD8(+) T cell immunity. Nat Immunol 5 (11):1143–1148. doi:10.1038/ni1129 ni1129 [pii]

Sobel ES, Kakkanaiah VN, Kakkanaiah M, Cheek RL, Cohen PL, Eisenberg RA (1994) T-B collaboration for autoantibody production in lpr mice is cognate and MHC-restricted. J Immunol 152(12):6011–6016

Soong RS, Trieu J, Lee SY, He L, Tsai YC, Wu TC, Hung CF (2013) Xenogeneic human p53 DNA vaccination by electroporation breaks immune tolerance to control murine tumors expressing mouse p53. PLoS One 8(2):e56912. doi:10.1371/journal.pone.0056912 PONE-D-12-35852 [pii]

Spears M, Taylor KJ, Munro AF, Cunningham CA, Mallon EA, Twelves CJ, Cameron DA, Thomas J, Bartlett JM (2012) In situ detection of HER2:HER2 and HER2:HER3 protein-protein interactions demonstrates prognostic significance in early breast cancer. Breast Cancer Res Treat 132(2):463–470. doi:10.1007/s10549-011-1606-z

Stevenson FK, Ottensmeier CH, Rice J (2010) DNA vaccines against cancer come of age. Curr Opin Immunol 22(2):264–270. doi:10.1016/j.coi.2010.01.019 S0952-7915(10)00020-8 [pii]

Stevenson FK, Mander A, Chudley L, Ottensmeier CH (2011) DNA fusion vaccines enter the clinic. Cancer Immunol Immunother 60(8):1147–1151. doi:10.1007/s00262-011-1042-2

Stewart TJ, Smyth MJ (2011) Improving cancer immunotherapy by targeting tumor-induced immune suppression. Cancer Metastasis Rev 30(1):125–140. doi:10.1007/s10555-011-9280-5

Stritesky GL, Jameson SC, Hogquist KA (2012) Selection of self-reactive T cells in the thymus. Annu Rev Immunol 30:95–114. doi:10.1146/annurev-immunol-020711-075035

Takenaka M, Seki N, Toh U, Hattori S, Kawahara A, Yamaguchi T, Koura K, Takahashi R, Otsuka H, Takahashi H, Iwakuma N, Nakagawa S, Fujii T, Sasada T, Yamaguchi R, Yano H, Shirouzu K, Kage M (2013) FOXP3 expression in tumor cells and tumor-infiltrating lymphocytes is associated with breast cancer prognosis. Mol Clin Oncol 1(4):625–632. doi:10.3892/mco.2013.107 mco-01-04-0625 [pii]

Thomas SK, Kwak LW (2012) Lymphoma vaccine therapy: next steps after a positive, controlled phase III clinical trial. Semin Oncol 39(3):253–262. doi:10.1053/j.seminoncol.2012.02.014 S0093-7754(12)00055-3

Viehl CT, Moore TT, Liyanage UK, Frey DM, Ehlers JP, Eberlein TJ, Goedegebuure PS, Linehan DC (2006) Depletion of CD4+CD25+ regulatory T cells promotes a tumor-specific immune response in pancreas cancer-bearing mice. Ann Surg Oncol 13(9):1252–1258. doi:10.1245/s10434-006-9015-y

Vogel CL, Cobleigh MA, Tripathy D, Gutheil JC, Harris LN, Fehrenbacher L, Slamon DJ, Murphy M, Novotny WF, Burchmore M, Shak S, Stewart SJ, Press M (2002) Efficacy and safety of trastuzumab as a single agent in first-line treatment of HER2-overexpressing metastatic breast cancer. J Clin Oncol 20(3):719–726

Walter S, Weinschenk T, Stenzl A, Zdrojowy R, Pluzanska A, Szczylik C, Staehler M, Brugger W, Dietrich PY, Mendrzyk R, Hilf N, Schoor O, Fritsche J, Mahr A, Maurer D, Vass V, Trautwein C, Lewandrowski P, Flohr C, Pohla H, Stanczak JJ, Bronte V, Mandruzzato S, Biedermann T, Pawelec G, Derhovanessian E, Yamagishi H, Miki T, Hongo F, Takaha N, Hirakawa K, Tanaka H, Stevanovic S, Frisch J, Mayer-Mokler A, Kirner A, Rammensee HG, Reinhardt C, Singh-Jasuja H (2012) Multipeptide immune response to cancer vaccine IMA901 after single-dose cyclophosphamide associates with longer patient survival. Nat Med 18(8):1254–1261. doi:10.1038/nm.2883 nm.2883 [pii]

Wolchok JD, Yuan J, Houghton AN, Gallardo HF, Rasalan TS, Wang J, Zhang Y, Ranganathan R, Chapman PB, Krown SE, Livingston PO, Heywood M, Riviere I, Panageas KS, Terzulli SL, Perales MA (2007) Safety and immunogenicity of tyrosinase DNA vaccines in patients with melanoma. Mol Ther 15(11):2044–2050. doi:10.1038/sj.mt.6300290 6300290 [pii]

Wong AL, Lee SC (2012) Mechanisms of resistance to trastuzumab and novel therapeutic strategies in HER2-positive breast cancer. Int J Breast Cancer 2012:415170. doi:10.1155/2012/415170

Wykosky J, Fenton T, Furnari F, Cavenee WK (2011) Therapeutic targeting of epidermal growth factor receptor in human cancer: successes and limitations. Chin J Cancer 30(1):5–12. doi:10.5732/cjc.010.10542 1944-446X2011015 [pii]

Yagi H, Nomura T, Nakamura K, Yamazaki S, Kitawaki T, Hori S, Maeda M, Onodera M, Uchiyama T, Fujii S, Sakaguchi S (2004) Crucial role of FOXP3 in the development and function of human CD25+CD4+ regulatory T cells. Int Immunol 16(11):1643–1656. doi:10.1093/intimm/dxh165 dxh165 [pii]

Yu WY, Chuang TF, Guichard C, El-Garch H, Tierny D, Laio AT, Lin CS, Chiou KH, Tsai CL, Liu CH, Li WC, Fischer L, Chu RM (2011) Chicken HSP70 DNA vaccine inhibits tumor growth in a canine cancer model. Vaccine 29(18):3489–3500. doi:10.1016/j.vaccine.2011.02.031 S0264-410X(11)00244-1

Yuan J, Ku GY, Gallardo HF, Orlandi F, Manukian G, Rasalan TS, Xu Y, Li H, Vyas S, Mu Z, Chapman PB, Krown SE, Panageas K, Terzulli SL, Old LJ, Houghton AN, Wolchok JD (2009) Safety and immunogenicity of a human and mouse gp100 DNA vaccine in a phase I trial of patients with melanoma. Cancer Immun 9:5 090505 [pii]

Yuan J, Adamow M, Ginsberg BA, Rasalan TS, Ritter E, Gallardo HF, Xu Y, Pogoriler E, Terzulli SL, Kuk D, Panageas KS, Ritter G, Sznol M, Halaban R, Jungbluth AA, Allison JP, Old LJ, Wolchok JD, Gnjatic S (2011) Integrated NY-ESO-1 antibody and CD8+ T-cell responses correlate with clinical benefit in advanced melanoma patients treated with ipilimumab. Proc Natl Acad Sci U S A 108(40):16723–16728. doi:10.1073/pnas.1110814108 1110814108 [pii]

Yuan J, Ku GY, Adamow M, Mu Z, Tandon S, Hannaman D, Chapman P, Schwartz G, Carvajal R, Panageas KS, Houghton AN, Wolchok JD (2013) Immunologic responses to xenogeneic tyrosinase DNA vaccine administered by electroporation in patients with malignant melanoma. J Immunother Cancer 1:20. doi:10.1186/2051-1426-1-202051-1426-1-20 2051-1426-1-20 [pii]

Zhang X, Smith DS, Guth A, Wysocki LJ (2001) A receptor presentation hypothesis for T cell help that recruits autoreactive B cells. J Immunol 166(3):1562–1571

Zinkernagel RM, Hengartner H (2001) Regulation of the immune response by antigen. Science 293(5528):251–253. doi:10.1126/science.1063005293/5528/251 293/5528/251 [pii]

Linked CD4 T Cell Help: Broadening Immune Attack Against Cancer by Vaccination

Natalia Savelyeva, Alex Allen, Warayut Chotprakaikiat, Elena Harden, Jantipa Jobsri, Rosemary Godeseth, Yidao Wang, Freda Stevenson and Christian Ottensmeier

Abstract In the last decade, immunotherapy with monoclonal antibodies targeting immunological check points has become a breakthrough therapeutic modality for solid cancers. However, only up to 50 % of patients benefit from this powerful approach. For others vaccination might provide a plausible addition or alternative. For induction of effective anticancer immunity CD4+ T cell help is required, which is often difficult to induce to self cancer targets because of tolerogenic mechanisms. Our approach for cancer vaccines has been to incorporate into the vaccine design sequences able to activate foreign T cell help, through genetically linking cancer targets to microbial sequences (King et al. in Nat Med 4(11):1281–1286, 1998; Savelyeva et al. in Nat Biotechnol 19(8):760–764, 2001). This harnesses the non-tolerized CD4 T cell repertoire available in patients to help induction of effective immunity against fused cancer antigens. Multiple immune effector mechanisms including antibody, CD8+ T cells as well as CD4 effector T cells can be activated using this strategy. Delivery via DNA vaccines has already indicated clinical efficacy. The same principle of linked T cell help has now been transferred to other novel vaccine modalities to further potentiate immunity against cancer targets.

Contents

N. Savelyeva (✉) · A. Allen · W. Chotprakaikiat · E. Harden · R. Godeseth · Y. Wang · F. Stevenson · C. Ottensmeier
Cancer Sciences Unit, Faculty of Medicine, University of Southampton, Tremona Road, Southampton SO16 6YD, UK
e-mail: N.Savelyeva@soton.ac.uk

W. Chotprakaikiat · J. Jobsri
Oral Biology Department, Naresuan University, Phitsanulok, Thailand

Current Topics in Microbiology and Immunology (2017) 405:123–143
DOI 10.1007/82_2016_500

Published Online: 05 October 2016

1 Introduction

Cancer vaccination aims to stimulate the patient's own immune system to fight tumours. The induced immunological response should be specific to the cancer cells, with minimal effect on normal tissues. Vaccines that have been approved by the FDA include prophylactic vaccines against viruses that cause malignancies, for example, the hepatitis B virus which drives hepatocellular carcinoma (Arbuthnot and Kew 2001) and the human papilloma virus (HPV) which causes cervical cancer (Mariani and Venuti 2010). Both vaccines are aimed at inducing antiviral antibody to prevent the infection that causes malignant transformation. The first therapeutic vaccine for patients with established cancer is Provenge® (Sipuleucel T) which has also been recently approved. This dendritic cell (DC) vaccine targets a protein expressed not by an infectious agent but by the cancer, prostate acid phosphatase (PAP). It is used for metastatic castration resistant prostate cancer patients (Kantoff et al. 2010). Several cancer vaccines are currently being developed or are in late stage clinical testing (Quoix et al. 2015) (NCT02187367).

For clinical success there are several major hurdles including tolerance and immunoregulation which must be overcome by vaccination.

1.1 Tolerogenic Pressure

1.1.1 T Cell Immunity

A number of mechanisms exist that prevent the immune system from attacking the host's own tissues, a concept defined as self-tolerance. Failure or deficiency of these mechanisms results in autoimmune responses. Central tolerance in the thymus and bone marrow ensures that newly formed T lymphocytes are not capable of recognizing self-peptides presented by MHC through positive and negative selection (reviewed in Xing and Hogquist 2012).

Although central tolerance is effective, it does not eliminate all potentially self-reactive T cells and hence a T cell repertoire against self-cancer targets is retained. To compensate, peripheral tolerogenic mechanisms act on mature lymphocytes that have escaped central tolerance. Regulatory T cells (Tregs) are crucial for maintaining peripheral tolerance; several subsets of Tregs exist. $Foxp3^+$ regulatory T cells can be induced in the periphery to control the response to tissue-restricted antigens not expressed by the thymus (Gregerson et al. 2009); these are known as iTregs (induced Tregs). A second type of Tregs derives from high-affinity self-reactive CD4 T cells, which are converted to $Foxp3^+$ Tregs in the thymus before exiting to the periphery (Martin et al. 2013). These cells are known as nTregs (natural Tregs) (Hsieh et al. 2012).

Tregs inhibit anti-self-immune responses in the secondary lymphoid organs, as well as within tumours, by a number of mechanisms involving secretion of suppressive cytokines IL-10 (Rubtsov et al. 2008) and tumour growth factor-β (TGF-β) (Wan and Flavell 2007), granzyme-dependent killing of responder cells (Cao et al. 2007), and others mechanisms (Bopp et al. 2007). Contact-dependent inhibition of DC activation through CTLA4 by binding to CD80 and CD86, and LAG-3 (lymphocyte activation gene-3) binding to MHC II have been described (Sansom 2000). Tregs can also operate directly in the tumour by delivering inhibitory signals to T cells (Facciabene et al. 2012; Weinberg et al. 2011).

Other components of the tumour microenvironment, as well as the tumour itself can exert tolerising pressure on T cells (Quail and Joyce 2013). Recently attention has focused on identification of mechanisms that contribute to a dysfunctional or exhausted phenotype of tumour-localized effector T cells (Wherry and Kurachi 2015). Targeting these inhibitory pathways, or so-called checkpoints molecules, is proving to be highly efficient for therapy of cancer (reviewed in Perez-Gracia et al. 2014).

1.1.2 B Cell Immunity

For induction of antibody, tolerogenic mechanisms will affect both the CD4 T cell compartment, essential for induction of antibody, and also B cells directly. Central tolerance will eliminate most self-reactive B cells through receptor editing, deletion and anergy (Nemazee 1996) but low avidity self-reactive B cells may survive. In the periphery self-reactive B cells are subjected to further regulation directly by antigen through the B cell receptor (BCR) and this can result in anergy (Goodnow et al. 1988; Merrell et al. 2006). In contrast to T cells, B cells can undergo affinity maturation in the germinal centre through the process of somatic hypermutation (MacLennan 1994). Therefore, there is a chance for low affinity B cells to increase their affinity in the germinal centre. However this requires functional non-tolerised CD4 T cells and a particular T cell subset, follicular T cells, are crucial (Vinuesa et al. 2005). Again there is an inhibitory counterpart for this process: follicular Tregs have been found to inhibit the germinal centre reaction and hence induction of high-affinity antibody (Chung et al. 2011).

1.2 Choice of Target Antigen: Specific, Neoantigens and Shared Antigens

The tumour antigen is the key component of a cancer vaccine. Tumour antigens (TAs) arise from viruses, mutated proteins or from overexpressed normal proteins (Stevenson et al. 2004b). The identification and characterisation of TAs was initially achieved using expression libraries of human tumours probed with autologous serum (SEREX) (Jager 2007). This led to the detection of anti-TA T cell responses in cancer patients (Jager 2007). Ideally, the antigen should only be found in the cancer cell and not expressed in any normal, healthy tissues to prevent autoimmunity. Tumour antigens can be broadly categorized into tumour-specific antigens (TSA) expressed only in cancer and tumour-associated antigens (TAA) with expression in cancer and other tissues.

The success of prophylactic vaccination against HPV with Cervarix (Monie et al. 2008) and Gardasil (Schiller et al. 2012) vaccines has raised the possibility of HPV as an attractive vaccine target post-infection. The HPV-derived oncoproteins E6 and E7 are cancer specific and also non-self (King et al. 2015). HPV infection causes cervical, ano-genital and head and neck squamous cell carcinoma with a large unmet clinical need and >500.000 deaths annually from HPV-driven malignancies worldwide (Warnakulasuriya 2010). DNA vaccination targeting E6 and E7 proteins has demonstrated induction of robust T cell responses followed by regression of precancerous cervical disease in a randomized phase II clinical trial (Trimble et al. 2015).

The idiotypic Ig of B cell malignancies arising as a result of variable Ig gene rearrangements and somatic hypermutation is unique for every B cell and is an excellent example of a TSA (McCarthy et al. 2003). Its identification several decades ago was followed by clinical targeting with vaccination (McCarthy et al. 2003; Villanueva et al. 2011). More recently novel technologies have allowed rapid manufacturing of these personalized vaccines for clinical application (McCann et al. 2015; Bendandi et al. 2010; Tuse et al. 2015). Mutated proteins such as K-Ras and p53 are another type of TSA (Abrams et al. 1996). These have been of interest as cancer targets for many years but have been difficult to deliver (Carbone et al. 2005).

Further advances in deep sequencing methods have permitted a rapid identification of novel antigens or neoantigens that arise from tumour-specific mutations (Schumacher and Schreiber 2015; Vigneron et al. 2013). Because these neoantigens arise within the tumour itself, the specific T cells are unlikely to have been subjected to central tolerance. In theory this means that there will be a wider T cell repertoire with a higher affinity for pMHC, which would be advantageous for any cancer vaccine. However, they are likely to be subjected to peripheral tolerance mechanisms. A surprising finding has been that neoantigenic peptides are not only restricted by MHC I but can also be MHCII restricted (Schumacher et al. 2014; Tran et al. 2014; Kreiter et al. 2015; Zanetti 2015). For only a small minority of these neoantigens T cell reactivities can be detected. This is presumably because the majority of reactive T cells have been tolerised in the periphery. Furthermore, owing to the fact that these novel sequences arise from within the tumour itself, they will rarely be shared among patients. Melanoma, colon, glioma and breast cancer are the examples of tumours where neoantigens have been found in humans (Schumacher et al. 2014; Tran et al. 2014; Linnemann et al. 2015; Kreiter et al. 2015). Both the financial and practical implications of 'personalized' cancer immunotherapy are a significant consideration, but intensive international efforts are underway to find technical solutions to this challenge. An important question also is how many of these mutated epitopes need to be targeted by one successful vaccine. The most likely scenario will be that a small number of targets may be enough to kick-start the immune system before 'epitope spreading' occurs (el-Shami et al. 1999; Ribas et al. 2003). Future experimental evidence will shed light on these important considerations.

TAA are expressed by both cancer and normal tissues and include cancer-testis antigens (CTAs), differentiation antigens and overexpressed antigens (reviewed in Buonaguro et al. 2011; Fratta et al. 2011). These antigens have received considerable attention in vaccine development over the years driven by the desire to vaccinate cohorts of patients in a consistent way. Where TAA are expressed in multiple types of tumour and in significant proportions or even in all patients with one cancer type, an off-the-self vaccine can be generated. The first approved cancer vaccine Provenge is the DC-based vaccine targeting TAA prostatic acid phosphatase (PAP) and is a successful example of this approach (Sonpavde et al. 2012). Several vaccines that target TAAs (hTERT, Her2, Muc1) are in late stage clinical trials with promising results (Acres et al. 2015; Quoix et al. 2015; Rochman 2015) (NCT02301754, NCT02327468, NCT02293707).

1.3 Activation of Relevant Immune Anticancer Mechanisms

Recognition of TAs by induced immune mechanisms is essential for cancer clearance. TAs are present on the cell surface, as soluble factors or located in the cytosol. Cell surface antigens such Her2-3, Id Ig, mammaglobin A (Tiriveedhi et al. 2014; Zuo et al. 2009), xCT (Lanzardo et al. 2016) and others can be recognized by antibody which in turn can induce several mechanisms of tumour elimination. Antibody-dependent cellular cytotoxicity, phagocytosis, direct antibody-induced apoptosis or cancer cell growth inhibition are the major mechanisms by which antibody causes tumour destruction (Weiner et al. 2009). Passive monoclonal antibody therapies targeting antigens on cancer cells have been very successful in the clinic demonstrating that this immune arm is effective for cancer elimination. Induction of potent antibody by active vaccination in clinical testing is equally desirable (Damodaran and Olson 2012). Vaccine CIMAvax-EGF targets a soluble antigen epidermal growth factor (EGF), the ligand for the EGF receptor which is overexpressed on lung cancer cells. This vaccine has been developed to induce neutralizing antibody against EGF to block its tumour growth-promoting effect (Rodriguez et al. 2010). Patients with high antibody responses had a remarkably better outcome than the control group of patients with IIIB/IV stage non-small cell lung carcinoma (Neninger Vinageras et al. 2008; Quaratino et al. 2014). From early 2016 patients in several centres in Europe and Asia are being recruited to test the vaccine in a phase III clinical trial for non-small cell lung carcinoma (NCT02187367).

The majority of antigens that have attracted attention so far, however, are intracellular proteins and hence will not be targeted by antibody. Immune attack relies instead on short, usually 9-mer, antigenic peptides presented in the context of MHC class I. These can be targeted by CD8+ cytotoxic T cells which will recognize the peptide MHC I complex and directly kill the target cell through perforins/granzyme or Fas-mediated mechanisms (Stevenson et al. 2013; Stevenson et al. 2004a). Most approaches to developing cancer vaccines have focused on activating this immune mechanism (Stevenson et al. 2013). A minority of cancers are MHCII positive including B cell lymphomas and some epithelial tumours. Here it is possible to direct targeting to peptides presented in the MHCII context by CD4 T cells (Savelyeva et al. 2001); (Savelyeva et al. 2003). Unlike the traditional helper function of CD4 T cells to CD8+ and B cells, cytolytic function of CD4+ T cells is less well defined. In this case, CD4 T cells are of the Th1 subset and direct killing is mediated through mechanisms involving Fas/FasL (Ju et al. 1994). Killing can also be mediated through other members of TNF-receptor ligand family, i.e. TRAIL, the ligand for Apo2 (TRAIL-R2 and R3, also known as DR4 and DR5, respectively) (Dorothee et al. 2002; Thomas and Hersey 1998) and TWEAK with Apo3 (DR3) as a receptor (Kaplan et al. 2000). Perforin/granzyme-mediated cytotoxity against MHC class II positive tumours has also been documented (Dorothee et al. 2002).

There are however only a few known MHC II positive cancers which can be targeted by CD4 T cells directly through recognition of tumour-specific peptides. For MHCII negative tumours CD4+ Th1 cells characterized by secretion of IFN-γ and TNF-a, can engage the effectors of the innate immune system. Killing of myeloma cells by Th1-activated macrophages is an example of where this mechanism has been very well defined (Haabeth et al. 2014). Natural killer (NK) cells can be also be engaged through similar mechanisms (Perez-Diez et al. 2007). Reprogramming the tumour microenvironment by Th1 cells may also lead to reduction of Tregs (Kreiter et al. 2015). MHCII positive APC such as macrophages or B cells have been found to provide the antigen specificity link by presenting the antigen to CD4 T cells (Haabeth et al. 2014; Tran et al. 2014). These previously underappreciated Th1 cells have now been found in several human tumours and their role in antitumour immunity is rapidly growing and their antitumour functions have been exploited in adoptive T cell therapies in metastatic cancer (Tran et al. 2014).

2 Targeting Cancer with Vaccination

A number of vaccine delivery vehicles have been explored to target cancer. They have been described in detail elsewhere (Melief et al. 2015). Here we will focus on genetic vaccines and include novel approaches to vaccination we have been developing.

2.1 DNA Vaccines

DNA vaccines are becoming promising modalities for cancer owing to their recent clinical advances (Trimble et al. 2015; Kraynyak et al. 2015). As with conventional vaccines, DNA vaccination aims to induce specific and durable humoral and cellular responses against TAs. A DNA cancer vaccine consists of a plasmid backbone acting as the natural adjuvant, the encoded specific cancer antigen and a strong viral promoter, usually CMV, is included to drive expression of the encoded tumour antigen. The adjuvant properties of plasmid DNA are linked to activation through TLR9 as well as cytoplasmic sensors of DNA (reviewed in Rice et al. 2008 and Barber 2011). Several immune sensors of plasmid DNA located in the cytoplasm, including Absent In Melanoma (AIM2), IFN-γ-inducible 16 (IFI16), DAI/ZBP and DNA-dependent protein kinase (DNA-PK), have been identified (Paludan and Bowie 2013). They all can contribute to adjuvant properties of plasmid DNA and promote the immune response to the encoded antigen. DNA vaccines can be easily manipulated by means of genetic engineering and additional sequences to improve immunogenicity of the target antigen, i.e. cytokines, chemokines or, as discussed below, a sequence for induction of linked T cell help, can be incorporated.

2.2 Fragment C of Tetanus Toxin in Fusion DNA Vaccines

TA often display similar properties to that of other self-proteins and, used alone, fail to induce adequate T cell responses owing to a low immunogenicity resulting from tolerogenic pressure. The DNA fusion vaccine concept was developed to overcome this barrier. Initial studies with protein vaccines focused on conjugating lymphoma-derived Id Ig antigen to the foreign protein keyhole limpet hemocyanin (KLH) (George et al. 1988; McCarthy et al. 2003). Unfortunately this had little success; first, the complex polymeric structure of KLH made it impractical within DNA vaccines and second, KLH induced a predominantly Th2 response, which we now know is not favourable for treating cancer (Timmerman 2009).

The carboxy-terminal fragment C (FrC) of tetanus toxin (TT) is a single polypeptide of approximately 50 kD. It is highly immunogenic and lacks the ability of whole TT to paralyze neuromuscular transmission, and hence lacks its toxicity

(Neubauer and Helting 1981; Cook et al. 2001). No undesirable clinical effects have been reported following its introduction into humans (Calvo et al. 2012).

Our laboratory first demonstrated the successful use of FrC for provision of linked CD4+ T cell help for poorly immunogenic cancer antigens in lymphoma (Spellerberg et al. 1997; King et al. 1998). We found that lymphoma-derived idiotypic (Id) Ig antigen by itself was unable to induce sufficient T cell help to drive the anti-Id antibody response. Protective anti-Id antibody was induced when we used a DNA fusion vaccine design consisting of V_H and V_L of Id Ig antigen assembled as scFv through a flexible linker and genetically linked to FrC (Id-FrC) (King et al. 1998). The Id-FrC fusion DNA vaccine was able to engage the non-tolerant CD4+ T cell repertoire available for FrC, to provide T cell help to Id-specific B cells to produce antibody (Fig. 1). Remarkably the vaccine was not only effective in the lymphoma model but the same design also generated protection against myeloma, which is Id surface-low/negative and hence not readily susceptible to targeting by antibody. The effectors which operated in this case were Id-specific CD4 Th1 cells capable of clearing Id Ig surface negative myeloma cells. Again only the Id-FrC fusion vaccine was effective; Id DNA vaccine without FrC failed to induce protection (King et al. 1998). We concluded that the Id-FrC design provided effective linked T cell help to both B cells and to weaker CD4 Th1 cells (Fig. 1). The study not only highlighted the requirement of foreign T cell help for antibody induction but also provided means of induction of CD4 Th mediated protective responses to weak cancer antigens. The latter was likely to involve the help-to-helper mechanism when DC activated by strong Th response are capable of activating weaker Th subsets in a similar way to how T-cell help operates for CTL induction (Gerloni et al. 2000).

The substantial immunological response achieved with this relatively simple constructed FrC fusion vaccine, led to early phase clinical trials of DNA Id-FrC fusion vaccines in patients with follicular lymphoma and multiple myeloma (MM). In the lymphoma study anti-Id antibody responses were seen in 38 % of patients (Rice et al. 2008) but problems with assessment of the efficacy of the vaccine arose because of the fact that the vaccine itself was patient-specific and therefore inter-patient comparisons could not be made. For MM we recently reported a Phase I clinical trial of an Id-FrC fusion DNA vaccine in patients with complete or partial responses following high-dose chemotherapy and autologous stem cell transplantation (McCann et al. 2015). The vaccine administered at least 6 months post-transplant was able to induce vaccine-specific CD4 T cell responses (McCann et al. 2015). Both FrC- and Id-specific CD4 T cells were detected in 29 % of patients, with 43 % of patients responding to FrC alone. These results are promising for a number of reasons. First, Id-FrC DNA vaccine can induce Id-specific CD4+ Th1 reactivity in the face of previous data indicating that patients with advanced MM shift towards a Th2 response (Yi et al. 1995). Second, the study demonstrated immune responses were observed even in patients previously treated with regimens reported to decrease the ability to mount an immunological response to vaccinations (Arrowood and Hayney 2002). Additionally, the study confirmed that Id-specific Th1 cells were not deleted in patients who, while they had a low burden disease at

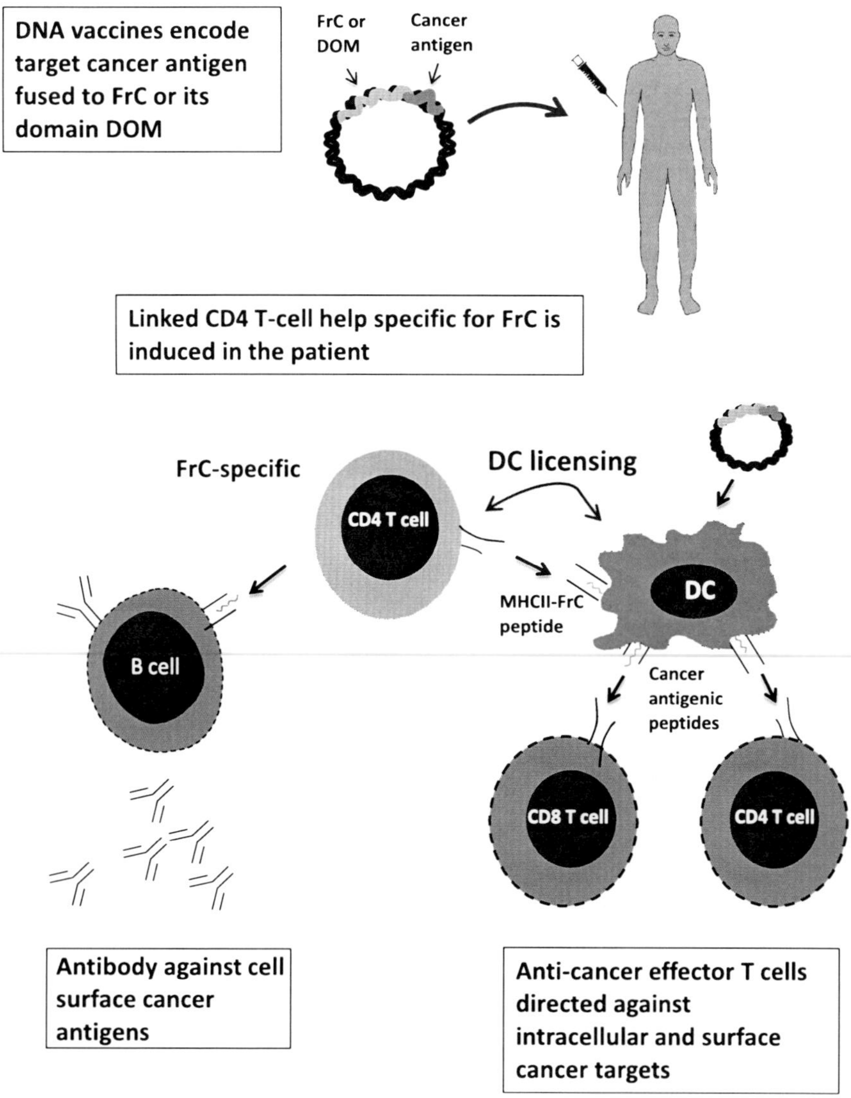

Fig. 1 Linked CD4+ T cell help induced by DNA vaccines encoding FrC or its domain DOM fused to target cancer antigen generates multiple immune mechanisms for cancer attack in patients. The key mechanism is induction of foreign FrC-specific T cell help which through licensing of dendritic cells (DC) leads to activation of CD8 and CD4 T cells specific for target cancer antigen. FrC-specific T cells also provide help to B cells to induce antibody against surface cancer targets

vaccination (with serum paraprotein below 50 g/L), previously had much higher levels of paraprotein. Deletion of Id-specific T cells (Bogen 1996) appears not to be an issue in our cohort therefore. Our data support that idiotypic vaccination is a valid concept for immunotherapy in this patient cohort.

2.3 *The p.DOM-Epitope Design to Induce CTL Responses*

As mentioned above most TA are intracellular and upon presentation in MHC I can be targeted by CD8 T cells. DNA vaccines are capable of inducing potent CD8+ T cell responses (Stevenson et al. 2013; Stevenson et al. 2004a). Lasting and efficient immunological responses require CD4 T cell help and FrC was expected to provide this. For cytotoxic responses however, a potential problem was identified. The natural CD8+ T cell response against viruses appears highly focused on only a few MHC Class I-binding epitopes, due to the phenomenon of immunodominance (Yewdell and Bennink 1999). This focus meant that delivery of cancer antigens via, for example, pox viral vectors, may fail due to competition from strong viral epitopes (Yewdell 2010). Failure has in fact been demonstrated in a clinical trial of an MVA-delivered melanoma antigen, where immune responses apparently focused on vector peptides rather than on the desired tumour peptides (Smith et al. 2005). We wondered therefore, whether FrC would also present strong epitopes for CD8 T cell attack and whether the immune response would focus on those rather than on the cancer-derived sequences. Indeed competitive epitopes were found in the C-terminal portion of FrC (Rice et al. 1999) therefore its subdomain, DOM was created through deletion of that portion (Rice et al. 2001). The DOM DNA fusion vaccine design decreased the potential competition from the carrier-derived MHC Class I-binding peptides (Rice et al. 2002). Tumour-derived peptide sequences have then been fused to the 3'-terminus of DOM to create the p.DOM-epitope design (Stevenson et al. 2004a). Using this design, we successfully demonstrated induction of high levels of epitope-specific CD8+ T cells in several preclinical models (Rice et al. 2008).

2.4 *Clinical Experience with the p.Dom-Epitope Design*

2.4.1 Induction of Immune Responses

Translation of preclinical studies of DNA vaccines to human patients initially appeared difficult. A hurdle for DNA cancer vaccines was the difficulty in scaling the amount and volume of the vaccine from mice to human subjects (Buchan et al. 2005). Since these initial attempts, there are now various methods to overcome this hurdle. Electroporation (EP) has emerged as a clinically viable method for DNA vaccination of cancer patients. The procedure is to pass an electric current across the tissue site at the same time as injection, or very soon after. The result is an increase in DNA transfection levels and therefore, antigen expression. Local inflammation was also increased through the electrical damage and also the activation of multiple sensors for dsDNA within the cell (Paludan and Bowie 2013). As a result, more antigen-presenting cells are attracted to the vaccination site, (Ahlen et al. 2007; Kraynyak et al. 2015) and significant immune responses can be induced even in large mammals.

Our own early experience evaluating immunogenicity of the p.Dom-PSMA epitope in patients with prostate cancer demonstrated low anti-DOM IgG antibody responses after i.m. delivery of DNA without EP (Low et al. 2009). In contrast, delivery of the vaccine with EP demonstrated significant levels of anti-DOM antibody and the responses were still seen after 18 months of follow up (Low et al. 2009). PSMA peptide-specific (PSMA27) responses were detected in 16 out of 30 vaccinated patients while 29 patients had DOM-specific Th1 responses. The clinical effects were visible as a significant increase of PSA doubling time in vaccinated patients (Chudley et al. 2012).

Clinical evaluation of a p.DOM-epitope fusion DNA vaccine without electroporation was carried out in 27 cancer patients in a multicenter clinical study (McCann et al. 2016). Patients were treated either with measurable disease after the failure of conventional treatment or in radiological remission. The vaccine targeted the HLA-A*0201 binding peptide CAP-1 from the carcinoembryonic antigen (CEA) linked to DOM. Both cellular responses against the CAP-1 peptide and humoral response against DOM were seen in patients without and with measurable disease. Mass-spectrometry confirmed that CAP-1 was expressed by cells in normal colon, primary colorectal tumour and metastatic colorectal tumour. ELISPOT and flow cytometry showed CAP-1 specific T cells in the peripheral blood confirming the immunogenicity of the vaccine. The vaccine was overall safe and well tolerated, but 48 % of patients reported diarrhoea. Interestingly, the bowel toxicity was linked to a better clinical outcome and immunological responses. Patients who reported diarrhoea were found to have higher DOM-specific responses with longer duration. Among patients with advanced cancer those with diarrhoea lived almost three times as long as those without diarrhoea, although the difference did not reach significance in this small cohort (McCann et al. 2016).

2.4.2 Understanding the Immunodominance Following p.DOM-Epitope Vaccine Delivery to Patients

One consideration we had in mind when designing the p.DOM-epitope vaccines was that the DOM portion should engage CD4 T cell help without inducing its own CD8 T cell responses. This was achieved by preserving Th epitopes and removing potential competitive CD8 epitopes including those restricted by HLA-A2 (Rice et al. 2001). Several studies in humanized HHD mice that are transgenic for the human HLA-A2 demonstrated lack of competition from DOM sequences and induction of robust CD8 responses to the chosen epitope (Joseph-Pietras et al. 2010; Campos-Perez et al. 2013).

Following DNA EP administration of p.DOM-epitope from WT-1 tumour antigen (WT1.37) to HLA-A2+ leukaemic patients, we were able to demonstrate induction of WT1.37-specific CD8+ CTL ex vivo. In parallel, using an overlapping peptide library to evaluate CD4 and CD8 responses to the DOM portion, we found not only robust CD4 T cell responses but unexpectedly also CD8 responses. When we next monitored the WT1 epitope and DOM CD8 T cell responses in patients over time we found simultaneously induced responses to both WT1 and DOM epitopes. Reactivity to a new HLA-A2-restricted epitope from DOM was detected in patients, but there was no antigenic competition with the tumour-derived epitope (manuscript submitted). These findings were retrospectively confirmed in patients vaccinated with DOM-PSMA27 with prostate cancer. Our data demonstrate that in a cancer setting there is an opportunity to deliver more than one epitope simultaneously, with a possibility of induction of a broader CTL immunity directed to multiple peptides.

2.5 Preexisting Immunity to TT Immunity and Performance of Vaccines Containing TT-Derived Fragments

One challenge faced by clinicians seeking to use TT-derived vaccines is the presence of preexisting antibodies to FrC, which might slow the induction of subsequent immunity when FrC is used as a carrier (Forconi et al. 2002). Such antibodies are highly prevalent across most patient populations, owing to the successful adoption of prophylactic vaccination against *C. tetani* and to the use of conjugate vaccines where TT acts as carrier for the bacterial polycaccharide (Miller et al. 2011). Our data suggest that antibody to DOM does not cross-react with those against TT protein (Low et al. 2009). It appears likely that for the humoral arm of the immune system DOM is perceived as a neoantigen, even after prior exposure to prophylactic TT vaccine. In contrast, preexisting TT-specific CD4 T cell immunity recognizes the epitopes in DOM sequence. This T cell memory can lead to accelerated responses to DOM-containing vaccines.

Interestingly pre-vaccination with TT has been recently observed to have unexpected enhancing effects on the subsequent efficacy of dendritic cell cancer vaccines in patients with glioblastoma. Preconditioning of the vaccination site with the conventional TT/DT vaccine led to improved migration of dendritic cells and improved patient survival. This phenomenon was mediated by CD4+ T cells induced by the conventional vaccine as their depletion led to significant decrease of the effect when the phenomenon was modelled in mice (Mitchell et al. 2015). This unexpected effect of CD4 T cell help is not fully understood but thought to be mediated at least in part by the pro-inflammatory chemokine CCL3. Combination of TT-specific linked T cell help through FrC or DOM-containing vaccines with preconditioning of the vaccination site might lead to further improvement of TA-specific cancer vaccines.

2.6 Novel Vaccination Approaches Based on FrC Linked T Cell Help

We have recently developed a novel FrC-based vaccine to target Her2+ve cancers via antibody. Her2 (ERBB2) is an excellent target as it is overexpressed on many solid cancers and its expression is associated with poor prognosis (Berchuck et al. 1990; Slamon et al. 1987). Passively transferred Mab Herceptin targeting Her2 has demonstrated efficacy in the clinic; a second monoclonal antibody pertuzumab has recently been approved (Hudis 2007; Swain et al. 2015).

However induction of potent anti-Her2 antibody by vaccination in patients is also attractive. To drive antibody responses to Her2 we used a novel truncated Her2 protein fragment ED44 which includes III and IV domains of Her2 (Chotprakaikiat et al. 2016). The ED44 fragment induced high levels of protective antibody against native Her2 in non-tolerant wild type mice. However in the tolerant preclinical model of spontaneous Her2 driven breast cancer, ED44 was effective only when it was conjugated to FrC. In this case, we demonstrated that conjugation not only significantly increased the levels of anti-Her2 antibody but led to increase of antibody affinity and additionally, broadened the spectrum of antibody isotypes. IgG2a, the most effective isotype for inducing ADCC and cancer attack through phagocytosis, was only induced by the FrC conjugate vaccine. These qualitative differences in the antibody response led to improved survival of mice with spontaneous metastatic Her2+ve breast cancer. We also demonstrated that FrC-induced T cell help was required for powerful antibody induction and could not be compensated for by TLR4 ligand adjuvant monophosphoryl lipid A. The latter is able to stimulate B cells directly and is a licensed adjuvant which is able to increase the antibody levels against targets from infectious diseases (Einstein et al. 2009). In our study in the tolerant setting it could increase the total levels of anti-Her2 antibody, however the antibody affinity was not increased. Importantly there was also a failure to induce ADCC and phagocytosis engaging IgG2a. Overall, despite the increase of total anti-Her2 IgG there was a minimal improvement in protection in the tolerant model in contrast to the FrC conjugate vaccine which induced a significant protection. This study was the first to demonstrate that foreign-linked T cell help induced through conjugation to FrC could not only impact the levels of antibody induced but also on the quality of the antibody against cancer targets.

2.7 mRNA Vaccines

mRNA vaccines are emerging as a promising vaccine modality and in the last five years clinical trials in metastatic melanoma, renal cell carcinoma, prostate cancer and other types of cancers targeting mutated and unmutated TA have been carried out (reviewed in Kreiter et al. 2011; Sahin et al. 2014). The idea behind mRNA vaccination is to inject RNA encoding TA, generated in vitro. The RNA is modified to improve stability and translation (reviewed in Kreiter et al. 2011) and additional means allowing to improve intracellular delivery are used including gene gun, electroporation, lipids and others (reviewed in Geall et al. 2013). Combining mRNA with liposomes also allows additional protection against nucleases and is becoming a preferred delivery method. After transfection the antigen is transcribed and presented to the immune system. Since RNA is the ligand for TLR7 and 8 (Diebold et al. 2004; Kariko et al. 2005) the vaccine is self-adjuvanting similar to DNA vaccines. Additional RNA sensors such as RNA-dependent protein kinases, in the cytoplasm could be also involved in the immune recognition of mRNA vaccines (Cohen-Chalamish et al. 2009). In addition to mRNA vaccines against TA, more recently mRNA vaccines have been used to deliver multi-epitope vaccines carrying a string of T cell epitopes from neoantigens identified in the tumour through the 'mutanome' approach (Boisguerin et al. 2014; Kreiter et al. 2015).

2.8 Plant Viral Particles: A Novel Platform for Induction of Immunity Against Cancer

Plant viral particles (PVP) are promising vaccine platforms for TAs. They are simultaneously able to provide linked T cell help through the viral coat protein (CP) and adjuvant usually through plant virus-derived genomic ssRNA (Jobsri et al. 2015). Additionally PVP are structurally analogous to virus-like particles and hence, factors such as dense antigen display and the particulate structure also contribute to their excellent immunogenicity (Lebel et al. 2015). Similar to ssRNA of human viruses and their synthetic analogues, native PVP ssRNA is a TLR7 ligand and hence serves as an adjuvant similar to RNA vaccines (Diebold et al. 2004; Jobsri et al. 2015). Individual epitopes or small fragments containing targeted epitopes can be linked to PVP both genetically and chemically. For longer antigenic fragments biotin-streptavidin or chemical linkage have been used (Lebel et al. 2015; Jobsri et al. 2015). Antigens linked to PVP mimic the structure of PVP and hence inherit the immunogenic properties of PVP. We have demonstrated these principles for the weak antigen of lymphoma, the idiotype (Jobsri et al. 2015). When conjugated to PVP idiotype induced potent protective anti-Id antibody responses superior to the 'gold standard' Id-KLH vaccine. Not only were the antibody levels higher but the induced linked CP specific T cell help was largely of Th1 bias in contrast to Th2 inducing KLH. The ability of PVP-based vaccines alone to induce strong Th1 bias has been also explored for induction of CD8+ T cells against cancer TAA. Specific CD8+ T cell responses and protection in a transplantable melanoma model was demonstrated using PVP-epitope vaccine (McCormick et al. 2006a, b). Further research is required to uncover the full potential of these powerful vaccine modalities for targeted cancer immunotherapy.

3 Concluding Remarks

DNA vaccines incorporating linked T cell help targeting conventional tumour antigens have demonstrated the ability to induce anti-tumour responses in patients with evidence of clinical benefit. This approach is promising for induction of diverse antitumour effector mechanisms in patients. Further extension of this approach to the newly discovered mutanome-derived neoantigens might offer an alternative approach to targeting cancer. Further work aiming to increase the potency of the induced responses through combinational approaches with checkpoint antibody inhibitors should benefit the cohorts of patients which are currently unresponsive to the checkpoint inhibitors alone.

References

Abrams SI, Hand PH, Tsang KY, Schlom J (1996) Mutant ras epitopes as targets for cancer vaccines. Semin Oncol 23(1):118–134

Acres B, Lacoste G, Limacher JM (2015) Targeted immunotherapy designed to treat MUC1-expressing solid tumour. Curr Top Microbiol Immunol. doi:10.1007/82_2015_429

Ahlen G, Soderholm J, Tjelle T, KjekenR, Frelin L, Hoglund U,… Sallberg M (2007) In vivo electroporation enhances the immunogenicity of hepatitis C virus nonstructural 3/4A DNA by increased local DNA uptake, protein expression, inflammation, and infiltration of $CD3^{+}$ T cells. J Immunol 179(7):4741–4753

Arbuthnot P, Kew M (2001) Hepatitis B virus and hepatocellular carcinoma. Int J Exp Pathol 82 (2):77–100

Arrowood JR, Hayney MS (2002) Immunization recommendations for adults with cancer. Ann Pharmacother 36(7–8):1219–1229

Barber GN (2011) Cytoplasmic DNA innate immune pathways. Immunol Rev 243(1):99–108. doi:10.1111/j.1600-065X.2011.01051.x

Bendandi M, Marillonnet S, Kandzia R, Thieme F, Nickstadt A, Herz S,… Gleba Y (2010) Rapid, high-yield production in plants of individualized idiotype vaccines for non-Hodgkin's lymphoma. Ann Oncol 21(12):2420–2427. doi:10.1093/annonc/mdq256 (mdq256 [pii])

Berchuck A, Kamel A, Whitaker R, Kerns B, Olt G, Kinney R et al (1990) Overexpression of HER-2/neu is associated with poor survival in advanced epithelial ovarian cancer. Cancer Res 50(13):4087–4091

Bogen B (1996) Peripheral T cell tolerance as a tumor escape mechanism: deletion of $CD4^{+}$ T cells specific for a monoclonal immunoglobulin idiotype secreted by a plasmacytoma. Eur J Immunol 26(11):2671–2679. doi:10.1002/eji.1830261119

Boisguerin V, Castle JC, Loewer M, Diekmann J, Mueller F, Britten CM,… Sahin U (2014) Translation of genomics-guided RNA-based personalised cancer vaccines: towards the bedside. Br J Cancer 111(8):1469–1475. doi:10.1038/bjc.2013.820

Bopp T, Becker C, Klein M, Klein-Hessling S, Palmetshofer A, Serfling E,… Schmitt E (2007) Cyclic adenosine monophosphate is a key component of regulatory T cell-mediated suppression. J Exp Med 204(6):1303–1310. doi:10.1084/jem.20062129

Buchan S, Gronevik E, Mathiesen I, King CA, Stevenson FK, Rice J (2005) Electroporation as a "prime/boost" strategy for naked DNA vaccination against a tumor antigen. J Immunol 174 (10):6292–6298

Buonaguro L, Petrizzo A, Tornesello ML, Buonaguro FM (2011) Translating tumor antigens into cancer vaccines. Clin Vaccine Immunol 18(1):23–34. doi:10.1128/CVI.00286-10

Calvo AC, Olivan S, Manzano R, Zaragoza P, Aguilera J, Osta R (2012) Fragment C of tetanus toxin: new insights into its neuronal signaling pathway. Int J Mol Sci 13(6):6883–6901. doi:10.3390/ijms13066883

Campos-Perez J, Rice J, Escors D, Collins M, Paterson A, Savelyeva N, Stevenson FK (2013) DNA fusion vaccine designs to induce tumor-lytic CD8+ T-cell attack via the immunodominant cysteine-containing epitope of NY-ESO 1. Int J Cancer 133(6):1400–1407. doi:10.1002/ijc.28156

Cao X, Cai SF, Fehniger TA, Song J, Collins LI, Piwnica-Worms DR, Ley TJ (2007) Granzyme B and perforin are important for regulatory T cell-mediated suppression of tumor clearance. Immunity 27(4):635–646. doi:10.1016/j.immuni.2007.08.014

Carbone DP, Ciernik IF, Kelley MJ, Smith MC, Nadaf S, Kavanaugh D,… Berzofsky JA (2005) Immunization with mutant p53- and K-ras-derived peptides in cancer patients: immune response and clinical outcome. J Clin Oncol 23(22):5099–5107. doi:10.1200/JCO.2005.03.158

Chotprakaikiat W, Allen A, Bui-Munh D, Harden E, Jobsri J, Cavallo F, Gleba Y, Stevenson FK, Ottensmeier C, Klimyuk V, Savelyeva N (2016) A plant expressed conjugate vaccine breaks CD4 tolerance and induces potent immunity againstmetastatic Her2+ breast cancer. Oncoimmunology. doi:10.1080/2162402X.2016.1166323

Chudley L, McCann K, Mander A, Tjelle T, Campos-Perez J, Godeseth R,… Ottensmeier C (2012) DNA fusion-gene vaccination in patients with prostate cancer induces high-frequency CD8(+) T-cell responses and increases PSA doubling time. Cancer Immunol Immunother 61 (11):2161–2170. doi:10.1007/s00262-012-1270-0

Chung Y, Tanaka S, Chu F, Nurieva RI, MartinezGJ, Rawal S,… Dong C (2011) Follicular regulatory T cells expressing Foxp3 and Bcl-6 suppress germinal center reactions. Nat Med 17 (8):983–988. doi:10.1038/nm.2426

Cohen-Chalamish S, Hasson A, Weinberg D, Namer LS, Banai Y, Osman F, Kaempfer R (2009) Dynamic refolding of IFN-gamma mRNA enables it to function as PKR activator and translation template. Nat Chem Biol 5(12):896–903. doi:10.1038/nchembio.234

Cook TM, Protheroe RT, Handel JM (2001) Tetanus: a review of the literature. Br J Anaesth 87 (3):477–487

Damodaran S, Olson EM (2012). Targeting the human epidermal growth factor receptor 2 pathway in breast cancer. Hosp Pract (1995) 40(4):7–15. doi:10.3810/hp.2012.10.997

Diebold SS, Kaisho T, Hemmi H, Akira S, Reis e Sousa C (2004). Innate antiviral responses by means of TLR7-mediated recognition of single-stranded RNA. Science 303(5663):1529–1531. doi:10.1126/science.1093616

Dorothee G, Vergnon I, Menez J, Echchakir H, Grunenwald D, Kubin M,… Mami-Chouaib F (2002) Tumor-infiltrating CD4+ T lymphocytes express APO2 ligand (APO2L)/TRAIL upon specific stimulation with autologous lung carcinoma cells: role of IFN-alpha on APO2L/TRAIL expression and -mediated cytotoxicity. J Immunol 169(2):809–817

Einstein MH, Baron M, Levin MJ, Chatterjee A, Edwards RP, Zepp F,… Group HPVS (2009) Comparison of the immunogenicity and safety of Cervarix and Gardasil human papillomavirus (HPV) cervical cancer vaccines in healthy women aged 18–45 years. Hum Vaccin 5(10):705–719

el-Shami K, Tirosh B, Bar-Haim E, Carmon L, Vadai E, Fridkin M,… Eisenbach L (1999) MHC class I-restricted epitope spreading in the context of tumor rejection following vaccination with a single immunodominant CTL epitope. Eur J Immunol 29(10):3295–3301. doi:10.1002/(SICI)1521-4141(199910)29:10<3295::AID-IMMU3295>3.0.CO;2-N

Facciabene A, Motz GT, Coukos G (2012) T-regulatory cells: key players in tumor immune escape and angiogenesis. Cancer Res 72(9):2162–2171. doi:10.1158/0008-5472.CAN-11-3687

Forconi F, King CA, Sahota SS, Kennaway CK, Russell NH, Stevenson FK (2002) Insight into the potential for DNA idiotypic fusion vaccines designed for patients by analysing xenogeneic anti-idiotypic antibody responses. Immunology 107(1):39–45

Fratta E, Coral S, Covre A, Parisi G, Colizzi F, Danielli R,… Maio M (2011) The biology of cancer testis antigens: putative function, regulation and therapeutic potential. Mol Oncol 5 (2):164–182. doi:10.1016/j.molonc.2011.02.001

Geall AJ, Mandl CW, Ulmer JB (2013) RNA: the new revolution in nucleic acid vaccines. Semin Immunol 25(2):152–159. doi:10.1016/j.smim.2013.05.001

George AJ, Folkard SG, Hamblin TJ, Stevenson FK (1988) Idiotypic vaccination as a treatment for a B cell lymphoma. J Immunol 141(6):2168–2174

Gerloni M, Xiong S, Mukerjee S, Schoenberger SP, Croft M, Zanetti M (2000) Functional cooperation between T helper cell determinants. Proc Natl Acad Sci USA 97(24):13269–13274. doi:10.1073/pnas.230429197

Goodnow CC, Crosbie J, Adelstein S, Lavoie TB, Smith-Gill SJ, Brink RA et al (1988) Altered immunoglobulin expression and functional silencing of self-reactive B lymphocytes in transgenic mice. Nature 334(6184):676–682. doi:10.1038/334676a0

Gregerson DS, Heuss ND, Lehmann U, McPherson SW (2009) Peripheral induction of tolerance by retinal antigen expression. J Immunol 183(2):814–822. doi:10.4049/jimmunol.0803748

Haabeth OA, Tveita AA, Fauskanger M, Schjesvold F, Lorvik KB, Hofgaard PO,… Bogen B (2014) How do CD4(+) T cells detect and eliminate tumor cells that either lack or express MHC class II molecules? Front Immunol 5:174. doi:10.3389/fimmu.2014.00174

Hsieh CS, Lee HM, Lio CW (2012) Selection of regulatory T cells in the thymus. Nat Rev Immunol 12(3):157–167. doi:10.1038/nri3155

Hudis CA (2007) Trastuzumab–mechanism of action and use in clinical practice. N Engl J Med 357(1):39–51. doi:10.1056/NEJMra043186

Jager D (2007) Potential target antigens for immunotherapy identified by serological expression cloning (SEREX). Methods Mol Biol 360:319–326. doi:10.1385/1-59745-165-7:319

Jobsri J, Allen A, Rajagopal D, Shipton M, Kanyuka K, Lomonossoff GP,… Savelyeva N (2015) Plant virus particles carrying tumour antigen activate TLR7 and induce high levels of protective antibody. PLoS One 10(2):e0118096. doi:10.1371/journal.pone.0118096

Joseph-Pietras D, Gao Y, Zojer N, Ait-Tahar K, Banham AH, Pulford K,… Sahota SS (2010). DNA vaccines to target the cancer testis antigen PASD1 in human multiple myeloma. Leukemia 24(11):1951–1959. doi:10.1038/leu.2010.196

Ju ST, Cui H, Panka DJ, Ettinger R, Marshak-Rothstein A (1994) Participation of target Fas protein in apoptosis pathway induced by CD4+ Th1 and CD8+ cytotoxic T cells. Proc Natl Acad Sci USA 91(10):4185–4189

Kantoff PW, Higano CS, Shore ND, Berger ER, Small EJ, Penson DF,… Investigators IS (2010) Sipuleucel-T immunotherapy for castration-resistant prostate cancer. N Engl J Med 363 (5):411–422. doi:10.1056/NEJMoa1001294

Kaplan MJ, Ray D, Mo RR, Yung RL, Richardson BC (2000) TRAIL (Apo2 ligand) and TWEAK (Apo3 ligand) mediate $CD4^+$ T cell killing of antigen-presenting macrophages. J Immunol 164 (6):2897–2904

Kariko K, Buckstein M, Ni H, Weissman D (2005) Suppression of RNA recognition by Toll-like receptors: the impact of nucleoside modification and the evolutionary origin of RNA. Immunity 23(2):165–175. doi:10.1016/j.immuni.2005.06.008

King CA, Spellerberg MB, Zhu D, Rice J, Sahota SS, Thompsett AR, Stevenson FK (1998) DNA vaccines with single-chain Fv fused to fragment C of tetanus toxin induce protective immunity against lymphoma and myeloma. Nat Med 4(11):1281–1286. doi:10.1038/3266

King E, Ottensmeier C, Pollock KG (2015) Novel approaches for vaccination against HPV-induced cancers. Curr Top Microbiol Immunol. doi:10.1007/82_2015_430

Kraynyak KA, Bodles-Brakhop A, Bagarazzi M (2015) Tapping the potential of DNA delivery with electroporation for cancer immunotherapy. Curr Top Microbiol Immunol. doi:10.1007/82_2015_431

Kreiter S, Diken M, Selmi A, Tureci O, Sahin U (2011) Tumor vaccination using messenger RNA: prospects of a future therapy. Curr Opin Immunol 23(3):399–406. doi:10.1016/j.coi.2011.03.007

Kreiter S, Vormehr M, van de Roemer N, Diken M, Lower M, Diekmann J,… Sahin U (2015) Mutant MHC class II epitopes drive therapeutic immune responses to cancer. Nature 520 (7549):692–696. doi:10.1038/nature14426

Lanzardo S, Conti L, Rooke R, Ruiu R, Accart N, Bolli E,… Cavallo F (2016). Immunotargeting of antigen xCT attenuates stem-like cell behavior and metastatic progression in breast cancer. Cancer Res 76(1):62–72. doi:10.1158/0008-5472.CAN-15-1208

Lebel ME, Chartrand K, Leclerc D, Lamarre A (2015) Plant viruses as nanoparticle-based vaccines and adjuvants. Vaccines (Basel) 3(3):620–637. doi:10.3390/vaccines3030620

Linnemann C, van Buuren MM, Bies L, Verdegaal EM, Schotte R, Calis JJ,… Schumacher TN (2015) High-throughput epitope discovery reveals frequent recognition of neo-antigens by CD4⁺ T cells in human melanoma. Nat Med 21(1):81–85. doi:10.1038/nm.3773

Low L, Mander A, McCann K, Dearnaley D, Tjelle T, Mathiesen I,… Ottensmeier CH (2009) DNA vaccination with electroporation induces increased antibody responses in patients with prostate cancer. Hum Gene Ther 20(11):1269–1278. doi:10.1089/hum.2009.067

MacLennan IC (1994) Germinal centers. Annu Rev Immunol 12:117–139. doi:10.1146/annurev.iy.12.040194.001001

Mariani L, Venuti A (2010) HPV vaccine: an overview of immune response, clinical protection, and new approaches for the future. J Transl Med 8:105. doi:10.1186/1479-5876-8-105

Martin B, Auffray C, Delpoux A, Pommier A, Durand A, Charvet C,… Lucas B (2013). Highly self-reactive naive CD4 T cells are prone to differentiate into regulatory T cells. Nat Commun 4:2209. doi:10.1038/ncomms3209

McCann KJ, Godeseth R, Chudley L, Mander A, Di Genova G, Lloyd-Evans P,… Ottensmeier CH (2015). Idiotypic DNA vaccination for the treatment of multiple myeloma: safety and immunogenicity in a phase I clinical study. Cancer Immunol Immunother 64 (8):1021–1032. doi:10.1007/s00262-015-1703-7

McCann KJ, Mander A, Cazaly A, Chudley L, Stasakova J, Thirdborough SM,… Ottensmeier CH (2016) Targeting carcinoembryonic antigen with DNA vaccination: on-target adverse events link with immunological and clinical outcomes. Clin Cancer Res. doi:10.1158/1078-0432.CCR-15-2507

McCarthy H, Ottensmeier CH, Hamblin TJ, Stevenson FK (2003) Anti-idiotype vaccines. Br J Haematol 123(5):770–781

McCormick AA, Corbo TA, Wykoff-Clary S, Nguyen LV, Smith ML, Palmer KE, Pogue GP (2006a) TMV-peptide fusion vaccines induce cell-mediated immune responses and tumor protection in two murine models. Vaccine 24(40–41):6414–6423. doi:10.1016/j.vaccine.2006.06.003

McCormick AA, Corbo TA, Wykoff-Clary S, Palmer KE, Pogue GP (2006b) Chemical conjugate TMV-peptide bivalent fusion vaccines improve cellular immunity and tumor protection. Bioconjug Chem 17(5):1330–1338. doi:10.1021/bc060124m

Melief CJ, van Hall T, Arens R, Ossendorp F, van der Burg SH (2015) Therapeutic cancer vaccines. J Clin Invest 125(9):3401–3412. doi:10.1172/JCI80009

Merrell KT, Benschop RJ, Gauld SB, Aviszus K, Decote-Ricardo D, Wysocki LJ, Cambier JC (2006) Identification of anergic B cells within a wild-type repertoire. Immunity 25(6):953–962. doi:10.1016/j.immuni.2006.10.017

Miller JM, Mesaros N, Van Der Wielen M, Baine Y (2011) Conjugate meningococcal vaccines development: GSK biologicals experience. Adv Prev Med 2011:846756. doi:10.4061/2011/846756

Mitchell DA, Batich KA, Gunn MD, Huang MN, Sanchez-Perez L, Nair SK, Sampson JH (2015) Tetanus toxoid and CCL3 improve dendritic cell vaccines in mice and glioblastoma patients. Nature 519(7543):366–369. doi:10.1038/nature14320

Monie A, Hung CF, Roden R, Wu TC (2008) Cervarix: a vaccine for the prevention of HPV 16, 18-associated cervical cancer. Biologics 2(1):97–105

Nemazee D (1996) Antigen receptor 'capacity' and the sensitivity of self-tolerance. Immunol Today 17(1):25–29

Neninger Vinageras E, de la Torre A, Osorio Rodriguez M, Catala Ferrer M, Bravo I, Mendoza del Pino M,… Lage Davila A (2008) Phase II randomized controlled trial of an epidermal growth factor vaccine in advanced non-small-cell lung cancer. J Clin Oncol 26(9):1452–1458. doi:10.1200/JCO.2007.11.5980

Neubauer V, Helting TB (1981) Structure of tetanus toxin: the arrangement of papain digestion products within the heavy chain-light chain framework of extracellular toxin. Biochim Biophys Acta 668(1):141–148

Paludan SR, Bowie AG (2013) Immune sensing of DNA. Immunity 38(5):870–880. doi:10.1016/j.immuni.2013.05.004

Perez-Diez A, Joncker NT, Choi K, Chan WF, Anderson CC, Lantz O, Matzinger P (2007) CD4 cells can be more efficient at tumor rejection than CD8 cells. Blood 109(12):5346–5354. doi:10.1182/blood-2006-10-051318

Perez-Gracia JL, Labiano S, Rodriguez-Ruiz ME, Sanmamed MF, Melero I (2014) Orchestrating immune check-point blockade for cancer immunotherapy in combinations. Curr Opin Immunol 27:89–97. doi:10.1016/j.coi.2014.01.002

Quail DF, Joyce JA (2013) Microenvironmental regulation of tumor progression and metastasis. Nat Med 19(11):1423–1437. doi:10.1038/nm.3394

Quaratino S, Forssmann U, Marschner J (2014) New approaches in immunotherapy for the treatment of lung cancer. Curr Top Microbiol Immunol. doi:10.1007/82_2014_428

Quoix E, Lena H, Losonczy G, Forget F, Chouaid C, Papai Z,… Limacher JM (2015) TG4010 immunotherapy and first-line chemotherapy for advanced non-small-cell lung cancer (TIME): results from the phase 2b part of a randomised, double-blind, placebo-controlled, phase 2b/3 trial. Lancet Oncology. doi:10.1016/S1470-2045(15)00483-0

Ribas A, Timmerman JM, Butterfield LH, Economou JS (2003) Determinant spreading and tumor responses after peptide-based cancer immunotherapy. Trends Immunol 24(2):58–61

Rice J, King CA, Spellerberg MB, Fairweather N, Stevenson FK (1999) Manipulation of pathogen-derived genes to influence antigen presentation via DNA vaccines. Vaccine 17(23–24):3030–3038

Rice J, Elliott T, Buchan S, Stevenson FK (2001) DNA fusion vaccine designed to induce cytotoxic T cell responses against defined peptide motifs: implications for cancer vaccines. J Immunol 167(3):1558–1565

Rice J, Buchan S, Stevenson FK (2002) Critical components of a DNA fusion vaccine able to induce protective cytotoxic T cells against a single epitope of a tumor antigen. J Immunol 169 (7):3908–3913

Rice J, Ottensmeier CH, Stevenson FK (2008) DNA vaccines: precision tools for activating effective immunity against cancer. Nat Rev Cancer 8(2):108–120. doi:10.1038/nrc2326 (nrc2326 [pii])

Rochman S (2015) New peptide vaccine for HER2-expressing breast tumors. J Natl Cancer Inst 107(2). doi:10.1093/jnci/djv022

Rodriguez PC, Rodriguez G, Gonzalez G, Lage A (2010) Clinical development and perspectives of CIMAvax EGF, Cuban vaccine for non-small-cell lung cancer therapy. MEDICC Rev 12 (1):17–23

Rubtsov YP, Rasmussen JP, Chi EY, Fontenot J, Castelli L, Ye X,… Rudensky AY (2008) Regulatory T cell-derived interleukin-10 limits inflammation at environmental interfaces. Immunity 28(4):546–558. doi:10.1016/j.immuni.2008.02.017

Sahin U, Kariko K, Tureci O (2014) mRNA-based therapeutics–developing a new class of drugs. Nat Rev Drug Discov 13(10):759–780. doi:10.1038/nrd4278

Sansom DM (2000) CD28, CTLA-4 and their ligands: who does what and to whom? Immunology 101(2):169–177

Savelyeva N, Munday R, Spellerberg MB, Lomonossoff GP, Stevenson FK (2001) Plant viral genes in DNA idiotypic vaccines activate linked $CD4^+$ T-cell mediated immunity against B-cell malignancies. Nat Biotechnol 19(8):760–764. doi:10.1038/90816 (90816 [pii])

Savelyeva N, Zhu D, Stevenson FK (2003) Engineering DNA vaccines that include plant virus coat proteins. Biotechnol Genet Eng Rev 20:101–114

Schiller JT, Castellsague X, Garland SM (2012) A review of clinical trials of human papillomavirus prophylactic vaccines. Vaccine 30(Suppl 5):F123–F138. doi:10.1016/j.vaccine.2012.04.108

Schumacher TN, Schreiber RD (2015) Neoantigens in cancer immunotherapy. Science 348 (6230):69–74. doi:10.1126/science.aaa4971

Schumacher T, Bunse L, Pusch S, Sahm F, Wiestler B, Quandt J,… Platten M (2014) A vaccine targeting mutant IDH1 induces antitumour immunity. Nature 512(7514):324–327. doi:10.1038/nature13387

Slamon DJ, Clark GM, Wong SG, Levin WJ, Ullrich A, McGuire WL (1987) Human breast cancer: correlation of relapse and survival with amplification of the HER-2/neu oncogene. Science 235(4785):177–182

Smith CL, Mirza F, Pasquetto V, Tscharke DC, Palmowski MJ, Dunbar PR,… Cerundolo V (2005) Immunodominance of poxviral-specific CTL in a human trial of recombinant-modified vaccinia Ankara. J Immunol 175(12):8431–8437

Sonpavde G, Di Lorenzo G, Higano CS, Kantoff PW, Madan R, Shore ND (2012) The role of sipuleucel-T in therapy for castration-resistant prostate cancer: a critical analysis of the literature. Eur Urol 61(4):639–647. doi:10.1016/j.eururo.2011.10.027

Spellerberg MB, Zhu D, Thompsett A, King CA, Hamblin TJ, Stevenson FK (1997) DNA vaccines against lymphoma: promotion of anti-idiotypic antibody responses induced by single chain Fv genes by fusion to tetanus toxin fragment C. J Immunol 159(4):1885–1892

Stevenson FK, Ottensmeier CH, Johnson P, Zhu D, Buchan SL, McCann KJ, Rice J (2004a) DNA vaccines to attack cancer. Proc Natl Acad Sci USA 101(Suppl 2):14646–14652. doi:10.1073/pnas.0404896101

Stevenson FK, Rice J, Ottensmeier CH, Thirdborough SM, Zhu D (2004b) DNA fusion gene vaccines against cancer: from the laboratory to the clinic. Immunol Rev 199:156–180. doi:10.1111/j.0105-2896.2004.00145.x

Stevenson FK, Di Genova G, Ottensmeier CH, Savelyeva N (2013) Genetic vaccines against cancer: design, testing and clinical performance. In: Prendergast GC, Jaffee EM (eds) Cancer immunotherapy immune suppression and tumor growth, 2nd edn. Elsevier, United States, pp. 223–233

Swain SM, Baselga J, Kim SB, Ro J, Semiglazov V, Campone M,… Group CS (2015) Pertuzumab, trastuzumab, and docetaxel in HER2-positive metastatic breast cancer. N Engl J Med 372(8):724–734. doi:10.1056/NEJMoa1413513

Thomas WD, Hersey P (1998) TNF-related apoptosis-inducing ligand (TRAIL) induces apoptosis in Fas ligand-resistant melanoma cells and mediates CD4 T cell killing of target cells. J Immunol 161(5):2195–2200

Timmerman JM (2009) Carrier protein conjugate vaccines: the "missing link" to improved antibody and CTL responses? Hum Vaccin 5(3):181–183

Tiriveedhi V, Tucker N, Herndon J, Li L, Sturmoski M, Ellis M,… Gillanders WE (2014) Safety and preliminary evidence of biologic efficacy of a mammaglobin-a DNA vaccine in patients with stable metastatic breast cancer. Clin Cancer Res 20(23):5964–5975. doi:10.1158/1078-0432.CCR-14-0059

Tran E, Turcotte S, Gros A, Robbins PF, Lu YC, Dudley ME,… Rosenberg SA (2014) Cancer immunotherapy based on mutation-specific CD4+ T cells in a patient with epithelial cancer. Science 344(6184):641–645. doi:10.1126/science.1251102

Trimble CL, Morrow MP, Kraynyak KA, Shen X, Dallas M, Yan J,… Bagarazzi ML (2015). Safety, efficacy, and immunogenicity of VGX-3100, a therapeutic synthetic DNA vaccine targeting human papillomavirus 16 and 18 E6 and E7 proteins for cervical intraepithelial neoplasia 2/3: a randomised, double-blind, placebo-controlled phase 2b trial. Lancet 386 (10008):2078–2088. doi:10.1016/S0140-6736(15)00239-1

Tuse D, Ku N, Bendandi M, Becerra C, Collins R Jr, Langford N, Butler-Ransohoff JE (2015) Clinical safety and immunogenicity of tumor-targeted, plant-made Id-KLH conjugate vaccines for follicular lymphoma. Biomed Res Int 2015:648143. doi:10.1155/2015/648143

Vigneron N, Stroobant V, Van den Eynde BJ, van der Bruggen P (2013) Database of T cell-defined human tumor antigens: the 2013 update. Cancer Immun 13:15

Villanueva H, de Cerio AL, Inoges S, Pastor F, Soldevilla MM, Bendandi M (2011) BiovaxID(R): a customized idiotype vaccine for the treatment of B-cell lymphoma. Expert Rev Vaccines 10 (12):1661–1669. doi:10.1586/erv.11.132

Vinuesa CG, Tangye SG, Moser B, Mackay CR (2005) Follicular B helper T cells in antibody responses and autoimmunity. Nat Rev Immunol 5(11):853–865. doi:10.1038/nri1714

Wan YY, Flavell RA (2007) 'Yin-Yang' functions of transforming growth factor-beta and T regulatory cells in immune regulation. Immunol Rev 220:199–213. doi:10.1111/j.1600-065X.2007.00565.x

Warnakulasuriya S (2010) Living with oral cancer: epidemiology with particular reference to prevalence and life-style changes that influence survival. Oral Oncol 46(6):407–410. doi:10.1016/j.oraloncology.2010.02.015

Weinberg AD, Morris NP, Kovacsovics-Bankowski M, Urba WJ, Curti BD (2011) Science gone translational: the OX40 agonist story. Immunol Rev 244(1):218–231. doi:10.1111/j.1600-065X.2011.01069.x

Weiner LM, Dhodapkar MV, Ferrone S (2009) Monoclonal antibodies for cancer immunotherapy. Lancet 373(9668):1033–1040. doi:10.1016/S0140-6736(09)60251-8

Wherry EJ, Kurachi M (2015) Molecular and cellular insights into T cell exhaustion. Nat Rev Immunol 15(8):486–499. doi:10.1038/nri3862

Xing Y, Hogquist KA (2012) T-cell tolerance: central and peripheral. Cold Spring Harb Perspect Biol 4(6). doi:10.1101/cshperspect.a006957

Yewdell JW (2010) Designing CD8+ T cell vaccines: it's not rocket science (yet). Curr Opin Immunol 22(3):402–410. doi:10.1016/j.coi.2010.04.002

Yewdell JW, Bennink JR (1999) Immunodominance in major histocompatibility complex class I-restricted T lymphocyte responses. Annu Rev Immunol 17:51–88. doi:10.1146/annurev.immunol.17.1.51

Yi Q, Osterborg A, Bergenbrant S, Mellstedt H, Holm G, Lefvert AK (1995) Idiotype-reactive T-cell subsets and tumor load in monoclonal gammopathies. Blood 86(8):3043–3049

Zanetti M (2015) Tapping CD4 T cells for cancer immunotherapy: the choice of personalized genomics. J Immunol 194(5):2049–2056. doi:10.4049/jimmunol.1402669

Zuo L, Li L, Wang Q, Fleming TP, You S (2009) Mammaglobin as a potential molecular target for breast cancer drug delivery. Cancer Cell Int 9:8. doi:10.1186/1475-2867-9-8

mRNA Cancer Vaccines—Messages that Prevail

Christian Grunwitz and Lena M. Kranz

Abstract During the last decade, mRNA became increasingly recognized as a versatile tool for the development of new innovative therapeutics. Especially for vaccine development, mRNA is of outstanding interest and numerous clinical trials have been initiated. Strikingly, all of these studies have proven that large-scale GMP production of mRNA is feasible and concordantly report a favorable safety profile of mRNA vaccines. Induction of T-cell immunity is a multi-faceted process comprising antigen acquisition, antigen processing and presentation, as well as immune stimulation. The effectiveness of mRNA vaccines is critically dependent on making the antigen(s) of interest available to professional antigen-presenting cells, especially DCs. Efficient delivery of mRNA into DCs in vivo remains a major challenge in the mRNA vaccine field. This review summarizes the principles of mRNA vaccines and highlights the importance of in vivo mRNA delivery and recent advances in harnessing their therapeutic potential.

Contents

Authors contributed equally to this work.

C. Grunwitz (✉) · L.M. Kranz (✉)
BioNTech RNA Pharmaceuticals GmbH, An der Goldgrube 12,
55131 Mainz, Germany
e-mail: christian.grunwitz@biontech.de

L.M. Kranz
e-mail: lena.kranz@biontech.de

Current Topics in Microbiology and Immunology (2017) 405:145–164
DOI 10.1007/82_2017_509

Published Online: 31 March 2017

1 Introduction

There was not much enthusiasm for mRNA in the scientific community back in the 1990s, and the emergence of messenger RNA (mRNA)-based therapeutics was hard to foresee. Although first reports of plasmid DNA (pDNA) and mRNA vaccines appeared around the same time (Tang et al.1992; Martinon et al. 1993), pDNA dominated the field for over a decade and the prevailing doctrine described mRNA as expensive, difficult to manufacture and notoriously unstable. Thus, 25 years ago, mRNA appeared to be anything but a worthwhile platform for the development of a new class of drug products.

Having experienced the difficulties and hurdles accompanied with large-scale production in a controlled environment, initial assumptions about the easy and cost-efficient production of pDNA were gradually disproven. Simultaneous improvements in the production, modification and stabilization of mRNA have nurtured the recognition of mRNA as a potential alternative. During the last decade, mRNA became increasingly recognized as a versatile tool for the development of new innovative therapeutics. Especially for vaccine development, mRNA is of outstanding interest as it maintains the key characteristics of pDNA, but with a superior safety profile. Similar to pDNA, mRNA vaccines lack MHC haplotype restriction, unlike peptide vaccination strategies. But in contrast to pDNA, mRNA does not require nuclear localization for translation of the encoded antigen. Moreover, it represents the minimal vector enabling transient protein expression and does not harbor the risk of insertional mutagenesis or permanent genomic alteration. Consequently, mRNA demonstrates inherent safety features optimal for therapeutic use.

Since 2008, numerous clinical trials have been initiated (Table 1) and consistently demonstrated the feasibility and suitability of mRNA vaccines for cancer treatment. One major challenge in the field is the efficient delivery of mRNA into DCs in vivo, as it significantly determines the quality and quantity of the desired immune response. This review summarizes the principles of mRNA vaccines and highlights the importance of optimal in vivo delivery for harnessing their therapeutic potential.

Table 1 mRNA cancer vaccine trials

Sponsor/Collaborator	Indication	Delivery route/format	Status	Reference/Clinical trial identifier
University Hospital Tuebingen CureVac	Melanoma	Intradermal/mRNA + GM-CSF	Completed	Weide et al. (2008)
University Hospital Tuebingen CureVac	Melanoma	Intradermal/protamine-complexed mRNA + GM-CSF, ± KLH	Completed	Weide et al. (2009) NCT00204607
University Hospital Tuebingen CureVac	Renal cell carcinoma	Intradermal (mRNA + GM-CSF)	Completed	Rittig et al. (2011, 2016)
CureVac	Nonsmall cell lung cancer	Intradermal/self-adjuvanted mRNA	Completed	Sebastian et al. (2011) NCT00923312
BioNTech RNA Pharmaceuticals	Melanoma	Intranodal/mRNA	Completed	NCT01684241
University of Florida CureVac	Prostate cancer	Intradermal/self-adjuvanted mRNA	Completed	NCT00906243
CureVac	Prostate cancer	Intradermal/self-adjuvanted mRNA	Completed	Kübler et al. (2015) NCT00831467
CureVac	Prostate cancer	Intradermal/self-adjuvanted mRNA	Ongoing	NCT01817738
BioNTech RNA Pharmaceuticals	Melanoma	Intranodal/poly-neo-epitopic mRNA	Ongoing	NCT02035956
BioNTech RNA Pharmaceuticals	Melanoma	Intravenous/liposome-formulated mRNA	Ongoing	Kranz et al. (2016) NCT02410733
BioNTech RNA Pharmaceuticals Seventh Framework Program	Triple Negative Breast Cancer	Intravenous/liposome-formulated mRNA	Recruiting	NCT02316457
University Hospital Southampton BioNTech RNA Pharmaceuticals Seventh Framework Program	HPV-induced cancers	Intravenous/liposome-formulated mRNA	Ongoing	EudraCT: 2014-002061-30

2 Concept of mRNA Vaccines

Induction of T-cell immunity is a multi-faceted process: antigen acquisition (active uptake, viral infection), antigen processing and presentation, and immune stimulation. The effectiveness of any vaccine intended to raise long-lasting virus- or tumor-specific T-cell responses, may it be peptide/protein, nucleic acids or cell-based, fully relies on making the antigen(s) of interest available to professional antigen-presenting cells, especially DCs. Their ability to convert antigenic information and accompanying danger signals into a format that can be recognized by T cells and that provides instructions about the type and extent of response is pivotal for vaccination purposes. The significance of DCs in mounting robust and long-lasting T cell immunity is well established and is reflected by the widespread use of ex vivo manipulated DCs for vaccination and FDA-approval of Sipuleucel-T in 2010.

mRNA vaccines are faced with another barrier. The mRNA molecule itself is not the pharmacologically active product but rather a vector encoding the relevant message. In contrast to peptide/protein vaccines, a crucial intermediate step is needed before the antigenic information can be made available to T cells: translation. The fundamental principle of mRNA therapeutics is 'hijacking' the cell's translational machinery to produce pharmacologically active proteins. In order to do so, synthetic mRNAs follow the blueprint of naturally occurring, mature and processed mRNA, and are exposed to the same regulatory mechanisms. Minimal structural requirements are a 5′ cap, a poly(A) tail, and an open reading frame (ORF) coding for the protein of interest, with a start codon in Kozak surrounding and flanked by a 5′ and 3′ untranslated region (UTR). Production in a cell-free system via in vitro transcription of a linearized pDNA or PCR product using a bacteriophage RNA polymerase is followed by DNase digestion and purification by standard methods (precipitation, bead-based methods, and chromatography).

Unlike cell-based vaccination where mRNA is electroporated directly into the cytoplasm of DCs ex vivo, direct mRNA vaccination faces various barriers that need to be overcome in order for this specialized molecule to perform as intended. These barriers can be summarized as (i) barriers encountered on the way from the injection site to the cell population of interest, i.e., DCs (extracellular barriers), (ii) barriers regarding active mRNA uptake by the target cell (endocytic barriers), and (iii) barriers affecting endosomal escape and mRNA release into the cytoplasm (intracellular barriers) (Fig. 1).

3 Antigen Acquisition

3.1 Uptake and Endosomal Release

Once mRNA has reached the close neighborhood of DCs (by any delivery route), the subsequent steps of cellular uptake and, importantly, access to the cytoplasm,

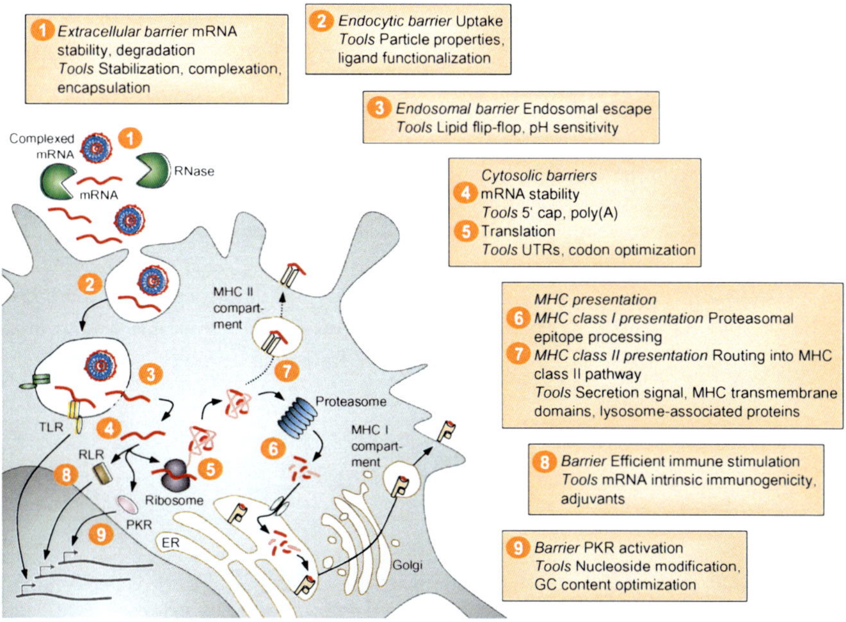

Fig. 1 Antigen-specific immunity, mRNA-specific barriers, and tools to evade them

are critical. Nonlipid nanoparticles may by highly protective of their cargo and easily coupled to targeting ligands, yet they are often confronted with the problem of efficient mRNA release once inside the cell. Incorporation of destabilizing or pH sensitive polymers is an option, although convincing vaccination studies have so far not been reported. Lipid-based nanoformulations, however, have a long record of being used for transfection of negatively charged biomolecules such as DNA, RNA, and oligonucleotides in vitro, and have been thoroughly investigated. The cationic lipids DOTMA and DOTAP have been the most extensively used transfection reagents due to their ability to facilitate membrane fusion (Felgner et al. 1987; Crook et al. 1998). Spontaneous fusion with cell membranes seemingly precludes its use for targeted in vivo applications, however, using these lipids in negatively charged complexes seems to prevent spontaneous, unspecific membrane fusion (Kranz et al. 2016), presumably due to electrostatic repulsion. Naked mRNA as well as negatively charged DOTMA or DOTAP containing mRNA-lipoplexes (~400 nm) have been shown to be internalized via macropinocytosis (Kranz et al. 2016; Diken et al. 2011), a mechanism constitutive in DCs as well as macrophages that covers a broad range of particle sizes (100 nm to 5 μm). Phagocytosis, restricted to macrophages, mainly deals with particles larger than 500 nm up to 10 μm, and clathrin- or caveolin-mediated endocytosis with particles smaller than 120 nm (Hirota and Terada 2012).

The exact nature of endosomal escape remains elusive, but depending on the formulation, a variety of concepts were proposed. DOPE, a zwitterionic phospholipid widely used in combination with cationic lipids as a helper lipid, is known to destabilize endosomal membranes (Zhou and Huang 1994; Farhood et al. 1995), as is cholesterol. For nucleic acid lipoplexes and especially those containing DOTAP and DOPE, a flip-flop mechanism has been proposed, where the positively charged lipids of the entrapped nanoformulations interact with anionic lipids present in the cytoplasm-facing endosomal monolayer. Lateral diffusion of the anionic lipids into the lipoplex generates neutrally charged ion pairs, leading to the displacement of nucleic acids from these cationic lipids and their release into the cytoplasm (Zelphati and Szoka 1996). Importantly, the lipid composition has a significant impact on the stability of the resulting mRNA-liposome complex, and the transfection rate.

3.2 Translation

When the interest into the use of mRNA as a gene delivery platform was eventually sparked, exploration of structural elements has led to engineered mRNA molecules highly optimized for stability and translational efficiency. pDNA templates encode all structural elements of functional mRNA except the 5′ cap, and sometimes the poly(A) tail.

The 5′ cap influences recognition by the translation initiation factor eIF4E and is the focus of numerous studies. Capping is achieved by the addition of a dinucleotide with a 5′-5′ triphosphate linkage during in vitro transcription, and is quite inefficient: Conventional caps (m^7GpppG) compete with GTP, and are incorporated into mRNA in both orientations, resulting in two RNA populations, Gpppm^{7}GpN, and m^7GpppGpN (Pasquinelli et al. 1995) (N: first template-encoded nucleotide). Consequently, one-half of the mRNA is improperly capped and will not be recognized by the translation initiation complex. The introduction of anti-reverse cap analogs (ARCA) solved the issue of reverse incorporation by the elimination of the 2′ or 3′ hydroxy group (to prevent nucleophilic attack by the RNA polymerase) through substitution of the 2′ or 3′ hydroxy group with a methoxy group ($m^{7,2'O}$GpppG and $m^{7,3'O}$GpppG, respectively) (Stepinski et al. 2001). Replacing a nonbridging oxygen in the phosphate moiety by sulfur resulted in ARCAs with improved resistance against 5′ to 3′ decay (β-S-ARCA), where one of the resulting ARCA diastereomers was superior over the other in terms of translational efficiency (Kuhn et al. 2010). Very recently, dithiodiphosphate (2S) analogs were introduced with high affinity for eIF4E and improved resistance against decapping enzymes (Strenkowska et al. 2016).

Both UTRs critically affect mRNA half-life and can serve as negative regulators as demonstrated for the integration of destabilizing AU-rich elements (Barreau et al. 2005) and miRNA binding sites (Fang and Rajewsky 2011). UTRs of human α- and β-globin have been most widely incorporated (based on historical use rather than substantial evidence), and provide options for improvement, for instance as reported by Holtkamp et al. (2006).

Translational efficiency can be further enhanced by replacing rarely used codons with frequent, synonymous codons. Although extensively described in the literature, coding sequence optimization appears to be a rather empirical process the necessity of which should be carefully evaluated case by case (reviewed in Mauro and Chappell 2014). A major caveat of codon optimization in the context of RNA vaccination is the elimination or introduction of potent cryptic T cell epitopes generated by ribosomal frameshifting or internal initiation of transcription (Saulquin et al. 2002; Schwab et al. 2003).

mRNA stability and protein expression are also improved by increasing the length of the poly(A) tail until around 120 adenosines (Holtkamp et al. 2006), presumably, because the formation of a circular structure through poly(A) binding proteins protects from decapping and deadenylating enzymes. 3′ extension should be avoided (unmasked poly(A) tail), for instance by pDNA linearization with type IIS restriction enzymes (Holtkamp et al. 2006). Encoding the poly(A) tail in the template vector is beneficial for its therapeutic use, yielding products with reproducible tail lengths compared to the enzymatic two-step method.

3.3 *Antigen Processing and Presentation*

After translation of the mRNA in the cytosol, the encoded protein will eventually be degraded into peptides by the proteasome, routed into the endoplasmic reticulum (ER) for loading onto MHC class I, and via the secretory pathway shuttled to the cell surface for presentation to CD8+ T cells. In contrast to peptide/protein vaccines, mRNA vaccines deliver antigen directly into the cytosol, facing the hurdle of intracellular proteins usually not entering the MHC class II pathway very efficiently (autophagy is one mechanism), with peptide loading taking place in MHC class II-containing secretory vesicles. In order to make mRNA-encoded protein eligible for MHC class II presentation, trafficking signals of endosomal or lysosomal proteins residing in MHC class II processing compartments have been fused to the encoded antigen, such as lysosome-associated membrane protein-1 (LAMP-1) (Bonehill et al. 2004; Bonini et al. 2001; Su et al. 2002), the chaperone calreticulin, MHC class II-associated invariant chain (Bonehill et al. 2003), and HIV TAT protein transduction domain (Kim et al. 2008). Kreiter et al. incorporated the secretion signal and the transmembrane as well as cytosolic domains of MHC class I at the N and C terminus, respectively, which improved both CD4+ and CD8+ T cell responses (Kreiter et al. 2007, 2008). Antigen routed into the secretory pathway may be reinternalized, and subsequently, enter the MHC class II presentation pathway, or, in the case of cross-presenting DCs, be processed for MHC class I presentation.

4 Immune Stimulation

T cell activation does not come easy, and presentation of antigen on MHC alone does not make a vaccine. Instead, the expression of costimulatory signals on the surface of antigen-presenting DCs needs to be actively induced and recognized by T cells, in the presence of a polarizing cytokine environment provided by mature DCs. Insufficient immune stimulation leads to the opposite effect, i.e., T cell deletion, anergy or tolerance towards the tumor. Adjuvants such as aluminum salts (alum), monophosphoryl lipid A or toll-like receptor (TLR) agonists stimulate 'danger signals' to provide immunostimulation when peptide or protein vaccines with low intrinsic immunogenicity are used. Synthetic mRNA, however, is recognized by pattern recognition receptors (PRRs) and functions per se immunostimulatory (Karikó et al. 2004; Ishii and Akira 2005; Reis e Sousa 2004). Ligation of endosomal TLR3, TLR7 or TLR8 with endocytosed mRNA in immune cells triggers the production of type I interferon (IFN), a master regulator of several inflammatory cytokines, Th cytokines, costimulatory molecules, chemokines, and receptors thereof. While TLR3 is activated by double-stranded RNA (dsRNA) (Alexopoulou et al. 2001) including double-stranded secondary structures (Karikó et al. 2004), TLR7 and 8 signal in response to ssRNA (Reis e Sousa 2004; Heil et al. 2004). Soluble cytoplasmic receptors trigger the expression of type I IFN and proinflammatory factors similar to TLRs (Yoneyama and Fujita 2007). The natural ligand for the retinoic acid-inducible gene-I (RIG-I) is short RNA with blunt-ended double-stranded base pairing and an uncapped 5′ triphosphate end (Hornung et al. 2006; Schlee et al. 2009), while activation of melanoma differentiation-associated antigen 5 (MDA5) has been reported to require much longer dsRNA than RIG-I (at least 2 kb) (Pichlmair et al. 2009), or viral mRNA lacking 2′-O-methylation (Züst et al. 2011).

In contrast, activation of dsRNA-recognizing protein kinase R (PKR) should be avoided, as triggering this signaling cascade would interfere with mRNA translation (Sahin et al. 2014). Incorporation of naturally occurring modified nucleosides, such as 2-thiouridine, N6-methyladenosines, 5-methylcytidine, or pseudouridine can suppress PKR activation (Anderson et al. 2010) by not forming dsRNA (2-thiouridine, N6-methyladenosine) or reducing dsRNA contaminants during in vitro transcription (5-methylcytidine, pseudouridine; Katalin Karikó, unpublished). HPLC purification alone was observed to abolish PKR activation. It has to be noted, however, that nucleoside modification, sophisticated purification as well as sequence optimization by maximizing GC content (Thess et al. 2015) are indeed valid methods for increasing translation, but come at the cost of immune activation. Consequently, caution should be taken when designing optimal mRNA, to fit it to the intended use: for cancer therapy, better immune activation may outweigh translation, whereas immune activation would be detrimental for other approaches such as protein replacement (Karikó et al. 2012), where high protein production is the primary aim.

Beneficial activation of combined innate and adaptive immunity has been recently reported for the systemic administration route. Systemic application of lymphoid-targeted mRNA formulated with liposomes induced strong upregulation of costimulatory molecules CD40 and CD86 on DCs (Kranz et al. 2016). Interestingly, maturation of DCs was not confined to the portion of DCs taking up mRNA, but was observed for the majority of splenic DCs, and especially for CD8α + DCs. Expression of early activation marker CD69 was similarly induced on all CD4+ and CD8+ T cells, in addition to NK cells. Concomitant type I IFN secretion by pDCs and macrophages led to considerable type I IFN serum levels, which was essential for generating this fundamentally stimulating environment, for T cells to differentiate into cytolytic effectors [confirmed by Broos et al. (2016)], and for the elimination of established tumors.

In this context, it is important to note that the carrier itself may be immunostimulatory to some extent, or may even be designed specifically for this purpose. DOTMA/DOPE or DOTMA/cholesterol liposomes are by themselves capable of inducing low systemic type I IFN when administered intravenously at high amounts (unpublished observation by the authors), and incorporation of LPS directly into the lipid shell of mRNA nanoformulations can improve the antitumoral response after subcutaneous injection, presumably due to generating inflammation at the injection site (Oberli et al. 2016). Protamine-stabilized mRNA constitutes a stronger danger signal compared to naked mRNA in vitro (Scheel et al. 2004, 2005). Intranodal administration [where type I IFN production is confined to the respective lymph node (unpublished observation by the authors)] has been demonstrated to profit from co-administration of mRNA-encoded active TLR4, CD40L, and CD70 (TriMix) which further improved antitumoral immunity (Van Lint et al. 2012). Other compounds reported to boost mRNA vaccine efficacy are the mTOR inhibitor rapamycin, increasing the quantity and quality of the memory pool (Diken et al. 2013), and Fms-like tyrosine kinase 3 ligand (FLT3L), which expands pDCs in the lymph node and promotes T cell homing into tumors (Kreiter et al. 2011).

5 Delivery

5.1 Delivery Route and Format: The Combination Matters

The modifications described above affect the mRNA molecule itself and become relevant once the mRNA molecule has entered the cytoplasm. With the mRNA molecule itself optimized, delivery has become the dominating field of mRNA research. Despite more than 20 years of exploring nucleic acid delivery and broadening our understanding of what these barriers are and how to tackle them, efficient targeting of mRNA into DCs specifically in vivo remains a problem. Apart from naked mRNA delivery, the field focused on complexation or encapsulation of mRNA to avoid excessive extracellular degradation and promote enhanced uptake by DCs. For mRNA in vivo delivery, lipid-based carrier systems have been used the

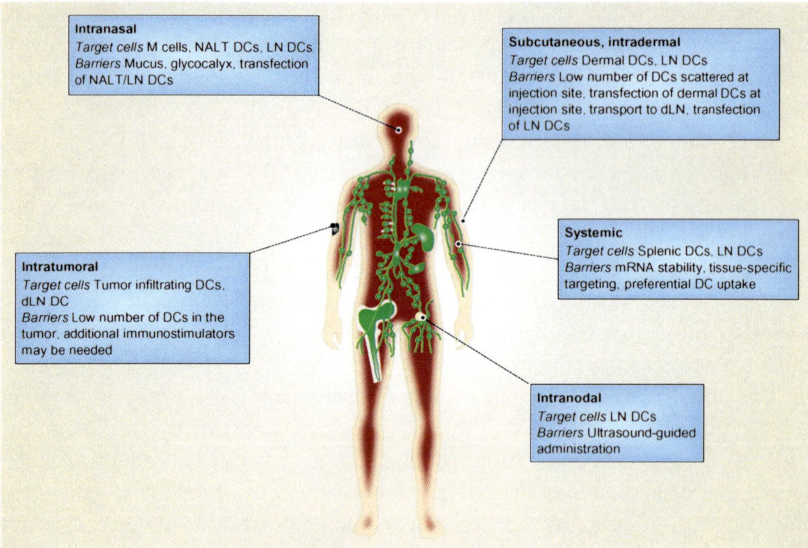

Fig. 2 mRNA delivery routes and associated barriers. *d* Draining. *LN* Lymph node. *NALT* Nasal-associated lymphoid tissue

most, building on extensive research on DNA gene transfer [reviewed in Phua et al. (2014), Phua (2015)], and among these also commercially available transfection reagents (such as Lipofectin, Lipofectamine, RNAiMAX, and Stemfect) have demonstrated in vivo transfection of DCs.

Two main factors are decisive when trying to solve the problem of delivery: delivery route (the way/site of entry into the body), and delivery format (naked, stabilized, adsorbed, complexed, encapsulated, etc.) (Fig. 2). We have learned that these two factors are interconnected, and need to be considered as a system. Each delivery route (subcutaneous, intradermal, intratumoral, intranasal, intranodal, intravenous) has to cope with its specific barriers, and these barriers will determine the adequate delivery format. In other words, a rational combination of delivery route and format should be the underlying motivation when designing vaccination concepts. Obtaining reasonable immune responses with a certain format and a certain delivery route does not necessarily mean that a certain delivery route is per se the better route, or that the format used will equally outperform other formats when injected at a different site.

5.2 *Subcutaneous and Intradermal Injection*

Although secondary lymphoid organs seem to be the obvious target tissues, many studies have focused on injection at distant sites, such as subcutaneous and intradermal application. Vaccination at these sites relies on the immediate presence of dermal DCs ready to take up antigen and migrate actively to the draining lymph node, or on passive transport to draining lymph nodes. Whereas both options are relevant for intradermal application, the subcutaneous space between the skin and underlying muscle tissue does not contain cells, impeding access to dermal DCs and making this vaccination strategy almost entirely dependent on the trafficking efficiency through the lymphatics to draining lymphoid tissue. Both naked and lipid-formulated mRNA injected s.c. lead to transfection of cells at the injection site, with naked mRNA outperforming lipid-formulated mRNA regarding translational efficiency (Phua et al. 2013). Induction of antigen-specific T cells in response to both formats was observed (Martinon et al. 1993; Pollard et al. 2013), although neither of them has been reported to transfect nodal cells (Phua et al. 2013; Kreiter et al. 2010). In contrast, a study using slightly negatively charged lipid nanoformulations of roughly 70–100 nm reported high and lasting translation at the injection site, much superior to naked mRNA, as well as in CD11c+ cells in draining lymph nodes (whether transfection occurred only at the transfection site or also directly in the node was not evaluated), leading to delayed growth of B16 melanoma (Oberli et al. 2016).

Intradermal vaccination with improved access to dermal DCs was predominantly advocated and advanced by the University of Tubingen spin-off biotech company CureVac. The discovery that antigen-specific T cell immunity was elicited after intradermal injection of naked or protamine-stabilized mRNA (Hoerr et al. 2000) initiated further characterization of the influence of protamine on stabilization and immune stimulation (Scheel et al. 2004, 2005; Carralot et al. 2004), and eventually led to the development of RNActive, a mixture of naked and protamine-stabilized mRNA. While the naked mRNA compound ensures translation of the antigen, the protamine-stabilized compound is poorly translated but functions as a TLR7 ligand (Fotin-Mleczek et al. 2011). This vaccine is internalized at the injection site predominantly by macrophages, neutrophils, and DCs, of which the majority take up both naked and protamine-stabilized mRNA, but uptake of naked mRNA is preferred (Kowalczyk et al. 2016). In addition, Selmi et al. showed naked mRNA was translated in the dermis rather than the epidermis (no translation), internalized mostly by dermal DCs independent of langerin expression, and that macropinocytosis by these cells was required for mounting T cell immunity (Selmi et al. 2016).

Induction of relevant immune responses in response to injection into nonlymphoid tissues seems to rely heavily on active cellular transport from the site of injection to draining lymphoid tissue. So far, seemingly contradictive data have been published about the capability of stabilizing polymers or nanoparticle formats to outperform naked mRNA, owing to the differences in particle characteristics. However, while naked mRNA will remain dependent on cellular transport as it may not stay intact during lymphatic trafficking, nanoformulations harbor great potential: Promoting efficient access to the lymphatics and increasing antigen availability to a larger reservoir of DCs may be achieved by rational design of carrier features such as particle size, charge, and colloidal stability. Achieving this would make distant injection an even more attractive delivery route for mRNA vaccines.

5.3 Intranasal Administration

The nasal cavity harbors lymphoid tissue, the nasal-associated lymphoid tissue (NALT) which is directly located under a thin layer of nasal epithelium intertwined with microfold (M) cells. These M cells can translocate particles from the epithelium to the NALT (Miller et al. 2007). Intranasal delivery takes advantage of this transport system to reach either NALT-resident DCs in close neighborhood with T cells or to drain passively from the NALT area to cervical lymph nodes through the lymphatics. The mucus layer covering the glycocalyx of the epithelium and the glycocalyx itself represent barriers for particle permission but also offer 'points of attack' for particle design. Promoting adhesion to the mucus may be one way to enhance uptake, while increased retention time should not come at the cost of impaired movement through the mucus. Small- to medium-sized lipid-formulated mRNA or mRNA adsorbed on pegylated core-shell nanoparticles were reported to elevate and prolong antigen expression when positively charged compared to naked mRNA (Phua et al. 2013; Su et al. 2011), while others find also negatively charged particles capable of transportation through the nasal epithelium (Rajapaksa et al. 2010), despite adjacent negatively charged glycocalyx. Pegylation may be one way to increase movement through the mucus, and larger particle sizes seem to be beneficial as well (Lai et al. 2009). Phua and colleagues have been doing intensive research on intranasal administration as a noninvasive needle-free mRNA cancer immunotherapy and were able to demonstrate for the first time antigen-specific immunity and delayed progression of subcutaneous tumors (Phua et al. 2014). Interestingly, these results were confined to positively charged lipid-formulated mRNA and were not achieved with naked mRNA, which is in line with previously reported lower antigen expression in response to naked mRNA.

Intranasal mRNA administration has proven to be a convenient method for antigen delivery to NALT DCs and induction of antitumoral immunity, provided that the mRNA is formulated. Further improvement of access to the NALT by facilitating the passage through the nasal epithelium through rational modification of particle properties seems feasible and holds promise for a noninvasive, broadly applicable tumor vaccine.

5.4 Intratumoral Injection

Tumor infiltrating DCs are in a unique position to prime T cells relevant for antitumoral immunity and aid to revert the 'corrupted' immunosuppressive tumor microenvironment. Using intratumoral mRNA administration, these DCs can be provided with (i) antigenic information to activate/re-activate antigen-specific T cells already present in the tumor, (ii) immunostimulatory molecules that trigger migration of tumor antigen-loaded DCs to draining lymph nodes, and/or (iii) immunomodulatory compounds (cytokines, decoy receptors, TLR agonists, antibodies, checkpoint inhibitors, etc.) fostering in situ vaccination and/or sustain T cell responses.

Intratumoral delivery to DCs has been most advanced by Thielemans and colleagues [reviewed in Van der Jeught et al. (2015)]. Their studies demonstrate that naked mRNA is taken up predominantly by cross-presenting CD8α+ DCs and that these cells can reactivate T cells at the tumor site, as well as migrate to the draining lymph node when in vivo transfected with TriMix (Van Lint et al. 2016). They further showed in a proof-of-concept study, that mRNA-encoded secreted proteins were able to lift some of the pressure off immune cells by reducing MDSC suppression, stimulating DCs and activating T cell lysis, which enhanced delay of tumor growth when combined with PD-1 blockade (Van der Jeught et al. 2014). Less immune-infiltrated tumors may not be quite as susceptible to intratumoral delivery; for these tumors, increasing the half-life of mRNA through stabilization or formulation may be an option. Nevertheless, utilizing DCs not only as antigen presenters but also as transient producers of mRNA-encoded immunomodulators at site and thus shapers of the tumor environment is another asset of mRNA immunotherapy.

5.5 *Intranodal Injection*

Injection directly into lymph nodes circumvents anatomical and physiological barriers associated with DC availability on site and migration/passive transport to draining lymphoid tissue, as discussed for intradermal and subcutaneous injection. A large DC reservoir at immediate disposal and close proximity between injected compound, target cell and immune effectors presumably supports rapid uptake in high numbers and minimizes loss of bioactive compound due to extracellular degradation, which is critical for naked, unprotected mRNA. Sahin and colleagues followed up on this hypothesis and described in 2010 that intranodal delivery of pharmacologically optimized naked antigen-encoding mRNA elicited potent anti-tumor immunity (Kreiter et al. 2010), and that mRNA was internalized and translated by lymph node resident conventional and cross-presenting CD8α+ DCs through macropinocytosis (Diken et al. 2011). Another study by Thielemans et al. confirmed the potency of this delivery route and format in additional tumor models (Van Lint et al. 2012). Expression and presentation of the encoded antigen in a costimulatory environment initiated by the mRNA itself induced protective immunity unattainable by subcutaneous, near-nodal or intradermal administration (Diken et al. 2011; Kreiter et al. 2010). Intranodal delivery is certainly not the most practical or comfortable route of injection, yet regarding immunological and anti-tumor responses, direct targeting of the lymphatic system seems to be the preferable route of injection for naked mRNA, compared to injection at distant sites.

5.6 Systemic Injection

The delivery problem is most apparent when it comes to intravenous administration. Precise and efficient delivery of mRNA-encoded antigen to secondary lymphoid compartments still constitutes a major challenge. How to stabilize mRNA during transit, how to avoid interaction with serum proteins (risk of aggregation) and at the same time guarantee release into the cellular interior? How to reach predominantly a certain tissue or cell type? Naked mRNA is instantly degraded and does not leave a lot of options for directed delivery. What is needed is a carrier for protection and direction. Lipid-based nonviral delivery systems have been exploited for efficient pDNA transfer since the late 1980s. Spleen and especially liver are favored for intravenous particle delivery as they can be reached through sinusoids and their large capillary endothelial fenestrations, where blood flow is slower and extravasation easier. The cells readily taking up particles are white pulp resident cells and hepatocytes, respectively. The majority of particles distributes to the liver, but mRNA is poorly translated (Kranz et al. 2016; Li et al. 1998) (presumably degraded by Kupffer cells), and even less mRNA is translated by splenic DCs. As it was repeatedly shown in vitro that positively charged pDNA-lipid complexes yielded much higher transfection efficiencies than neutral or negatively charged particles, mostly positively charged pDNA-LPX were investigated for their gene transfer capability in vivo. Upon intravenous injection of these particles, researchers found high reporter gene expression in the lungs (Canonico et al. 1994a, b; Lee et al. 1996; Liu et al. 1997), and although some expression was observed in the spleen when decreasing the positive charge of the complex, a systematic analysis of the charge-biodistribution relationship was not seriously pursued at that time. Instead, developments focused almost stringently on functionalization of liposomes and other nanoparticles with molecular ligands to reroute pDNA or mRNA nanoparticles to lymphoid tissues and DCs (Phua 2015; Tacken et al. 2007; Mitragotri et al. 2014). Intravenous delivery of positively charged lipid mRNA formulations produced from Stemfect transfection reagent also led to antigen expression in the spleen, lungs and liver (Phua et al. 2013). However, Midoux and colleagues demonstrated that mRNA encoding MART1 complexed with cationic histidylated PEG-polylysine (PEG-HpK) and further encapsulated in histidine-containing HDHE/cholesterol liposomes (so-called lipopolyplexes), delayed melanoma progression in a prophylactic setting (Mockey et al. 2007). Another study from the same group, this time using PEG-HpK-mRNA complexes encapsulated with mannosylated liposomes, demonstrated increased antigen expression in splenic DCs compared to nonmannosylated particles (no data was provided regarding transfection of nonDCs). However, therapeutic efficacy was not tested (Perche et al. 2011).

In principle, induction of tumor-specific immunity is feasible via this delivery route, but the transfection efficiency of DCs still appeared far too low to be of therapeutic relevance. Very recently, Sahin and colleagues reported that delivery of mRNA can be achieved without the need of highly functionalized, complex and costly delivery formats. By systematic in vivo assessment of antigen expression delivered from mRNA-lipoplexes made from different cationic lipids and uncharged helper lipids, they discovered that the mRNA-to-lipid ratio of lipid-formulated, tumor antigen-encoding mRNA determined the biodistribution of mRN-lipoplexes, and that a slightly negative particle net charge was the key feature for targeting DCs in vivo (Kranz et al. 2016) (confirmed with the commercial transfection reagent RNAiMAX [unpublished and Broos et al. (2016)]. Besides the primary target spleen, they managed to transfect CD11c+ cells in the bone marrow, an important tissue for T cell memory homing, and surprisingly, antigen expression was also detectable in the lymph nodes which for the major portion did not originate from blood-borne infiltrating cells. Expanding the targeted DC reservoir this way, strong effector and memory CD8+ and CD4+ T cell immunity was elicited against viral, mutant neo-antigens or self-antigens, and progressive tumors in therapeutic mouse models of melanoma, colon carcinoma and human papillomavirus (HPV)-associated cancer were rejected. Toxicities have not been observed in mice and cynomolgus monkeys, and a first-in-human clinical study for melanoma is currently ongoing.

When drawing our attention particularly to clinically approved drugs, it is remarkable that despite enormous experimental efforts, only for a limited number of drugs nanoformulations are used. These are nonfunctionalized and composed of materials with a long record of medicinal use. Notably, almost all of the approved drug nanoformulations are composed of well-known biomaterials (e.g., phosphatidylcholine, cholesterol and phosphatidylethanolamine), solely relying on passive targeting. Having the complexity of scale-up processes, GMP production and the regulatory framework in mind, it appears that newly developed mRNA vaccine formulations should be as simple as possible and only as complex as necessary to serve their ultimate purpose—protection of mRNA, fostering efficient engulfment by professional antigen-presenting cells and enabling efficient antigen processing and presentation.

6 Conclusion

Nowadays the great flexibility of mRNA is well appreciated. In the vaccine field, first clinical studies are completed and several others ongoing. Strikingly, all of these studies have proven that large-scale GMP production of mRNA is feasible and concordantly report a favorable safety profile of mRNA vaccines. By now, multiple mRNA vaccine projects are at late clinical stage of development. Undoubtedly, the efficient delivery of mRNA to specific organs, tissues or cell types is a major obstacle in the field. The current strategy of evaluating and optimizing formulations for nucleic acid delivery is highly debatable and it needs to be noted that isolated in vitro studies are not expedient. The studies mentioned above highlight that especially for systemic targeting, in vitro transfection efficiencies of specific cell types are not particularly helpful for predicting effectiveness in vivo, since in vitro studies cannot, by any means, foresee distribution behavior in complex organisms. There is already a plethora of published studies reporting highly functionalized and complex particles with an outstanding transfection rate in vitro. In spite of it all, only a handful of formulations is applicable in vivo. By now several studies have shown that characteristics, such as negative surface charge and a particle size larger than 200 nm, foster uptake by DCs while reducing unspecific uptake by nontarget cells. The potential of lipid-based mRNA vaccines for cancer immunotherapy has long been acknowledged, but it was not until recently that discoveries in this field have brought significant advances.

Beside vaccines, mRNA is taking hold in other fields, underpinning its role as a multipurpose platform. This is reflected by a continuously increasing number of new companies on the scene (Table 2). Notably, the medicinal portfolios of these

Table 2 Company overview: mRNA vaccines and mRNA-based therapeutics

Company	Research focus	Industry partners	Location	Year of foundation
Arcturus Therapeutics	Protein replacement Rare diseases	Ultragenyx Pharmaceutical	San Diego, USA	2013
BioNTech RNA Pharmaceuticals	Cancer Infectious disease	Genentech Sanofi-Aventis Bayer Healthcare	Mainz, Germany	2008
CureVac	Infectious disease Cancer	Boehringer Ingelheim Sanofi Pasteur Acuitas Therapeutics In-cell-Art	Tuebingen, Germany	2000 (Weide et al. 2008)
eTheRNA Immunotherapies	Cancer Infectious disease		Niel, Belgium	2013
Ethris	Rare diseases Protein replacement Regenerative medicine	Shire Pharmaceuticals	Planegg, Germany	2009
Eukarÿs	Protein replacement		Évry, France	2010
GlaxoSmithKline	Infectious disease		Brentford, UK	2000
In-cell-Art	Infectious disease Protein replacement	Sanofi Pasteur CureVac	Nantes, France	2005
Moderna[a]	Cardiometabolic disease Cancer Rare diseases Infectious disease	AstraZeneca MSD Sharp & Dohme Alexion Vertex	Cambridge, USA	2010
Novartis	Infectious disease		Basel, Switzerland	1996
PhaseRX	Protein replacement Rare diseases		Seattle, USA	2006
Silence Therapeutics	Protein replacement		London, UK	1994

[a]Including all Moderna proprietary venture companies

companies lean towards another high impact field: gene therapy with a focus on rare genetic disorders. While mRNA vaccines very much depend on efficient immunostimulation and less on translational yield per cell, the opposite is desired for gene therapy. For such purposes, modified 'stealth' mRNA is optimized for low immunogenicity and high translation since high protein yield is the primary aim. In 2016, AstraZeneca and Moderna filed the first-in-human clinical trial (NCT02935712) using modified mRNA encoding vascular endothelial growth factor-A (VEGF-A).

Given that the mRNA field is moving beyond 'simple' vaccines, challenges associated with tissue- or cell-specific targeting still need to be faced. In cases where high protein yield in the circulation is the goal, the specificity of the producing cell type will be less critical, and passive targeting strategies might be sufficient. Nevertheless, in cases such as genome engineering (e.g., CRISPR/Cas9) and genetic reprogramming, selective mRNA delivery will have a detrimental impact on therapy safety and might be only feasible by introducing new mRNA formulations with active targeting components.

Acknowledgements We gratefully acknowledge helpful discussions with Katalin Karikó and Ugur Sahin.

References

Alexopoulou L, Holt AC, Medzhitov R, Flavell RA (2001) Recognition of double-stranded RNA and activation of NF-kappaB by Toll-like receptor 3. Nature 413:732–738

Anderson BR et al (2010) Incorporation of pseudouridine into mRNA enhances translation by diminishing PKR activation. Nucleic Acids Res 38:5884–5892

Barreau C, Paillard L, Osborne HB (2005) AU-rich elements and associated factors: are there unifying principles? Nucleic Acids Res 33:7138–7150

Bonehill A et al (2003) Efficient presentation of known HLA class II-restricted MAGE-A3 epitopes by dendritic cells electroporated with messenger RNA encoding an invariant chain with genetic exchange of class II-associated invariant chain peptide. Cancer Res 63:5587–5594

Bonehill A et al (2004) Messenger RNA-electroporated dendritic cells presenting MAGE-A3 simultaneously in HLA class I and class II molecules. J Immunol 172:6649–6657

Bonini C, Lee SP, Riddell SR, Greenberg PD (2001) Targeting antigen in mature dendritic cells for simultaneous stimulation of CD4+ and CD8+ T cells. J Immunol 166:5250–5257

Broos K et al (2016) Particle-mediated intravenous delivery of antigen mRNA results in strong antigen-specific T-cell responses despite the induction of Type I interferon. Off J Am Soc Gene Cell Ther 38:1–11

Canonico A, Plitman J, Conary J, Meyrick B, Brigham K (1994a) No lung toxicity after repeated aerosol or intravenous delivery of plasmid-cationic liposome complexes. J Appl Physiol 77:415–419

Canonico A, Conary J, Meyrick B, Brigham K (1994b) Aerosol and intravenous transfection of human alpha 1-antitrypsin gene to lungs of rabbits. Am J Respir Cell Mol Biol 10:24–29

Carralot J-P et al (2004) Polarization of immunity induced by direct injection of naked sequence-stabilized mRNA vaccines. Cell Mol Life Sci 61:2418–2424

Crook K, Stevenson BJ, Dubouchet M, Porteous DJ (1998) Inclusion of cholesterol in DOTAP transfection complexes increases the delivery of DNA to cells in vitro in the presence of serum. Gene Ther 5:137–143
Diebold SS, Kaisho T, Hemmi H, Akira S, Reis e Sousa, C (2004) Innate antiviral responses by means of TLR7-mediated recognition of single-stranded RNA. Science 303:1529–1531
Diken M et al (2011) Selective uptake of naked vaccine RNA by dendritic cells is driven by macropinocytosis and abrogated upon DC maturation. Gene Ther 18:702–708
Diken M et al (2013) mTOR inhibition improves antitumor effects of vaccination with antigen-encoding RNA. Cancer Immunol Res 1:386–392
Fang Z, Rajewsky N (2011) The impact of miRNA target sites in coding sequences and in 3'UTRs. PLoS ONE 6:e18067
Farhood H, Serbina N, Huang L (1995) The role of dioleoyl phosphatidylethanolamine in cationic liposome mediated gene transfer. Biochim Biophys Acta 1235:289–295
Felgner PL et al (1987) Lipofection: a highly efficient, lipid-mediated DNA-transfection procedure. Proc Natl Acad Sci U S A 84:7413–7417
Fotin-Mleczek M et al (2011) Messenger RNA-based vaccines with dual activity induce balanced TLR-7 dependent adaptive immune responses and provide antitumor activity. J Immunother 34:1–15
Heil F et al (2004) Species-specific recognition of single-stranded RNA via toll-like receptor 7 and 8. Science 303:1526–1529
Hirota K, Terada H (2012) Endocytosis of particle formulations by macrophages and its application to clinical treatment
Hoerr I, Obst R, Rammensee HG, Jung G (2000) In vivo application of RNA leads to induction of specific cytotoxic T lymphocytes and antibodies. Eur J Immunol 30:1–7
Holtkamp S et al (2006) Modification of antigen-encoding RNA increases stability, translational efficacy, and T-cell stimulatory capacity of dendritic cells. Blood 108:4009–4017
Hornung V et al (2006) 5′-Triphosphate RNA is the ligand for RIG-I. Science 314:994–997
Ishii KJ, Akira S (2005) TLR ignores methylated RNA? Immunity 23:111–113
Karikó K, Ni H, Capodici J, Lamphier M, Weissman D (2004) mRNA is an endogenous ligand for Toll-like receptor 3. J Biol Chem 279:12542–12550
Karikó K, Muramatsu H, Keller JM, Weissman D (2012) Increased erythropoiesis in mice injected with submicrogram quantities of pseudouridine-containing mRNA encoding erythropoietin. Mol Ther 20:948–953
Kim S-G et al (2008) Modification of CEA with both CRT and TAT PTD induces potent anti-tumor immune responses in RNA-pulsed DC vaccination. Vaccine 26:6433–6440
Kowalczyk A et al (2016) Self-adjuvanted mRNA vaccines induce local innate immune responses that lead to a potent and boostable adaptive immunity. Vaccine 34:3882–3893
Kranz LM et al (2016) Systemic RNA delivery to dendritic cells exploits antiviral defence for cancer immunotherapy. Nature 534:396–401
Kreiter S et al (2007) Simultaneous ex vivo quantification of antigen-specific CD4+ and CD8+ T cell responses using in vitro transcribed RNA. Cancer Immunol Immunother 56:1577–1587
Kreiter S et al (2008) Increased antigen presentation efficiency by coupling antigens to MHC class I trafficking signals. J Immunol 180:309–318
Kreiter S et al (2010a) Intranodal vaccination with naked antigen-encoding RNA elicits potent prophylactic and therapeutic antitumoral immunity. Cancer Res 70:9031–9040
Kreiter S et al (2010b) Intranodal vaccination with naked antigen-encoding RNA elicits potent prophylactic and therapeutic antitumoral immunity. Cancer Res 70:9031–9040
Kreiter S et al (2011) FLT3 ligand enhances the cancer therapeutic potency of naked RNA vaccines. Cancer Res 71:6132–6142
Kübler H et al (2015) Self-adjuvanted mRNA vaccination in advanced prostate cancer patients: a first-in-man phase I/IIa study. J Immunother Cancer 3:26
Kuhn A et al (2010) Phosphorothioate cap analogs increase stability and translational efficiency of RNA vaccines in immature dendritic cells and induce superior immune responses in vivo. Gene Ther 17:961–971

Lai SK, Wang Y-Y, Hanes J (2009) Mucus-penetrating nanoparticles for drug and gene delivery to mucosal tissues. Adv Drug Deliv Rev 61:158–171

Lee E et al (1996) Detailed analysis of structures and formulations of cationic lipids for efficient gene transfer to the lung. Hum Gene Ther 7:1701–1717

Li S, Rizzo MA, Bhattacharya S, Huang L (1998) Characterization of cationic lipid-protamine-DNA (LPD) complexes for intravenous gene delivery. Gene Ther 5:930–937

Liu Y et al (1997) Factors influencing the efficiency of cationic liposome-mediated intravenous gene delivery. Nat Biotechnol 15:167–173

Martinon F et al (1993) Induction of virus-specific cytotoxic T lymphocytes in vivo by liposome-entrapped mRNA. Eur J Immunol 23:1719–1722

Mauro VP, Chappell SA (2014) A critical analysis of codon optimization in human therapeutics. Trends Mol Med 20:604–613

Miller H, Zhang J, Kuolee R, Patel GB, Chen W (2007) Intestinal M cells: the fallible sentinels? World J Gastroenterol 13:1477–1486

Mitragotri S, Burke PA, Langer R (2014) Overcoming the challenges in administering biopharmaceuticals: formulation and delivery strategies. Nat Rev Drug Discov 13:655–672

Mockey M et al (2007) mRNA-based cancer vaccine: prevention of B16 melanoma progression and metastasis by systemic injection of MART1 mRNA histidylated lipopolyplexes. Cancer Gene Ther 14:802–814

Oberli MA et al (2016) Lipid nanoparticle–Assisted mRNA delivery for potent cancer immunotherapy. Nano Lett acs.nanolett.6b03329. doi:10.1021/acs.nanolett.6b03329

Pasquinelli AE, Dahlberg JE, Lund E (1995) Reverse 5′ caps in RNAs made in vitro by phage RNA polymerases. RNA 1:957–967

Perche F et al (2011) Enhancement of dendritic cells transfection in vivo and of vaccination against B16F10 melanoma with mannosylated histidylated lipopolyplexes loaded with tumor antigen messenger RNA. Nanomedicine 7:445–453

Phua KKL (2015) Towards targeted delivery systems : Ligand conjugation strategies for mRNA nanoparticle tumor vaccines. J Immunol Res 2015

Phua KKL, Leong KW, Nair SK (2013) Transfection efficiency and transgene expression kinetics of mRNA delivered in naked and nanoparticle format. J Control Release 166:227–233

Phua KKL, Nair SK, Leong KW (2014a) Messenger RNA (mRNA) nanoparticle tumour vaccination. Nanoscale 6:7715–7729

Phua KKL, Staats HF, Leong KW, Nair SK (2014b) Intranasal mRNA nanoparticle vaccination induces prophylactic and therapeutic anti-tumor immunity. Sci Rep 4:5128

Pichlmair A et al (2009) Activation of MDA5 requires higher-order RNA structures generated during virus infection. J Virol 83:10761–10769

Pollard C et al (2013) Type I IFN counteracts the induction of antigen-specific immune responses by lipid-based delivery of mRNA vaccines. Mol Ther 21:251–259

Rajapaksa TE et al (2010) Intranasal M cell uptake of nanoparticles is independently influenced by targeting ligands and buffer ionic strength. J Biol Chem 285:23739–23746

Rittig SM et al (2011) Intradermal vaccinations with RNA coding for TAA generate CD8+ and CD4+ immune responses and induce clinical benefit in vaccinated patients. Mol Ther 19:990–999

Rittig SM et al (2016) Long-term survival correlates with immunological responses in renal cell carcinoma patients treated with mRNA-based immunotherapy. Oncoimmunology 5:e1108511

Sahin U, Karikó K, Türeci Ö (2014) mRNA-based therapeutics—developing a new class of drugs. Nat Rev Drug Discov 13:759–780

Saulquin X et al (2002) +1 Frameshifting as a novel mechanism to generate a cryptic cytotoxic T lymphocyte epitope derived from human interleukin 10. J Exp Med 195:353–358

Scheel B et al (2004) Immunostimulating capacities of stabilized RNA molecules. Eur J Immunol 34:537–547

Scheel B et al (2005) Toll-like receptor-dependent activation of several human blood cell types by protamine-condensed mRNA. Eur J Immunol 35:1557–1566

Schlee M et al (2009) Recognition of 5′ triphosphate by RIG-I helicase requires short blunt double-stranded RNA as contained in panhandle of negative-strand virus. Immunity 31:25–34
Schwab SR, Li KC, Kang C, Shastri N (2003) Constitutive display of cryptic translation products by MHC class I molecules. Science 301:1367–1371
Sebastian M et al (2011) Messenger RNA vaccination in NSCLC: findings from a phase I/IIa clinical trial. J Clin Oncol 29:2584
Selmi A et al (2016) Uptake of synthetic naked RNA by skin-resident dendritic cells via macropinocytosis allows antigen expression and induction of T-cell responses in mice. Cancer Immunol Immunother 65:1075–1083
Stepinski J, Waddell C, Stolarski R, Darzynkiewicz E, Rhoads RE (2001) Synthesis and properties of mRNAs containing the novel 'anti-reverse' cap analogs 7-methyl(3′-O-methyl)GpppG and 7-methyl (3′-deoxy)GpppG. RNA 7:1486–1495
Strenkowska M et al (2016) Cap analogs modified with 1,2-dithiodiphosphate moiety protect mRNA from decapping and enhance its translational potential. Nucleic Acids Res 44:9578–9590
Su Z et al (2002) Enhanced induction of telomerase-specific CD4(+) T cells using dendritic cells transfected with RNA encoding a chimeric gene product. Cancer Res 62:5041–5048
Su X, Fricke J, Kavanagh DG, Irvine DJ (2011) In vitro and in vivo mRNA delivery using lipid-enveloped pH-responsive polymer nanoparticles. Mol Pharm 8:774–787
Tacken PJ, de Vries IJM, Torensma R, Figdor CG (2007) Dendritic-cell immunotherapy: from ex vivo loading to in vivo targeting. Nat Rev Immunol 7:790–802
Tang DC, DeVit M, Johnston SA (1992) Genetic immunization is a simple method for eliciting an immune response. Nature 356:152–154
Thess A et al (2015) Sequence-engineered mRNA without chemical nucleoside modifications enables an effective protein therapy in large animals. Mol Ther. doi:10.1038/mt.2015.103
Van der Jeught K et al (2014) Intratumoral administration of mRNA encoding a fusokine consisting of IFN-β and the ectodomain of the TGF-β receptor II potentiates antitumor immunity. Oncotarget 5:10100–10113
Van der Jeught K, Van Lint S, Thielemans K, Breckpot K (2015) Intratumoral delivery of mRNA: overcoming obstacles for effective immunotherapy. Oncoimmunology 4:e1005504
Van Lint S et al (2012) Preclinical evaluation of TriMix and antigen mRNA-based antitumor therapy. Cancer Res 72:1661–1671
Van Lint S et al (2016) Intratumoral delivery of TriMix mRNA results in T-cell activation by cross-presenting dendritic cells. Cancer Immunol Res 4:146–156
Weide B et al (2008) Results of the first phase I/II clinical vaccination trial with direct injection of mRNA. J Immunother 31:180–188
Weide B et al (2009) Direct injection of protamine-protected mRNA: results of a phase 1/2 vaccination trial in metastatic melanoma patients. J Immunother 32:498–507
Yoneyama M, Fujita T (2007) Function of RIG-I-like receptors in antiviral innate immunity. J Biol Chem 282:15315–15318
Zelphati O, Szoka FC (1996) Mechanism of oligonucleotide release from cationic liposomes. Proc Natl Acad Sci U S A 93:11493–11498
Zhou X, Huang L (1994) DNA transfection mediated by cationic liposomes containing lipopolylysine: characterization and mechanism of action. Biochim Biophys Acta 1189:195–203
Züst R et al (2011) Ribose 2′-O-methylation provides a molecular signature for the distinction of self and non-self mRNA dependent on the RNA sensor Mda5. Nat Immunol 12:137–143

The Use of Anti-CD40 mAb in Cancer

Marcus Remer, Ann White, Martin Glennie, Aymen Al-Shamkhani and Peter Johnson

Abstract Immunomodulatory monoclonal antibody (mAb) therapy is at the forefront of developing cancer therapeutics with numerous targeted agents proving highly effective in selective patients at stimulating protective host immunity, capable of eradicating established tumours and leading to long-term disease-free states. The cell surface marker CD40 is expressed on a range of immune cells and transformed cells in malignant states whose signalling plays a critical role in modulating adaptive immune responses. Anti-CD40 mAb therapy acts via multiple mechanisms to stimulate anti-tumour immunity across a broad range of lymphoid and solid malignancies. A wealth of preclinical research in this field has led to the successful development of multiple anti-CD40 mAb agents that have shown promise in early-phase clinical trials. Significant progress has been made to enhance the engagement of antibodies with immune effectors through their interactions with Fcγ receptors (FcγRs) by the process of Fc engineering. As more is understood about how to best optimise these agents, principally through the fine-tuning of mAb structure and choice of synergistic partnerships, our ability to generate robust, clinically beneficial anti-tumour activity will form the foundation for the next generation of cancer therapeutics.

Contents

M. Remer (✉) · A. White · M. Glennie · A. Al-Shamkhani · P. Johnson
Cancer Sciences Unit, Faculty of Medicine, University of Southampton, Southampton General Hospital, Southampton SO16 6YD, UK
e-mail: m.e.remer@soton.ac.uk

Current Topics in Microbiology and Immunology (2017) 405:165–207
DOI 10.1007/82_2014_427

Published Online: 05 February 2015

1 Introduction

A revolution in cancer immunotherapy has recently emerged with the development of novel immunomodulatory antibodies, classified as immunostimulatory agonist mAb or checkpoint blocking mAb. Noteworthy clinical trial response rates and survival outcomes have been described with anti-CTLA-4 and anti-PD-1 mAb checkpoint blockers across a range of predominantly solid tumours, such as lung cancers and melanoma, in heavily pretreated patients with advanced disease associated with very poor prognoses. The fully human IgG1 anti-CTLA-4 mAb ipilimumab was approved by the FDA in March 2011 after several large phase III trials demonstrated prolonged overall survival (OS) in advanced melanoma (Hodi et al. 2010; Robert et al. 2011). Metastatic melanoma has been historically associated with particularly poor outcomes, with 2-year survival being between 10 and 20 % prior to immunotherapy (Falkson et al. 1998; Middleton et al. 2000). The addition of ipilimumab to the conventional cytotoxic agent dacarbazine improved the median duration of best overall response (ORR) from 8.1 to 19.3 months (Robert et al. 2011). However, 2-year OS was 24.2 % with ipilimumab monotherapy (Hodi et al. 2010). Essentially, the survival benefit was being driven by a small subpopulation of roughly 10 % who were achieving significant prolonged long-term survival. The emergence of the fully human IgG4 anti-PD-1 mAb nivolumab has enabled 1-year and 2-year OS to reach 62 and 43 %, respectively, in melanoma with an ORR of 31 % (Topalian et al. 2014). The combination of ipilimumab with nivolumab produced an additive effect with an ORR of 53 % and 1- and 2-year OS of 85 and 79 %, respectively (Wolchok et al. 2013; Sznol et al. 2014). These achievements are matched with other anti-PD-1 mAbs, such as pembrolizumab (formerly lambrolizumab) with an ORR of 52 % in its highest dosing cohort in metastatic melanoma (Hamid et al. 2013), and pidilizumab for relapsed/refractory diffuse large B cell lymphoma (DLBCL) achieving an ORR of 51 % (Armand et al. 2013). Immunomodulatory antibody research has garnered interest in the ability to stimulate immune responsiveness to induce robust anti-tumour immunity.

Although less developed than the antagonistic immune checkpoint blocking mAb, the agonistic immunostimulatory mAb also shows great promise as cancer therapeutics (Melero et al. 2007; Lee et al. 2013). One target under active investigation is the costimulatory receptor CD40. CD40 is a member of the tumour necrosis factor (TNF) superfamily of receptors and ligands (Smith et al. 1994) that are critical mediators of multiple physiological processes involved in immune cell function and apoptosis. CD40 is a 277-amino acid, 45–50 kDa transmembrane glycoprotein that is principally expressed on antigen-presenting cells (APCs) (Clark and Ledbetter 1986; Hart and McKenzie 1988; Schriever et al. 1989). B lymphocytes, dendritic cells (DCs), and monocytes/macrophages are professional APCs that constitutively express CD40 where it acts as a key regulator of humoral and cellular immunity (Grewal and Flavell 1998). CD40 is also expressed on a plethora of non-immune cells including endothelial cells, epithelial cells, haematopoietic progenitors, and platelets (Galy and Spits 1992; Yellin et al. 1995). CD40 expression was first described on normal and malignant B cells and human urinary bladder carcinomas (Paulie et al. 1985). Subsequently, it has been described on virtually all B cell malignancies (e.g. non-Hodgkin's lymphoma) and numerous solid epithelial tumours (e.g. breast, lung, ovary, melanoma, and bladder). The CD40 ligand (CD40L), originally termed CD154, is primarily expressed by activated CD4+ T helper (Th) lymphocytes and is transiently induced under inflammatory conditions (Armitage et al. 1992).

Agonistic anti-CD40 monoclonal antibody (mAb) therapy is an emerging immunotherapy with much promise of offering clinical benefit through its role in activating a variety of immune cells to generate effective anti-cancer immune responses. Extensive research has provided convincing evidence that CD40 signalling regulates tumour survival and is critical in tumour antigen presentation to the immune system. Early pivotal studies demonstrated that anti-CD40 antibodies can be used to eradicate lymphomas in murine models and provide protection against tumour rechallenge through rapid induction of anti-tumour cytotoxic T cells that occurs independently of CD4+ T cell help (French et al. 1999; Todryk et al. 2001; Nowak et al. 2003). CD40-activated DCs can overcome tolerance to restore antigen-specific cytotoxic T lymphocyte (CTL) responses in mice depleted of CD4 + T cells (Ridge et al. 1998). Depletion of CD8+ T cells abrogates anti-tumour immunity, exposing the central role of CTL-mediated tumour eradication in solid tumours (Todryk et al. 2001).

The application of cancer immunotherapy strategies to target CD40 aims to effectively boost anti-tumour immunity and abrogate the multitude of cancer host immune evasion mechanisms. Tumours proliferate and metastasise by escaping immune surveillance by a variety of means including down-regulation of antigen processing and presentation by reduced expression of essential costimulatory molecules e.g. B7 family members, loss of MHC or tumour antigens, and deletion of T cells which lack the optimal activation signals (Chen et al. 1992; Restifo et al. 1993; Gajewski et al. 2006). A key mechanism by which CD40 stimulation improves immune recognition is through upregulation of adhesion and costimulatory molecules on the tumour cell surface. Whilst in normal B cells, CD40 signalling augments proliferation, differentiation, and survival, it induces apoptosis in many transformed cells in vitro and in vivo, such as breast carcinomas and aggressive lymphomas (Costello et al. 1999; Ziebold et al. 2000). To date, there are a number of existing anti-CD40 mAb that have been developed and are undergoing early-phase clinical trials as monotherapies and in combination with conventional chemotherapy. Anti-CD40 mAb therapy enhances natural endogenous CD40/CD40L interactions facilitating CD40-conditioned DCs to generate antigen-specific effector CD8+ CTLs leading to tumour destruction.

2 Normal Physiological Role of CD40

Contact-dependent CD40-CD40L cross-linking mediates a broad spectrum of systemic immune and inflammatory responses including T cell-dependent humoral responses, B cell proliferation, differentiation, adhesion and survival, memory B cell and germinal centre development, immunoglobulin class switching and affinity maturation, and interleukin (IL)-6 secretion (Noelle et al. 1992; Tsubata et al. 1993; Klaus et al. 1994; van Kooten and Banchereau 2000; Dadgostar et al. 2002). The critical role of CD40 in humoral immunity is demonstrated by the inability of immunoglobulin class switching, formation of germinal centres, and failure to develop B cell memory in individuals with X-linked hyper-IgM syndrome, whereby a defective CD40L gene leads to a breakdown of crosstalk between B and T cells (Hill and Chapel 1993). Such individuals are markedly immunocompromised and susceptible to opportunistic infections. A similar phenotype is seen in mice engineered to have defective CD40 or CD40L genes, with the mutant mice being unable to mount non-IgM responses (e.g. IgG, IgA and IgE) to thymus-dependent antigens and dysfunctional germinal centre formation, suggesting ineffective memory B cell development (Kawabe et al. 1994; Xu et al. 1994). These mice were capable of generating T cell-independent responses to thymus-independent antigens, highlighting the essential role of CD40 in T cell-mediated B cell immunity. Aside from the setting of genetic immunodeficiency, the consequences of CD40 signalling are best understood when appreciated in the context of the cell type expressing CD40 and the characteristics of the microenvironment in which it operates.

The key functions of CD40 are mediated through its expression on APC. CD40 is expressed on B cells from the early pro-B stage through to the terminally differentiated secreting plasma cell or memory B cell (van Kooten and Banchereau 2000). B cell activation through CD40 enables clonal proliferation and differentiation into antibody-secreting plasma cells and memory B cells although distinct biological effects are dependent on the stage of B cell maturation. CD40L has been shown to preferentially direct the terminal differentiation of germinal centre B cells to become memory B cells rather than plasma cells (Arpin et al. 1995). In addition,

CD40-stimulated B cells have been shown to prolong memory B cell lifespan in vitro through upregulation of telomerase activity (Hu et al. 1997).

On DCs, CD40 signalling contributes to CD4+ helper function and enables functional maturation of DCs. Licensed DCs upregulate expression of costimulatory ligands, such as CD80 (B7-1), CD86 (B7-2), and CD70, and downregulate inhibitory molecules, such as programmed cell death ligand (PD-L1) (Kurts et al. 2010). Through cross-priming, these licensed mature DCs process and present exogenous antigens in bound complexes with MHC I molecules to naive CD8+ T cells, mediating their inauguration into effector CTLs with potent cytotoxic potential and capacity for memory differentiation (Schoenberger et al. 1998; Heath and Carbone 1999). CD40 signalling amplifies the cytotoxic response and prevents tolerance induction or energy.

CD40 stimulation on macrophages enhances APC function promoting cytokine release (IL-12) and upregulating costimulatory molecules (CD80 and CD86) to augment T cell responses (Kurts et al. 2010). In addition, in vitro CD40 activation on macrophages leads to the production of the inflammatory cytokine TNF-α, nitric oxide, and TNF-related apoptosis-inducing ligand (TRAIL), which mediates macrophage cytotoxic function (van Kooten and Banchereau 1997; Griffith et al. 1999; Klimp et al. 2002). CD40-activated macrophages and monocytes can exert direct pro-apoptotic anti-tumour effects enabling them be become tumouricidal with the self-generation of the pro-inflammatory cytokine IFN-γ, in turn leading to further macrophage activation (Alderson et al. 1993; Buhtoiarov et al. 2005).

3 CD40 Intracellular Signalling

CD40 engagement with the multimeric extracellular CD40L initiates receptor trimeric clustering leading to a conformational change and CD40 localisation to membrane lipid rafts that recruit cytoplasmic adapter molecules known as TNF receptor-associated factors (TRAFs) to distinct binding sites on the CD40 cytoplasmic tail (McWhirter et al. 1999). The TRAF trimers initiate rapid protein phosphorylation by recruiting specific tyrosine and serine/threonine kinases that activate well-characterised signal transduction pathways, which include the phosphoinositide 3-kinase (PI-3K), nuclear factor-κB (NF-κB), p38/mitogen-activated protein kinase (MAPK), and c-Jun-NH2-kinase (JNK)/stress-activated protein kinase (SAPK) pathways (Berberich et al. 1994, 1996; Ren et al. 1994; Li et al. 1996). These pathways modulate targeted gene expression through activation of selective transcription factors which regulate apoptosis, cell cycle progression, survival, cytokine production, expression of costimulatory molecules, and sustained MHC/peptide complex presentation (Quezada et al. 2004; Vonderheide 2007). CD40 intracellular signalling is cell-type specific, resulting in differential signalling between B cells and DCs, controlled at the level of TRAF selection, leading to diversity of downstream pathway recruitment, and thereby resulting in distinctive phenotypes, such as B cells with enhanced affinity maturation (Ahonen et al. 2002).

Ligation of CD40/CD40L on DCs activates the NF-κB pathway whose gene product includes the anti-apoptotic protein BCL-2 in human DCs and Bcl-X_L in mice, responsible for DC maturation and survival (Quezada et al. 2004). DC maturation enables prolonged antigen presentation to cognate T cells, which in turn become activated, differentiate and undergo clonal expansion (Miga et al. 2001).

In the context of malignancy, high-grade B cell non-Hodgkin's lymphoma (NHL) cells show constitutive expression of NF-κB due to the sustained presence of an assembled large scaffold-like signalling structure called a signalosome within the membrane lipid raft (Pham et al. 2002). This unique signalling mechanism is initiated through autochthonous or ectopic production of CD40L, enabling the neoplastic B cell to bypass external accessory signals required by normal B cells. The lymphoma cells become autonomous, self-sustaining with continuous cell-cycling growth. The CD40 signalosome represents a therapeutic target with in vitro studies demonstrating disappearance of the CD40 signalosome, downregulation of NF-κB expression, growth inhibition, and lymphoma cell death with anti-CD40 and anti-CD40L antibody therapy (Pham et al. 2002).

4 CD40 Expression in Cancer

CD40 expression has been identified on a wide range of tumour cells, comprising almost 100 % of B cell neoplasms and approaching 70 % of solid malignancies (Vonderheide 2007). CD40 expression is likely to reflect pre-existent expression on non-transformed precursor cells. CD40 is also expressed on the majority of multiple myeloma (MM) cells, in contrast to low expression levels of CD20 in MM (Pellat-Deceunynck et al. 1994). Examples of epithelial tumours expressing CD40 include breast, lung, ovarian, melanoma, renal, cervical, nasopharyngeal, and bladder malignancies (Thomas et al. 1996; Wingett et al. 1998; Cooke et al. 1999; Sabel et al. 2000; Gallagher et al. 2002).

4.1 Effect of CD40 Activation in Malignancy

The effect of CD40 pathway activation in B cell malignancies is heterogenous, with the effect of inducing apoptosis and inhibition of cell growth in some xenograft tumour models and B cell lines in vitro (Funakoshi et al. 1994; Planken et al. 1996). This anti-tumour effect is seen in high-grade NHLs, such as Burkitt's lymphoma or EBV-driven lymphomas. Anti-CD40 mAb augments human B cell responses through enhanced secondary IgG antibody responses and can prevent lymphomatous transformation of EBV-positive cells, which would otherwise occur spontaneously (Funakoshi et al. 1995; Murphy et al. 1999). When combined, these early studies showed that anti-CD40 mAb could promote normal B cell function and is selective in inhibiting malignant cells. Growth inhibition is presumed to be a function of activation-induced cell death (AICD)—apoptosis, cell cycle arrest or necrosis mediated by Fas/FasL interactions that negatively regulate activated T cells to maintain peripheral tolerance. CD40 activation upregulates surface expression of the death receptor Fas leading to pro-apoptotic triggering (Wang et al. 1997). CD40 pathway activation mediates AICD in aggressive lymphomas through upregulated expression of Bax, a pro-apoptotic member of the Bcl-2 gene family, which translocates to the mitochondria mediating mitochondrial outer membrane permeabilisation, cyctochrome c release, and activation of caspases (Hengartner 2000; Szocinski et al. 2002). In contrast, CD40 stimulation promotes malignant transformation, tumour proliferation, and lymphomagenesis in other lymphoma subtypes, particularly low-grade indolent lymphomas, such as follicular NHL, CLL, and hairy cell leukaemia (Fluckiger et al. 1994; Voorzanger-Rousselot et al. 1998; Castillo et al. 2000; Homig-Holzel et al. 2008; Kusam et al. 2009). This differential outcome to CD40 activation in B cell malignancies may correlate with the stage of B cell maturation at which transformation occurred.

Gene expression analysis has identified the pre-existing status of CD40 signalling in lymphoma cells as an important predictor of response to anti-tumour CD40 therapy (Burington et al. 2011; Shi and Dornan 2012). Sensitivity to stimulatory anti-CD40 mAb (SGN-40) is associated with p53 mutation and BCL6 expression with higher levels of intrinsic DNA damage. NHL cell lines with constitutively activated CD40 signalling were more resistant to anti-CD40 mAb (SGN-40) whilst cells with inactive CD40 were more sensitive to SGN-40. A 15-gene expression signature panel has been validated using DLBCL tumours demonstrating a majority (88 %) of the 39 specimens predicted to be resistant to CD40 activation failed to respond to SGN-40 (Burington et al. 2011).

Similarly to lymphoid malignancies, CD40 activation in MM also produces differential responses with studies reporting both MM proliferation and apoptosis/growth arrest in response to CD40 ligation (Teoh et al. 2000). CD40L upregulates IL-6 secretion, a paracrine and autocrine growth factor, which has been shown in some studies to negatively modulate the disease and effect prognosis (Urashima et al. 1995). Anti-CD40 mAb is able to specifically block this effect reducing IL-6 secretion. IL-6 activity is regulated by the cell cycle regulatory protein p53, expressed by the TP53 gene—'the guardian of the genome'. CD40 activation directly modulates p53-dependent cell cycle regulation in MM cell lines and can induce either proliferation or growth arrest depending on p53 status (Teoh et al. 2000).

In metastatic melanoma, CD40 expression is downregulated during melanoma progression enabling tumour escape, with a differential level of expression seen in the primary tumour to that of the metastases (Thomas et al. 1996). CD40 expression is only seen in a minority of cell lines derived from metastases. The net result of CD40 activation in immunogenic metastatic melanoma is tumour-specific CTL-mediated cell lysis and apoptosis (von Leoprechting et al. 1999). The upregulation of MHC class I molecules, enabling tumour antigen recognition, is thought to be responsible for the enhanced susceptibility of specific CTL-mediated destruction.

Ligation of CD40 in CD40-expressing breast carcinomas cell lines leads to increased MHC class II expression resulting in growth inhibition and Fas-mediated apoptosis (Wingett et al. 1998). Early in vivo studies demonstrated this growth inhibition and prolonged survival through AICD, with the administration of soluble recombinant human CD40L in SCID mice challenged with human breast tumours (Hirano et al. 1999). The significantly higher expression level of CD40 in breast tumour cells compared to normal breast epithelial cells has been demonstrated in both nuclear and cytoplasmic CD40 expression (83 versus 30 % and 53 versus 30 %, respectively; where n = 181), with improved survival associated with cytoplasmic CD40 expression (Slobodova et al. 2011).

5 Antibody Mechanism of Action

The goal of immunostimulatory antibodies is indirect tumour cell eradication by triggering immune receptors to stimulate an immune response against cancer cells (Melero et al. 2007). Agonist antibodies provide a therapeutic strategy to boost anti-tumour immunity that can augment natural immune responses or as potential adjuvants alongside cancer vaccines. Anti-CD40 mAb has several potential mechanisms of action, which include tumour eradication through recruitment of immune effectors and antibody-dependent cell-mediated cytotoxicity (ADCC), cell signalling to induce direct apoptosis or growth arrest, and crucially, through licensing of APCs to stimulate an anti-cancer immune response. Cross-linked anti-CD40 mAbs can trigger CD40 on APCs to prime effector CTLs, release pro-inflammatory cytokines such as IL-2, and indirectly activate NK cells (Turner et al. 2001). The different mechanisms of anti-CD40 mAb therapy were not identified simultaneously. Initial development was driven by an understanding that direct apoptotic signalling on CD40+ tumours could represent an alternative target in rituximab-resistant lymphoid malignancies. Direct apoptotic signalling targets CD40-expressing cells and is a non-immune-mediated mechanism of tumour killing. Interest in targeting the tumour indirectly, through immune stimulation to generate an anti-tumour response, has led to the emergence of new clinical trials and shaped the field of agonist anti-CD40 mAb therapy.

5.1 Direct Apoptotic Signalling

Early studies demonstrated that direct targeting of CD40+ tumours by ligation of anti-CD40 mAb or soluble recombinant CD40L induced pro-apoptotic signalling and growth arrest (Funakoshi et al. 1994; von Leoprechting et al. 1999; Eliopoulos et al. 2000; Ghamande et al. 2001). This has been observed in various lymphoid and solid tumours (Pellat-Deceunynck et al. 1996; Wang et al. 1997; Hirano et al. 1999). Cell growth could be inhibited by specific anti-CD40 mAb both in vitro and in vivo in Burkett's lymphoma cell lines (Funakoshi et al. 1994). A total of 40–60 % growth inhibition was achieved in the Daudi BL cell line in vitro.

No inhibition was seen in the Raji BL line with soluble anti-CD40 mAb. However, cross-linking the anti-CD40 mAb with a secondary antibody led to significant growth inhibition. This effect was further characterised highlighting a possible direct mechanism by demonstrating that growth inhibition could still be maintained despite the concurrent use of mAb against the Fc receptor which blocks ADCC (Funakoshi et al. 1996). This was in contrast to anti-CD20 mAb which despite greater efficacy than anti-CD40 mAb, its effect was fully abrogated by inhibiting ADCC. Nonetheless, the growth inhibitory effect of anti-CD40 mAb is primarily mediated through Fc receptor-dependent mechanisms, namely ADCC, as opposed to direct apoptotic signalling. The direct anti-tumour activity of anti-CD40 mAb is not the same for all CD40-expressing tumours, with CD40+ melanoma cell lines being insensitive to direct targeting with the immunostimulatory anti-CD40 IgG2 mAb CP-870,893 (Kalbasi et al. 2010).

5.2 *T Cell-Dependent Cytotoxicity*

Anti-CD40 mAb send a 'licence to kill' signal by activating CD40-expressing APCs, which in turn cross-primes tumour-specific CTLs in the tumour, peripheral blood and spleen, capable of eradicating even CD40-negative solid tumours in vivo (Todryk et al. 2001; van Mierlo et al. 2002). Thus, a key cellular target of anti-CD40 mAb is a CD40-expressing DC which becomes activated upon stimulation leading to CTL cross-priming and migration from the periphery to draining lymph nodes. This results in increased tumour antigen presentation in tumour-draining lymph nodes.

In preclinical murine studies in vivo, agonistic anti-CD40 mAbs (rat anti-mouse IgG2a FGK45 and 3/23) produced robust therapeutic efficacy leading to the complete eradication of multiple CD40+ B cell lymphomas and were resistant to tumour rechallenge with the same lymphoma (French et al. 1999). Depletion studies confirmed that treatment is CD8+ T cell dependent through APC activation, occurring in the absence of CD4+ T cell help. Efficacy was also dependent on a sufficient tumour burden of viable lymphoma cells, achieved through either larger inoculum of tumour cells or delayed antibody administration to permit tumour growth pre-treatment. The hypothesis to explain this phenomenon was the requirement of sufficient tumour-associated antigen to prime CD40–activated APCs. These findings were reproduced in follow-up studies that confirmed that anti-CD40 mAb therapy could eradicate B cell lymphomas even after widespread dissemination throughout secondary lymphoid organs, liver, and bone marrow (Tutt et al. 2002). Anti-CD40 mAb therapy led to an early rapid NK cell cytotoxic response; however, upon NK cell depletion, this effect was not required for therapeutic efficacy, which again was solely CD8+ CTL dependent—both in the primary response and in the secondary response with tumour rechallenge. This suggests that CD8+ T cell memory provides long-term protection; however, this does decline over time.

5.3 T Cell-Independent Cytotoxicity

A considerable body of research has focused on anti-CD40 mAb ability to directly kill CD40-expressing tumour (e.g. via ADCC) or though T cell-mediated cytotoxicity; however, CD40 ligation has been shown to activate innate immune cells such as NK cells and macrophages which are capable of anti-tumour activity in their own right. One group showed that anti-CD40 ligation indirectly activated NK cells through secretion of Th1 cytokines (IL-12 and IFN-γ), as opposed to via ADCC and that the anti-tumour response was reduced by NK cell depletion in murine melanomas, colon adenocarcinomas, and neuroblastomas (Turner et al. 2001). Furthermore, anti-CD40 mAb administration after CD8+ T cell depletion produced an anti-tumour effect, attributed to NK cell-mediated cytolysis. Other immune mechanisms of action, independent of T cell-mediated cytotoxicity, include tumouricidal macrophages that induce the depletion of tumour stroma leading to tumour breakdown and subsequent regression, as described in pancreatic tumours (Beatty et al. 2011). This is thought to be a key mechanism of action behind the strong agonistic anti-CD40 mAb CP-870,893. Macrophages act as APCs and express CD40, which can be directly activated by anti-CD40 mAb to secrete IFN-γ and mediate tumour cell destruction, as described in melanomas both in vitro and in vivo (Buhtoiarov et al. 2005). Finally, CD40-activated follicular B cells may function both as APCs and antibody-secreting plasma cells directed at tumour-specific antigens after protective immunity was demonstrating against mesotheliomas in vivo (Jackaman et al. 2011).

5.4 Recruitment of Immune Effectors

Therapeutic cancer antibodies are capable of utilising various effector mechanisms to mediate cytotoxicity in order to achieve efficacy. These include ADCC, complement-dependent cytotoxicity (CDC), and antibody-dependent cell-mediated phagocytosis (ADCP). ADCC is the process where non-specific cytotoxic effector cells (NK cells and macrophages/monocytes) ubiquitously express membrane-bound FcγRs that cross-link with the Fc region of the IgG antibody molecule, which is attached to a specific target cell, i.e. CD40-positive lymphoma cell. FcγRs provide the physical connection between the specificity of the adaptive immune system and the potent innate immune system that executes cytotoxic effector responses. FcγR binding increases the metabolic activity of the cytotoxic cell facilitating the release of cytoplasmic lytic enzymes, granzymes, perforin-containing granules and TNF that induce cell lysis of the antibody-targeted cell. FcγRs are also present on DCs with activatory signalling resulting in cross-presentation of antigens to CD8+ CTLs, CD4+ Th cells, and Treg cells that recognise MHC-restricted peptides triggering activation of various effector functions, cross-signalling, and regulation of peripheral tolerance.

A substantial body of research has investigated the critical interactions between the Fc portion of therapeutic antibodies and FcγRs of immune cells. The characteristics of these interactions, including the antibody isoforms, glycoform, variants, binding affinity, avidity, structural motifs, orientation, and immobilisation are important determinants of the amplitude of the cytotoxic effector response generated in addition to the duration of the response is maintained. Manipulation of these factors through Fc engineering has significantly increased the binding affinities for activating FcγRIIIa and FcγRIIa, giving rise to optimised ADCC and ADCP. It is important to note that human FcγRs are not fully analogous with their orthologous murine counterparts. For instance, the affinity of the human FcγRs for the different IgG isotypes is significantly lower than is the case in mice. The use of mouse models to investigate the mechanisms governing immune regulation and the therapeutic potential of novel antibodies remains invaluable; however, these effects are not always directly transferable to humans.

5.5 *Fcγ Receptor Interactions*

There are two functional classes of FcγRs—activating receptors (human FcγRI, FcγRIIa,c, and FcγRIIIa,b) and their murine orthologues (FcγRI, FcγRIII, and FcγRIV) and inhibitory receptors (FcγRIIb) (Nimmerjahn and Ravetch 2008). Differences in their molecular structure confer distinct antibody binding affinities and cellular distribution, acting as discriminators of their functional capacity. Intracellular signalling of antibody-bound FcγRs is regulated in activatory receptors via an immunoreceptor tyrosine-based activation motif (ITAM) comprised of a specific amino acid sequence within the intracellular tail of the receptor. Phosphorylation of tyrosine kinases induce an activatory signalling cascade with a functional outcome determined by the type of cell expressing the FcγR. Inhibitory FcγRIIb signalling is regulated via an immunoreceptor tyrosine-based inhibitory motif (ITIM) in its cytoplasmic domain. Phosphatase enzymes that remove phosphate groups from tyrosine residues inhibit FcγR signalling. A fundamental aspect of the FcγR system is the coexpression of both activatory and inhibitory receptors on an individual cell regulating signalling thresholds for activation. The ratio of activating-to-inhibiting receptor binding (A/I ratio) has been shown to predict in vivo mAb activity and determines isotype dominance (Nimmerjahn and Ravetch 2005). The exceptions to this rule are B cells which only expresses the low-affinity inhibitory FcγRIIb, regulating BCR activation, and NK cells which only express the activating FcγRIII. With the exception of the high-affinity FcγRI, all other receptors bind with low-medium affinities, which reduce binding of background monomeric antibody molecules thereby preventing non-specific triggering of pro-inflammatory responses.

The Fc portion on the constant region of therapeutic antibodies comprises of one of the four IgG isotypes in humans (IgG1–IgG4) and mice (IgG1, IgG2a, IgG2b, and IgG3). The differential specificity and binding affinity of IgG isotypes for each FcγR, which is different between humans and mice, entrench a high degree of complexity at the interface of FcγR interactions. This complexity is compounded by many nuanced caveats woven into the FcγR system. In humans, IgG1 and IgG3 are the most pro-inflammatory isotypes, whilst in mice, IgG2a and IgG2b are the most pro-inflammatory with greatest activity (Nimmerjahn and Ravetch 2006). Mouse IgG1 antibodies have an A/I ratio less than one, which suggests their activity is critically influenced by the inhibitory FcγRIIb (Nimmerjahn and Ravetch 2005). As a result, mouse IgG1 preferentially binds to inhibitory FcγRIIb conferring minimal ADCC activity. By contrast, mouse IgG2a and IgG2b antibodies had much higher A/I ratios (70 and 7, respectively) and are therefore under less control by the inhibitory FcγRIIb. Mouse IgG2a is the most potent mouse IgG isotype in mediating ADCC due to its efficient engagement with activating FcγRIV. These factors are important considerations in the design of therapeutic antibodies, especially when human antibodies have been derived from murine antibodies. That withstanding, the A/I ratios between the human IgG isotypes are different, relative to one another, with human IgG1 mAb binding with a high A/I ratio to a broad range of FcγRs, thereby augmenting ADCC. By contrast, human IgG2 mAb has minimal FcγR binding other than to an allelic variant of FcγRIIa and does not potentiate ADCC. Allelic variants or polymorphisms of activatory FcγRs can give rise to differences in A/I ratios and hence alter the affinity for certain antibody isotypes. Analysis of FcγR polymorphisms demonstrated that differences in molecular structure modulate antibody–receptor binding affinity, characterising the strength of ADCC. NHL patients carrying the FcγRIIIa allotype resulted in high affinity for anti-CD20 IgG1 rituximab, leading to improved clinical efficacy compared with the low-affinity allelic variant (Cartron et al. 2002).

Therapeutic antibodies that deplete target cells via ADCC demonstrate enhanced tumour protection in FcγRIIb-deficient mice in xenograft models of breast cancers treated with trastuzumab (Clynes et al. 2000). ADCC was abrogated in mice deficient in activating Fc receptors resulting in loss of anti-tumour activity. Agonistic FcγRIIb-specific mAbs have been shown to induce programmed cell death in vitro (Williams et al. 2012) but failed to produce tumour protection in vivo due to receptor internalisation on target cells, in addition to consumption by host cells (Williams et al. 2013).

Pivotal studies addressing the role of isotype selection of anti-CD40 mAb have highlighted the key role of the inhibitory receptor FcγRIIb in regulating antibody agonist activity (Li and Ravetch 2011; White et al. 2011). In the first pivotal study, rat anti-mouse CD40 mAb (3/23) with engineered mouse IgG1 or mouse IgG2a Fc constant regions were given alongside immunisations with OVA to mice adoptively transferred with OVA-specific CD4+ and CD8+ T cells enabling an OVA-specific T cell response to be interrogated (White et al. 2011). 3/23 mouse IgG1 vaccination with OVA produced a dramatic increase in anti-OVA Ab levels and expansion of peripheral and splenic CD4+ and CD8+ T cells, indicating that the IgG1 isotype was able to induce both humoral and cell-mediated immune stimulation. Conversely, 3/23 mouse IgG2a was not an immunostimulator, being unable to induce an Ab or CD8+ T cell response. In addition, the mouse IgG1 Ab and parental rat IgG2a activated APCs (splenic DCs) in vitro and in vivo as evidenced by increased expression of CD70 (the TNF receptor ligand expressed on APCs—which provides T cell costimulation, via it receptor CD27) and induced robust B cell activation, proliferation, and prosurvival intracellular signalling, consistent with strong agonistic activity. This was again in contrast to the mouse IgG2a Ab. Experiments involving activatory and inhibitory FcγR knockout mice demonstrated that mouse IgG1 anti-CD40 mAb increased anti-OVA Ab responses and splenic B cell proliferation in wild-type mice and mice lacking activatory FcγRs. In mice lacking the inhibitory FcγRIIb, mouse IgG1 failed to produce anti-OVA Ab responses and failed to stimulate B cell proliferation. Mouse IgG2a anti-CD40 mAb produced only low-level B cell proliferation in wild-type and knockout mice. These findings indicate that engagement with the inhibitory FcγRIIb is responsible for the agonistic ability of the anti-CD40 mAb whilst activatory FcγRs are not required. Therefore, the choice of antibody Fc isotype, which confers differing binding affinities to inhibitory FcγRIIb, has a critical role in determining overall anti-CD40 mAb activity.

In the second pivotal study, a mouse model was set up that enabled the interrogation of an OVA-specific CD8+ T cell response activated by OVA presentation on a DC receptor (DEC205-positive cells) triggered by a chimeric antibody with fused human IgG1 Fc region [DEC-OVA(hIgG1)] (Li and Ravetch 2011). This mAb alongside an agonistic anti-CD40 mAb was then injected into mice whose FcγRs were selectively knocked out or manipulated to provide insights into relationships between FcγR and the final T cell response generated, via a CD40-licensed DC. Mice lacking in activating FcγRs were still able to produce OVA-specific T cells upon OVA-targeting and anti-CD40 mAb stimulation. In contrast, mice lacking the inhibitory FcγRIIb were unable to generate OVA-specific T cell responses with anti-CD40 mAb. With the addition of the immunostimulant Toll-like receptor 3 (TLR3) agonist, poly I:C, OVA-specific T cells were activated indicating the critical requirement of agonistic anti-CD40 mAb to engage with inhibitory FcγRIIb to generate an antigen-specific CD8+ T cell response. This finding demonstrated a potential mechanism to enhance the efficacy of agonistic anti-CD40 mAb by manipulating its Fc region to optimise binding with inhibitory FcγRIIb. Anti-CD40 mAb with Fc isotypes that preferentially bind the inhibitory FcγRIIb (mouse IgG1 and human IgG1) led to expansion, activation and effector activity (IFN-γ secretion), whilst mouse IgG2a, which has 10-fold less affinity to inhibitory FcγRIIb failed to augment a T cell response. A human IgG1 variant with enhanced affinity for inhibitory FcγRIIb further potentiated the T cell response. The anti-tumour activity of these modified anti-CD40 mAb were investigated in an OVA-expressing CD40-negative melanoma mouse model with either mouse FcγRIIb (in wild-type mice) or human FcγRIIb (in humanised transgenic mice). T cell-mediated anti-tumour activity was significantly enhanced by Fc isotypes that preferentially bind the inhibitory FcγRIIb (mouse IgG1 and human IgG1). These findings were replicated in a CD40-negative B cell lymphoma model in the absence of immunisation with a tumour-expressed antigen, with the additional demonstration of resistance to tumour rechallenge at 10 weeks indicating the presence of a memory T cell response. These findings show that T cell-dependent anti-tumour immunity is optimised by anti-CD40 mAb that preferentially binds the inhibitory

FcγRIIb. However, anti-CD40 mAb activity also functions via ADCC, which is driven by activating FcγRs on innate immune effectors (NK cells and monocytes/macrophages) in response ligation with CD40 on CD40-expressing cells. These two mechanisms would appear to be in conflict with one another with respect to which Fc isotype choice is most effective, i.e. one that favours inhibitory FcγRs vs. activatory FcγRs. When the above model was repeated in two CD40+ tumour models, treatment with anti-CD40 mAb enhanced for ADCC (mouse IgG2a) significantly depleted peripheral CD40+ cells but only led to a minor survival advantage in one CD40+ tumour. This was in stark contrast to anti-CD40 mAb enhanced for inhibitory FcγRIIb binding (mouse IgG1), which significantly expanded peripheral CD8+ T cells, resulting in growth arrest in one CD40+ tumour model and long-term survival in the other. The interpretation of these findings is that T cell-dependent cytotoxicity mediated via CD40-induced APC licensing is a more potent anti-tumour effect than ADCC mediated via the recruitment of immune effectors.

The immunostimulatory activity of anti-CD40 mAb is driven by antibody cross-linking mediated by FcγRIIb, which is located on neighbouring cells to antibody-ligated CD40+ cells. Cross-linking of anti-CD40 mAb results in enhanced CD40 receptor clustering and activation, which mimics the effect of endogenous multimeric CD40L (Li and Ravetch 2013). Furthermore, it is the FcγRIIb bioavailability—level of surface expression and its biodistribution that is important for cross-linking and hence in vivo activity, rather than intracellular signalling effects or binding affinity (White et al. 2011). Significantly, the binding affinities of specific FcγR do not directly correlate with their ability to induce anti-CD40 mAb antibody cross-linking. The key immune cells expressing FcγRIIb are most likely DCs and B cells. Mouse DCs express both activating and inhibiting FcγRs whilst B cells exclusively express FcγRIIb. This could suggest that B cells are more important determinants of anti-CD40 mAb activity, through activation of humoral responses and as APCs, stimulating cellular T cell-mediated responses.

Recently, White et al. demonstrated anti-CD40 mAb isotype being a critical determinant of therapeutic activity, correlating with the degree of FcγRIIb engagement, with mouse IgG1 conferring long-term tumour protection in a syngeneic B cell lymphoma model, in contrast to the inactive mouse IgG2a (White et al. 2014). In contrast with direct-targeting anti-CD20 mAb, complete responses were achieved in large established tumours with relatively small doses of agonistic anti-CD40 mAb, highlighting the effectiveness of immunostimulation. Anti-tumour immunity was dependent on FcγRIIb engagement on the tumour cell itself and not on host cells. This dependence on FcγRIIb may in part reflect its high expression levels on B cells, facilitating the critical cross-linking needed for agonistic activity, since therapeutic efficacy can be reproduced when cross-linking is mediated through upregulated activatory FcγRs or chemically induced independent of FcγR expression. That withstanding, transcoengagement with FcγRIIb successfully mediates receptor cross-linking, whilst barring ADCC-induced depletion of CD40+ targets cells and promoting T cell-mediated tumour protection. These findings are supported by data showing that cross-linking anti-CD40 mAb FGK45 (rat anti-mouse IgG2a) is required to induce B cell activation in vitro and that optimal agonistic activity is FcγRIIb dependent in vitro (Richman and Vonderheide 2014).

Most human anti-cancer mAb are IgG1 isotypes, intentionally selected because of their ability to augment cytotoxic activity with stronger binding to activating FcγR and higher A/I ratios. However, in mice, IgG2a isotypes most share these functional characteristics and represent the appropriate choice when cytotoxic activity is required. Nonetheless, mouse IgG1 isotypes serve as the most potent anti-CD40 mAb agonists for the reasons described. These differences in FcγR coengagement are unique to mouse IgG1/IgG2a and rat IgG2a isotypes and do not exist in human Fc isotypes, particularly with reference to the preferential binding of mouse IgG1 to FcγRIIb. Fc engineering would be a strategy to generate human IgG1 anti-CD40 mAb that have the greatest affinity for FcγRIIb to promote agonistic activity (Vonderheide and Glennie 2013). However, the assumption is that the superior cross-linking ability of FcγRIIb is the same in humans as mice. Furthermore, there may be an ultimate trade-off between enhanced adaptive immunity, principally T cell effector responses, and cytotoxicity mediated by innate immune mediators.

5.6 Fc Engineering

The goal of Fc engineering is to manipulate coengagement between an antibody Fc region and FcγRs on immune effector cells. FcγRIIb-targeted Fc engineering has been shown to potentiate apoptosis and increase anti-tumour activity (Li and Ravetch 2012, 2013; Tobinai et al. 2012).

Considerable progress has been made in generating optimised antibody Fc binding affinity for activating FcγRs, principally FcγRIIIa and FcγRIIa, resulting in enhanced ADCC and ADCP (Desjarlais et al. 2007; Stavenhagen et al. 2007). Antibodies which have been successfully Fc engineered include anti-CD20 mAb, rituximab; anti-Her2/neu mAb, trastuzumab; anti-EGFR mAb, cetuximab; anti-CD52 mAb, alemtuzumab; anti-CD30 mAb, and anti-CD19 mAb (Lazar et al. 2006; Horton et al. 2008). Fc engineering of anti-CD40 mAb that optimises ADCC has been shown to enhance anti-tumour immunity, which is primarily mediated through FcγR-dependent mechanisms (Horton et al. 2010). The Fc-engineered humanised anti-CD40 antibody (XmAbCD40) possessed increased binding affinity for activating FcγRIIIa producing significantly increased NK cell-mediated ADCC, whilst only modestly enhanced FcγRIIa binding produced a smaller increased macrophage-mediated ADCP. XmAbCD40 resulted in almost complete tumour regression in Ramos lymphoma xenograft models in vivo. With a smaller tumour load given intraperitoneally, in contrast to intravenous administration, XmAbCD40 therapy completely eradicated all tumours (n = 15), whilst rituximab eradicated none (P = 0.000076). Despite the anti-tumour effect of XmAbCD40 being statistically significant compared to the non-Fc-engineered anti-CD40 mAb IgG1 analogue, the relative difference was not dramatic with the IgG1 analogue still able to induce tumour shrinkage. Understanding what these results might mean for human patients is not straightforward due to the inherent differences between the human and mouse FcγR systems. XmAbCD40 enhanced binding to mouse-activating FcγRI and FcγRIV, which are expressed on mouse DCs and macrophages but not NK cells. NK cells exclusively express activating FcγRIII in humans and mice. The enhanced binding of XmAbCD40 to mouse FcγRIII or human FcγRIIIa, expressed on NK cells, is much higher in humans relative to mice, suggesting that NK cell-mediated ADCC is of greater importance in humans than mice. Conversely, in mice, macrophage-mediated cellular immunity could be more important with another study demonstrating that the anti-tumour activity of the anti-CD40 mAb SGN-40 occurs via FcγR coengagement on macrophages that mediate ADCP (Oflazoglu et al. 2009). Fc engineering has the potential to optimise Fc-FcγR interactions such that the ability to recruit immune effectors is of greater consequence than the cell surface expression level of the target antigen or antibody epitope specificity.

6 Developed Anti-CD40 mAbs with Early Clinical Trial Data

To date, three agonistic and one antagonistic anti-CD40 mAb (SGN-40, CP-870,893, ChiLob 7/4, and lucatumumab, respectively) have been investigated in early human clinical trials in a range of lymphoid and solid tumours, as monotherapies and in combination with other agents (Tables 1, 2, 3, 4 and 5). These antibodies show marked heterogeneity of activity ranging from strong agonism to antagonism with dose-escalated infusions administered at doses as low as 0.01 mg/kg and as high as 16 mg/kg. The agonistic strength of anti-CD40 is determined either by their ability to stimulate B cell proliferation or their ability to activate B cells through upregulation of costimulatory molecules and cytokine secretion (Carpenter et al. 2009; Rakhmilevich et al. 2012). Concerns about potential toxicity due to autoimmune reactions, severe cytokine release syndrome (CRS), hyper-immune stimulation syndrome leading to AICD, thromboembolic disease (since CD40 is expressed on endothelial cells and platelets), tumour proliferation or angiogenesis have not been realised in early-phase clinical trials in a clinically relevant way. The incidence of severe CRS was observed with the most potent agonist, CP-870,893, in 11 % of patients when administered with weekly dosing; however, this was manageable with no cases of hospitalisation (Ruter et al. 2010). Severe autoimmune reactions, which are associated with approved immunomodulatory antibodies (e.g. anti-CTLA-4 mAb, ipilumumab), have not been observed. Transient, asymptomatic, but occasionally dose-limiting, transaminitis, and thrombocytopenias have been observed but with no suggestion of liver failure, bleeding or disseminated intravascular coagulation (Vonderheide et al. 2007; Advani et al. 2009; Furman et al. 2010; Hussein et al. 2010; Bensinger et al. 2012). Overall, toxicity of

Table 1 Summary of phase I trials of SGN-40 anti-CD40 mAb therapy

Author	Patient characteristics	Anti-CD40 mAb	Treatment arms (n)	Adverse events (n)		Antidrug antibodies (%)	Response (n)	
Hussein et al (2010) Phase I USA NCT00079716 Completed	44 Patients Relapsed/ Refractory advanced MM	SGN-40 Dacetuzumab Humanised mAb Murine CDRs Weak Agonist Fc Region IgG1	**Single-agent SGN-40** 11 cohorts; 1 cycle 0.5–8 mg/kg IV Day 1 0–8 mg/kg Day 4 0.5–16 mg/kg Days 8, 15, and 22 0–16 mg/kg Day 29 MTD 12 mg/kg with steroid premedication	6 DLTs Commonest AEs: • Fatigue 57 % Headache 43 % • CRS 1st dose 41 % • Transaminitis 41 % • Lymphopenia 27 % • Nausea 23 % • Anaemia 21 %	≥G3 SAEs (18 %): • G4 Aseptic meningitis 1 patient • G4 Hyperviscosity syndrome 1 patient • G3 Thrombocytopenia 7 % • G3 anaemia, headache, hypercalcaemia, neutropaenia, renal failure 5 %	1 Patient HAHA Low titre	**OR**	**0/44**
							Best response	SD 9/44 (20 %)
							PD	5/44 (115)
Advani et al. (2009) Phase I USA NCT00103779 Completed	50 Patients Relapsed/ Refractory NHL (DLBCL 42 %) (FL 24 %) (MCL 20 %) (MZL 6 %) (SLL/CLL 2 %) (Others 6 %)		**Single-agent SGN40** 6 Cohorts; 1–2 cycles 1 mg/kg IV Day 1 0–2 mg/kg Day 4 2–4 mg/kg Day 8 3–8 mg/kg Days 15, 22 and 29 MTD not reached	Commonest AEs: • Fatigue 34 % • Pyrexia 22 % • Headache 20 % • Inflammatory eye disorders 12 %	≥G3 SAEs (26 %): • Lymphopenia 18 % • Hyperuricaemia 14 % • Malignant neoplasm progression 10 % • Anaemia 6 % • Pleural effusion 6 % • Thrombocytopenia 4 % • Cardiotoxicity 4 %	None detected	**OR**	**6/50 (12 %)**
							CR	1/50 (2 %)
							PR	5/50 (10 %)
							SD	13/50 (26 %)
							PD	29/50 (58 %)

(continued)

Table 1 (continued)

Author	Patient characteristics	Anti-CD40 mAb	Treatment arms (n)	Adverse events (n)		Antidrug antibodies (%)	Response (n)	
Furman et al. (2010) Phase I USA NCT0028310 Completed	12 Patients Relapsed CLL Prior purine-analogue containing regimen		**Single-agent SGN40** 4 Cohorts; 1–2 cycles 1–4 mg/kg IV Days 1, 4 and 8 3–8 mg/kg Days 15, 22 and 29 of cycle 1 and Days 1, 15, 29 and 43 of cycle 2 MTD not reached	1 DLT Commonest AEs: • Fatigue 50 % • Headache 33 % • Anorexia 25 % • Conjunctivitis 17 %	≥G3 AE: • G3–4 Thrombocytopenia 17 % • G3 Neutropaenia 8 %	None detected	**OR**	**0/12**
							Best response	SD 5/12 (42 %)
							PD	7/12 (58 %)

MM multiple myeloma; *CDR* complimentarity-determining region; *DLT* dose-limiting toxicities; *MDT* maximum-tolerated dose; *AE* adverse event; *SAE* serious adverse event; *CRS* cytokine release syndrome; *HAHA* human anti-human antibodies; *γ-GTP* γ-glutamyl transpeptidase; *OR* objective response; *CR* complete response; *PR* partial response; *SD* stable disease; *PD* progressive disease; *NHL* non-Hodgkin's lymphoma; *DLBCL* Diffuse large B cell lymphoma; *FL* follicular lymphoma; *MCL* mantle cell lymphoma; *MZL* marginal zone lymphoma; *SLL* small lymphocytic lymphoma; *CLL* chronic lymphocytic lymphoma; *VTE* venous thromboembolism; *PE* pulmonary embolus; *RCC* renal cell carcinoma

Table 2 Summary of Phase I trials of CP-870,893 anti-CD40 mAb therapy

Author	Patient characteristics	Anti-CD40 mAb	Treatment arms (n)	Adverse events (n)		Antidrug antibodies (%)	Response (n)	
Vonderheide et al. (2007) Phase I Completed	29 Patients Advanced solid tumours: Melanoma 52 % NSCLC 17 % Sarcoma 10 % Cholangioncarcinoma 7 % Breast cancer 3 % + others	CP-870,893 Human mAb No murine sequences Agonist Fc Region IgG2	**Single-agent CP-870,893** Redosing for responders 6 dose levels (mg/kg): 0.01, 0.03, 0.06, 0.1, 0.2, 0.3 MTD 0.2 mg/kg	3 DLT Commonest AEs: • G1-2 CRS 55 %	≥G3 AE: G3-4 Lymphopenia 45 % G3 Electrolyte disturbance 24 % G3 Transaminitis 10 % <1 %: G3 Pericardial effusion, G3 Pneumonia, G4 Seizure, G3 Headache, G4 PE, G3 Bone pain	None detected	**OR**	**4/29 (14 %)**
							Best response	PR 4/29 (14 %) (Melanoma)
							SD	7/29 (24 %)
							PD	18/20 (62 %)
Ruter et al. (2010) Phase I Completed	27 Patients Advanced solid tumours: Melanoma 41 % Breast cancer 11 % Mesotheioma 7 % RCC 7 % + others (13 in total)		**Single-agent CP-870,893** Weekly administration 4 dose levels (mg/kg): 0.05, 0.1, 0.2, 0.25 MTD 0.2mg/kg	2 DLT (CRS, urticaria) Commonest AEs: • CRS any grade (56 %)	≥G3 AE: G3 Abdominal pain 7 % G3 CRS 11 % G4 PE 1 patient G3 Autoimmune diabetes 1 patient	None detected	**OR**	**0/27**
							Best response	SD 7/27 (26 %)
							PD	20/27 (74 %)

NSCLC Non-small cell lung cancer; *RCC* renal cell carcinoma; *VTE* venous thromboembolism; *PE* pulmonary embolus

Table 3 Summary of phase I/II trials of Lucatumumab anti-CD40 mAb therapy

Author	Patient characteristics	Anti-CD40 mAb	Treatment arms (n)	Adverse events (n)		Antidrug antibodies (%)	Response (n)	
Bryd et al. (2012) Phase I NCT00108108 Completed	26 Patients Symptomatic CLL Relapsed/ refractory to fludarabine-based regimen(s)	Lucatumumab (HCD122) Human Ab Strong Antagonist Fc Region: IgG1	**Single-agent Lucatumumab** Weekly ×4 5 dose levels (mg/kg): 0.3, 1.0, 3.0, 4.5, 6.0 MTD 3.0 mg/kg	4 DLT (fat enzyme elevation): Commonest AEs Chills (54 %), Nausea (46 %), Hypotension (35 %), Arthralgia, Pyrexia (27 %), Diarrhoea, Vomiting, Fatigue (23 %)	≥G3 AE: Elevated lipase 19 % Neutropaenia 11 % Dyspnoea, elevated amylase, pneumonia 8 %	None detected	**OR**	**1/26 (3.8 %)**
							Best response	PR 1/26 (3.8 %)
							SD	17/26 (65 %)
							Mean duration	76 days (range 29–504)
							PD	5/26 (19 %)
Bensinger et al. (2012) Phase I NCT00231166 Completed	28 Patients Relapsed/ Refractory MM		**Single-agent Lucatumumab** Weekly ×4 for 1–2 cycles 4 dose levels (mg/kg): 1.0, 3.0, 4.5, 6.0 MTD 4.5 mg/kg	3 DLT Commonest AEs: Infusion reactions (71 %) Chills (54 %), Hypoalbuminaemia, Hyperglycaemia (75 %), Hypophosphataemia (50 %), Transaminitis (43 %), Elevated lipase, Hypokalaemia (39 %), Hyponatraemia (36 %), Elevated Creatinine, Headache, Hypotension, Pyrexia (32 %), Fatigue (29 %)	Commonest ≥G3 AE: Lymphopenia (93 %), Leucopenia (25 %), Anaemia (21 %), Neutropaenia (18 %), Thrombocytopenia (11 %), Elevated lipase (11 %), Hypophosphataemia (11 %)	n/a	**OR**	**1/28 (4 %)**
							Best response	PR 1/28 (4 %)
							SD	12/28 (43 %)
							Mean duration	61 days (range 17–798)
							PD	10/28 (36 %)

(continued)

Table 3 (continued)

Author	Patient characteristics	Anti-CD40 mAb	Treatment arms (n)	Adverse events (n)		Antidrug antibodies (%)	Response (n)	
Fanale et al. (2014) Phase Ia/II NCT00670592 Completed	111 Patients Relapsed/ Refractory lymphomas FL (19 %) DLBCL (30 %) MALT (6 %) MCL (11 %) HL (33 %)		**Single-agent Lucatumumab** Weekly ×4 of 8 week cycle Retreatment for ≥SD 2 dose levels: 3–4 mg/kg MTD 4 mg/kg	6 DLT Commonest AEs: Chills (39 %) Pyrexia (34 %) Fatigue (25 %) Nausea (23 %) Dyspnea (22 %)	Commonest ≥G3 AE: Lipase increased (25 %)	n/a[a]	**FL OR**	**7/21 (33 %)**
							FL CR	1/21 (4.8 %)
							FL PR	6/21 (28.6 %)
							FL SD	11/21 (52 %)
							FL PD	3/21 (14 %)
							DLBCL OR	**4/34 (11.8 %)**
							DLBCL CR	2/34 (5.9 %)
							DLBCL PR	2/34 (5.9 %)
							DLBCL SD	11/34 (32 %)
							DLBCL PD	15/34 (44 %)
							HL OR	**5/37 (13.5 %)**
							HL CR	0/37
							HL PR	5/37 (13.5 %)
							HL SD	12/37 (32 %)
							HL PD	14/37 (37.8 %)
							Best response MCL SD	5/12 (41.7 %)

DLBCL diffuse large B cell lymphoma; *FL* follicular lymphoma; *HL* Hodgkin lymphoma; *MALT* mucosa-associated lymphatic tissue lymphoma; *MCL* mantle cell lymphoma

[a] anti-lucatumumab antibodies were measured however no results provided

Table 4 Summary of combination therapy trials with anti-CD40 mAb therapy

Author	Patient characteristics	Anti-CD40 mAb	Treatment arms (n)	Adverse events (n)		Antidrug antibodies (%)	Response (n)	
Fayad et al. (2011) Phase IIb NCT00529503 Terminated	151 Patients with refractory DLBCL Futility analysis lead to early trial termination as response rate was not improved with SGN-40	SGN-40 Dacetuzumab Humanised mAb Murine CDRs Weak Agonist Fc Region IgG1	**R-ICE +/− SGN-40** SGN-40 2–8 mg/kg IV; D-1, 3, 8, 15 of Cycle 1, and D1, 8, 15 of Cycles 2, 3 Rituximab 375 mg/m^2 IV; D-2 of Cycle 1, and D1 Cycles 2, 3; Etoposide 100 mg/m^2 IV; D1-3 of Cycles 1–3; Carboplatin AUC = 5 mg/mL min IV; D2 of Cycles 1–3 Ifosfamide 5 g/m^2 24 h. IV; D2 of Cycles 1–3				R-ICE + SGN-40	ORR 64 % CR 36 %
							R-ICE alone	ORR 68 % CR 42 %
Beatty et al. (2013) Phase I NCT00711191 Completed	22 Patients Advanced chemotherapy-naive pancreatic ductal adenocarcinoma	CP-870,893 Human mAb No murine sequences Agonist Fc Region IgG2	**Gemcitabine + CP-870,893** CP-870,893 0.1–0.2 mg/kg D3 Gemcitabine 1000 mg/m^2 IV weekly ×3 4-week cycles CP-870,893 MTD 0.2 mg/kg	1 DLT (stroke) Commonest AEs: CRS (85 %) Fatigue (85 %) Transaminitis (85 %) Hyperglycaemia (85 %) Anaemia (77 %) Hypocalcaemia (77 %) Nausea (77 %) Lymphopenia (54 %) Vomiting (46 %) Pyrexia (46 %) Constipation (46 %)	Commonest ≥G3 AE: Lymphopenia (23 %) Hyperglycaemia (18 %) Neutropaenia (14 %) CRS 1 patient Stroke 1 patient	n/a	**OR**	**4/22 (19 %)**
							Best response	PR 4/22 (19 %)
							SD	11/22 (50 %)
							Median PFS	5.2 months [95 % CI, 1.9–7.4]
							Median OS	8.4 months [95 %CI, 5.3–11.8]
							1-year OS	28.6 %

(continued)

Table 4 (continued)

Author	Patient characteristics	Anti-CD40 mAb	Treatment arms (n)	Adverse events (n)		Antidrug antibodies (%)	Response (n)	
Vonderheide et al. (2013) Phase I NCT00607048 Completed	32 Patients Advanced solid tumours: Melanoma 78 % + others (7 in total)	CP-870,893 Human mAb No murine sequences Agonist Fc Region IgG2	**Paclitaxel + Carboplatin + CP-870,893** Paclitaxel 175 mg/m^2 IV D1 Carboplatin AUC6 IV D1 CP-870,893 0.1–0.2 mg/kg IV D3 OR D8 21-day cycles MTD 0.2 mg/kg	2 DLTs Commonest AEs: Fatigue (81 %) Peripheral neuropathy (46 %) CRS (42 %) Neutropaenia (38 %)	SAEs G5 intracranial haemorrhage 1 patient G4 Febrile neutropaenia 1 patient	None detected	**OR**	**6/30 (20 %)**
							Best response	PR 6/30 (20 %)
							Mean duration	75 days [50–96]
							SD	12/30 (40 %)
							PD	12/30 (40 %)
Forero-Tores et al. (2013) Phase Ib NCT00655837 Completed	33 Patients Relapsed/Refractory DLBCL 61 % Transformed 30 % Follicular G3 9 %	SGN-40 Dacetuzumab Humanised mAb Murine CDRs Weak agonist Fc Region IgG1	**SGN-40 + Rituximab + Gemcitabine** SGN-40 4–12 mg/kg IV; Days 1, 4, 8, 15 and 22 of Cycle 1 and Days 1, 8 and 15 of Cycles 2–8. Rituximab 375 mg/m^2 IV; Days 2, 8, 15 and 22 of Cycle 1 and Day 1 of Cycles 2–8. Gemcitabine 1000 mg/m^2 IV; Days 1 and 15 of all Cycles	Commonest AEs: CRS (61 %) Nausea (42 %) Fatigue (36 %) Thrombocytopenia (36 %) Headache (30 %)	SAEs (45 %) Commonest ≥G3 AE: Thrombocytopenia (36 %) Hypokalaemia (18 %) Neutropaenia (15 %) Pneumonia (15 %) G3 Cardiomyopathy 1 patient G5 Pneumonitis 1 patient	None detected	OR	14/30 (47 %)
							CR	6/30 (20 %)
							PR	8/30 (27 %)
							Median PFS	25 weeks [95 % CI.15–36.6]

NSCLC non-small cell lung cancer; *RCC* renal cell carcinoma; *VTE* venous thromboembolism; *PE* pulmonary embolus

Table 5 Active trials with anti-CD40 mAb therapy at the time of writing (epub 5/2/2015)

Anti-CD40 mAb	Study type	Tumour type	Cotreatment	Sample size	Clinical trials.gov identifier
Chi Lob 7/4	Phase I	NHL	None	30	NCT01561911
CP-870,893	Phase I	Metastatic melanoma	Tremelimumab	32	NCT01103635
	Phase I	NHL	Rituximab	22	NCT00556699
	Phase II	NHL	None	46	NCT00435916
Dacetuzumab (SGN-40)	Phase I	MM	Lenalidamide and Dexamethasone	38	NCT00525447
	Phase Ib	MM	Bortezomib	18	NCT00664898
Lucatumumab (HCD122)	Phase I	NHL	Bendamustine	50	NCT01275209

NHL non-Hodgkin's lymphoma; *MM* multiple myeloma

anti-CD40 mAb has been acceptable, including in combination with multi-agent chemotherapy.

Immune pharmacodynamic analysis of patients treated with the IgG1 chimeric agonistic anti-CD40 mAb—ChiLob7/4 failed to produce an augmented response in combination with DC-activating TLR ligands (LPS and CpG) (Chowdhury et al. 2014). Notably, the IgG2 fully human agonistic anti-CD40 mAb—CP-870,893 has produced augmented B cell activation in combination with CpG TLR9 stimulation (Carpenter et al. 2009). Similarly, the cytokines TNF-α and IL-6, associated with a classical cytokine storm, were not detected in ChiLob 7/4-treated patients but have been in CP-870,893-treated patients (Vonderheide et al. 2007). These differences suggest that the antibody FcγR isotypes are important determinants of biologic activity and the potential for toxicity. Equally, the choice of antibody IgG isotype is critical to its function with anti-CD40 IgG2 mAb (CP-870,893) principally mediating its effects via DC and macrophage activation, whilst anti-CD40 IgG1 mAbs (SGN-40, ChiLob7/4) principally augment ADCC and CDC (Vonderheide and Glennie 2013). Interestingly, FcγR, both activating and inhibiting, bind IgG1 with greater affinity than IgG2 isotypes, with the inhibitory FcγRIIb binding to IgG2 with the lowest affinity compared to all other Fc isotypes (Bruhns et al. 2009; Bruhns 2012).

6.1 Dacetuzumab (SGN-40)

SGN-40, developed by Seattle Genetics Inc., is a humanised anti-CD40 IgG1 mAb with murine complementarity-determining regions (CDRs) that target CD40. Through multiple discrete mechanisms, SGN-40 is capable of inducing apoptosis in cultured NHL cells in vivo by augmenting effector CTL responses, ADCC, ADCP, and direct apoptotic signalling (Law et al. 2005; Oflazoglu et al. 2009). The humanised SGN-40 was developed from the chimeric anti-CD40 mAb SGN-14, which itself was derived from the murine mAb S2C6 (Francisco et al. 2000). Both murine and humanised antibodies recognise the same epitope. In contrast to other anti-CD40 mAbs, SGN-14, and SGN-40 are weak or partial agonists (K_d of ~ 1 nmol/L) for resting B cells and do not block CD40/CD40L interactions in vitro. Preclinical studies have identified immune effector functioning via ADCC and direct apoptotic signalling via caspase-3 activation as key mechanisms responsible for SGN-40 anti-tumour activity. The precise pathway leading to caspase-3-mediated apoptosis has not been elucidated, with neutralising anti-FasL antibodies failing to suppress apoptosis of lymphomatous B cells treated with SGN-40, suggesting a Fas-independent pathway. The combination use of SGN-40 with cycloheximide (CHX), a protein synthesis inhibitor, sensitises MM cell lines to CD40-mediated apoptosis (Tai et al. 2004). Specifically, SGN-40 led to downregulation of the IL-6 receptor and upregulation of multiple cytotoxic TNF ligands (FasL, TRAIL, and TNF-α). Utilising multiple death signals results in apoptosis mediated by several pathways that activate specific caspases. CHX blocks the anti-apoptotic protein FLIP (FLICE (FADD-like IL-1β-converting enzyme) inhibitory protein). These findings suggested a role for combination therapy with SGN-40. Proliferation assays have shown that SGN-40 does not stimulate resting B cells and is therefore unlikely to lead to an expansion of normal circulating haematopoietic CD40+ cells (Law et al. 2005).

The first-in-human phase I trial examining SGN-40 was conducted in 44 patients with recurrent/refractory advanced MM that had a median number of 5 previous systemic therapies (Table 1) (Hussein et al. 2010). This multicentre trial utilised a 3 + 3 conventional study design with patient cohorts receiving weekly or initial biweekly SGN-40 with sequential intrapatient dose escalation for 4–5 weeks in total. The dosing range was broad between 0.5 mg/kg weekly ×4 up to 8–16 mg/kg weekly ×5, with a corresponding C_{max} between 12.1 and 636 μg/mL. Treatment was generally well tolerated, 41 % developed CRS associated with first infusion, which reduced with subsequent treatments and steroid premedication. 6 patients experienced dose-limiting toxicity (DLT), no objective responses (OR) were observed and the best clinical response was stable disease (SD) in 20 %, which was unrelated to dose. 12 % of patients had 1-level improvement in ECOG performance status. The maximum-tolerated dose (MTD) was 12 mg/kg/week with dose escalation and steroid premedication.

The phase I trial of SGN-40 in relapsed/refractory NHL subtypes was performed in 50 patients using a dose escalation schedule over 5 weeks with a maximum weekly dose of 8 mg/kg (Advani et al. 2009). 13 patients (26 %) achieving stable disease or better went on to receive a second cycle of 4 infusions of SGN-40. The MTD was not established at the doses tested, and there was no dose-response relationship, with responses seen at 3 mg/kg and higher. The ORR was 12 % with one DLBCL patient achieving a durable CR for greater than a year. Two patients who discontinued the study due to adverse events went on to have delayed and durable CRs. Variable degrees of elevation were observed in the concentration of plasma cytokines IL-1β, IL-6, IL-10, and TNF-α in response to SGN-40. The degree of CD40 expression was not correlated with clinical response. SGN-40 was generally tolerable with adverse events being less frequent in cycle 2 suggesting tolerability with extended therapy.

A small 12-patient phase I trial of SGN-40 was conducted in patients with CD40-positive CLL with a median of 4 prior systemic therapies (range 2–11) (Furman et al. 2010). The study design was similar to other SGN-40 phase I trials with 3 patient cohorts following intrapatient dose escalation of 3–8 mg/kg/week for up to 9 weeks (equivalent to 2 cycles). The aim of this design was to reduce first dose CRS, alongside paracetamol/antihistamine premedication. No SAEs were observed, Grade 4 thrombocytopenia was the only DLT, and the MTD was not reached. There were no objective responses with the best clinical response being SD in 42 %. The study authors postulated that prior immunosuppressive therapies and the burden of disease are possible factors that negatively affected efficacy to SGN-40. Based on these modest results, the investigators documented that phase II monotherapy of SGN-40 in CLL would not be pursued.

Overall, SGN-40 is well tolerated with mild side effects, unrelated to dose, which most commonly reflect mild, self-limiting CRS symptoms (e.g. headache, fatigue, fever, etc.) or non-infectious inflammatory eye disorders such as conjunctivitis and blepharitis. Drug-related side effects such as conjunctivitis and mild asymptomatic transaminitis are likely to reflect CD40 expression on conjunctiva and hepatic Kuppfer cells, respectively. The efficacy of SGN-40 as a monotherapy is modest across the tumour types tested.

6.2 CP-870,893

CP-870,893 (Pfizer) is a fully human anti-CD40 IgG2, kappa, mAb that binds human CD40 with sub-nanomolar affinity (K_d of 0.4 nmol/L) augmenting DC costimulatory molecule expression and cytokine secretion. CP-870,893 has poor complement activation and minimal FcR binding on effector cells due to its IgG2 isotype and does not block CD40L binding (Bedian et al. 2006). Recent data have confirmed that CP-870,893 does not elicit ADCC or CDC in $CD40^{hi}$ cancer cell lines in vitro and is not dependent on FcγR interactions or antibody cross-linking for it biologic activity (Richman and Vonderheide 2014). Thus, its mechanism of action is not to kill by direct targeting and cell deletion, but rather through indirect activation of DCs and macrophages (Kalbasi et al. 2010; Vonderheide and Glennie 2013). Agonist activity was determined as CP-870,893 upregulates MHC Class II, CD80, CD86, CD23, and ICAM-1 surface molecules when incubated with human whole blood, with an EC50 of 5–50 ng/ml. High levels of IL-12, a T cell stimulating factor, were secreted when human monocyte-derived DCs were stimulated with CP-870,893. In vitro and primate studies with CP-870,893 demonstrated activation of APCs, a rapid depletion in circulating B cells, upregulated B cell surface markers and enhanced immunogenicity of CD40-positive tumour cells susceptible to eradication by human CTLs. One hypothesis for the rapid but transient reduction of circulating B cells is that CP-870,893 increases expression of the adhesion molecule ICAM-1 and chemokine CCR7, driving B cells into the tumour and secondary lymphoid organs (Carpenter et al. 2009). However, no lymphadenopathy or acute splenomegaly was seen in the phase I trial (Vonderheide et al. 2007). Single intraperitoneal injections of CP-870,893 into CD40-positive human tumours in SCID beige mice induced growth arrest of B cell lymphomas, the breast carcinoma BT-474, and the prostate tumour PC-3 (Gladue et al. 2006). Additional in vitro studies further demonstrated the agonist ability of CP-870,893 with activation of both naive CD19+ and memory CD19+CD27+ B cells triggering the expression of immunostimulatory molecules (CD86, CD70, CD40, and MHC class I and II), with B cells acting as conditioned APCs leading to activation of reactive T cells with effector cytokine secretion (IL-2 and IFN-γ) (Carpenter et al. 2009). The half-life of CP-870,893 was found to be less than 24 h in two human studies. Tumour regression was seen in combination with a sub-optimal dose of cisplatin chemotherapy. Modest objective anti-tumour activity was seen in the first phase I trial (Table 2); however, weekly dosing resulted in little efficacy which may reflect immune overstimulation and subsequent relative immunosuppression (Vonderheide et al. 2007; Ruter et al. 2010).

The first human phase I clinical trial of CP-870,893 monotherapy was performed in 29 patients with advanced solid malignancies, which included melanoma, non-small cell lung cancer (NSCLC), sarcoma, cholangiocarcinoma, and several others (Vonderheide et al. 2007). Six single-dose levels were explored between 0.01 and 0.3 mg/kg, with repeat dosing available for responders. Three patients experienced DLT with a MTD established at 0.2 mg/kg. Pharmacodynamic testing showed a rapid but transient, dose-dependent reduction in circulating CD19+ B cells and up to 10-fold increase in CD86 costimulatory molecule expression. CP-870,893 was well tolerated, with the commonest adverse event being mild transient CRS associated with elevated serum TNF-α and IL-6 in some patients. Normal serum tryptase levels were used to indicate that CRS was not an anaphylactic or allergic reaction. Two melanoma patients developed widespread vitiligo, suggestive of T cell-dependent autoimmunity. The best responses were seen in four patients with advanced melanoma achieving partial responses, one of which continued to respond beyond 14 months from first dose and has been described separately as achieving complete remission after 5 years (Vonderheide and Glennie 2013).

Due to the encouraging results of CP-870,893, a second phase I trial was conducted with weekly administration in 27 patients with multiple advanced solid tumours (Ruter et al. 2010). The weekly dosing schedule was designed according to the pharmacodynamics profile of CP-870,893 with effects such as transaminitis resolving within 1 week from administration. Overall, good tolerability was observed, with an MTD of 0.2 mg/kg, the same established in the initial phase I trial and defined by a similar incidence of CRS with typical transient self-limiting symptoms such as rigours, fever, and chills. Grade 3 CRS was used to describe prolonged or recurrent symptoms; however, no patients required hospitalisation. Lymphocytes, monocytes, and platelets were transiently depleted, returning to normal 24–48 h after infusion of CP-870,893; however, platelet recovery was slower. This reflects CD40 expression on these cell populations. Elevated liver enzymes returned to baseline prior to the next infusion. The best response observed was SD in 26 %, seen at all dosing levels, with a median time to progression of just over 4 months in these patients. Weekly dosing of CP-870,893 is feasible; however, no objective clinical responses were observed. Similar to previous in vitro and in vivo data, there was upregulation of B cell costimulatory and adhesion molecules, consistent with B cell activation, which was sustained above baseline levels and observed with each dose. There was inter-patient variation of baseline peripheral T cell populations; however, 50 % of patients tested post-treatment had marked depletion of CD4+ and CD8+ T cell subsets with inconsistent functional capability as determined by IFN-γ and perforin expression, respectively. These findings are consistent with mouse melanoma models where anti-CD40 mAb treatment alone accelerated depletion of tumour-specific CD8+ T cells producing a negative effect of cancer therapy (Kedl et al. 2001). These tumour-specific CD8+ T cells could be rescued when anti-CD40 mAb was given with selective tumour antigen vaccination. In another study, mice immunised with agonistic anti-CD40 mAb with IL-2 or IL-15 (an important cytokine for memory T cell development) had significant primary anti-tumour response but subsequently developed marked CD4+ T cell apoptosis with impaired secondary memory responses, succumbing to secondary tumour challenge (Berner et al. 2007). Despite the ability of CP-870,893 to activate B cells with APC capacity, the induction of specific anti-tumour T cells was not observed. The study authors concluded that the lack of clinical responses observed may reflect to frequent dosing of CP-870,893, leading to immune hyperstimulation with counterproductive peripheral T cell depletion and persistent B cell stimulation. This is supported by the immunosuppressive effect seen with daily agonistic anti-CD40 mAb administration used to treat chronic autoimmune inflammatory rheumatoid arthritis in mouse models (Mauri et al. 2000).

6.3 ChiLob 7/4

ChiLob 7/4 is an IgG1 chimeric agonistic anti-CD40 mAb (K_d of 0.2 nmol/L) developed by the University of Southampton. The phase I trial of ChiLob 7/4 monotherapy is currently ongoing (Table 5), involving a dose-escalation study design of 4 weekly IV infusions at a range from 0.5 to 240 mg/dose in 28 CD40-positive patients with a range of solid (n = 26) and lymphoid malignancies (DLBCL; n = 2) (Johnson et al. 2010, 2013). Preliminary data reported the best clinical responses observed have been stable disease, seen in 11 of the first 21 patients, with one mesothelioma patient achieving prolonged disease stabilisation after receiving a single 1.6 mg initial dose. The same patient was retreated after more than 3 years with a 240 mg dose achieving ongoing stable disease in excess of 17 months. ChiLob 7/4 was tolerable, with infusion reactions prevented by steroid premedication and dose-limiting Grade 3 hepatic transaminitis observed in two patients at 240 mg single dose. Human anti-chimeric antibody (HACA) responses were common at low doses (5–50 mg) but absent at higher doses (160–240 mg), corresponding with dose-dependent partial depletion of peripheral blood CD19+ B cells. Activation of innate immune effectors, NK cells and monocytes, was detected by elevated CD54 expression at doses of 160 mg or above, but there was no consistent change in T cell markers suggestive of activation.

Alongside the phase I study, investigators monitored the effects of ChiLob 7/4 on the activation of myeloid dendritic cells (mDC1), plasmacytoid dendritic cells (pDC) and cytokine profiles by performing ex vivo whole-blood stimulation assays on the peripheral blood of study participants (Chowdhury et al. 2014). When ChiLob 7/4 was cross-linked with a goat anti-human IgG Fcγ-specific antibody, it was able to upregulate CD83 on pDCs and mDC1s in a dose-dependent manner, indicating early dendritic cell activation. Similarly, increases in various Th1 cytokines (IL-12, MIP1a, MIP1b, IL-8, IL-6, and TNF-α) were detected with increasing concentration of Fc receptor cross-linked ChiLob 7/4. The activation capacity of ChiLob 7/4 to induce dendritic cell maturation and migration, as evidenced by the upregulation of the chemokine receptor CCR7, was quantified by comparison with known DC-activating TLR ligands. When cross-linked, ChiLob 7/4 showed near-equivalent levels in activating DCs when compared to the potent TLR ligand LPS, but occurred more rapidly, with mDC1 CCR7 upregulation detectable after 4 h. A similar cytokine profile was generated with cross-linked ChiLob 7/4 to that of LPS; however, IL-6 expression was significantly lower with ChiLob 7/4 suggesting an overall lower pro-inflammatory response. The fact that ChiLob 7/4 has a human IgG1 Fc portion and relatively low binding affinity to inhibitory FcγRIIb, thus limiting the opportunity for cross-linking, may be suggestive that IgG1 is not the ideal isotype to exploit its immunostimulatory activity.

In vivo effects of ChiLob 7/4 on circulating DCs and cytokine expression were investigated through sequential blood sampling of study participants. Two of the cytokines that are frequently associated with a cytokine storm (TNFa and IL-6) were not detectable in samples from ChiLob 7/4-treated patients. However, this may reflect missed detection due to time point sampling or steroid-induced cytokine suppression. Overall, stronger CD40 stimulation was required to trigger cytokine production than DC activation. Despite the heterogenous patient population producing a mixed pattern of DC activation kinetics, similarities were observed with higher ChiLob 7/4 doses in the ex vivo analysis with artificial cross-linking. This suggests that some degree of antibody cross-linking may be occurring in vivo after administration with the soluble non-cross-linked drug. The biologic activity of agonistic anti-CD40 mAb is dependent on FcγR cross-linking which provides a structural scaffold to enable CD40 signalling.

7 Antagonistic Anti-CD40 mAb

7.1 Lucatumumab (HCD122)

Lucatumumab (Novartis) is a fully humanised anti-CD40 IgG1 mAb that augments ADCC and blocks the ligation of CD40L with CD40. Lucatumumab binds to CD40 with high affinity (K_d of 0.5 nmol/L) has a slow 'off-rate' with preclinical studies showing lucatumumab to be a potent CD40L antagonist inhibiting signalling pathways, secretion of cytokines, differentiation, proliferation and survival (Luqman et al. 2008). Lucatumumab inhibits CD40L-mediated growth of normal B cells, NHL cells and CLL cells in vitro (Byrd et al. 2012). Lucatumumab, formerly named CHIR-12.12, binds to CD138-expressing MM lines, inhibiting PI3K/AKT, NF-κB, and ERK activation induced by CD40L, antagonising CD40L-induced proliferation and triggering lysis via ADCC in CD40-positive cells (Tai et al. 2005a, b). Lucatumumab was shown to have strong antagonistic activity in B cell CLL tumour cells causing ADCC mediated lysis more efficiently than rituximab in vitro, despite nearly sixfold higher CD20 cell surface binding sites compared to CD40. This effect was thought to be because lucatumumab, unlike rituximab, is not internalised but remains uniformly distributed on the cell surface and therefore more responsive to interact with NK cells or other effector cells that mediate ADCC (Luqman et al. 2008). Lucatumumab has potent activity in MM cells in vitro and xenograft models in vivo, significantly prolonging the survival in tumour-bearing mice with tumour regression seen in 63 % ($p < 0.01$) (Long et al. 2005).

A first-in-man phase I trial of lucatumumab monotherapy was conducted in 26 patients with symptomatic, fludarabine-experienced CLL with five dose cohorts between 0.3 and 6.0 mg/kg, receiving weekly infusions for 4 weeks (Table 3.) (Byrd et al. 2012). A MTD was established at 3.0 mg/kg due to four DLTs from asymptomatic elevated lipase/amylase levels with no clinical or radiological evidence of pancreatitis. This effect most likely represented CD40 expression within pancreatic tissue, a phenomenon previously reported (Vosters et al. 2004). Overall, lucatumumab had acceptable tolerability and a half-life of approximately 7 days. The best objective response was a nodular PR in one patient, whilst 65 % of participants achieved SD for a mean duration of 76 days (range 29–504 days). The study authors summarised these results as representing minimal single-agent activity, advising future studies to focus on combination approaches.

A phase I trial of lucatumumab monotherapy was performed in 28 patients with relapsed/refractory MM with four dose levels of 1.0–6.0 mg/kg in weekly infusions for 4–8 weeks (Bensinger et al. 2012). Three DLTs were observed establishing an MTD of 4.5 mg/kg. Numerous AEs were reported, frequently related to infusion reactions that were generally mild to moderate in severity. SAEs included haematological, biochemical and electrolyte disturbances with 14 % of participants discontinuing the study drug as a result of AEs. The ORR was 4 % due to one PR. 43 % of patients achieved SD, lasting on average just over 2 months. The study authors reflect on these modest results by highlighting that the study population was heavily pretreated with a median of eight prior MM therapies and that the 11-week follow-up period may fail to document delayed responders. They postulate potential synergy could exist between lucatumumab and approved agents such as lenalidomide or bortezomib for MM.

A larger phase Ia/II trial of single agent lucatumumab was conducted in 111 patients with multiple NHL subtypes and HD (Fanale et al. 2014). The six DLTs consisted of asymptomatic elevated lipase and transaminitis resulting in a MTD of 4 mg/kg. The half-life at 4 mg/kg was approximately 4.5 days. SAEs occurred in 27.9 % with the most common being secondary to dyspnoea, fever, and chills. Efficacy was subtype specific with an ORR for MALT, FL, HD, and DLBCL of 42.9, 33.3, 13.5, and 11.8 %, respectively. Lucatumumab has overall modest activity as a single agent with several potential mechanisms of action; however, further investigation is required to establish an optimal treatment setting within a particular tumour subtype.

8 CD40 Combination Therapy

As with the monotherapy clinical trials, dacetuzumab causes direct killing of tumour cells whilst CP-870,893 exploits the immunostimulatory capacity of anti-CD40 activation. Overall, the combination studies demonstrate modest clinical efficacy; however, activity in pancreatic cancer by immune stimulation represents a role for immunotherapy in a cancer frequently associated with resistance to conventional cytotoxic chemotherapy. Combining immunotherapy with non-immunoablative chemotherapy has the aim of chemotherapy-induced tumour cell killing leading to increased tumour antigen available for cross-presentation, which when combined with immunomodulatory antibodies increases cross-priming of tumour-specific CTLs (Lake and Robinson 2005). Chemotherapy-induced apoptosis of large murine tumours loads APCs with tumour antigens and sensitises them to CD40 signalling. One study demonstrated that gemcitabine chemotherapy which induced apoptosis in established murine solid tumours (mesothelioma) enabled subsequent synergy with an anti-CD40 mAb (FGK45) leading to long-term tumour remission and resistance to tumour rechallenge indicative of established immunological memory (Nowak et al. 2003). Exogenous CD40 ligation was associated with both CD4+ and CD8+ T cell infiltration into the tumours. However, depletion studies demonstrated that unlike the pivotal role of CD8+ effectors, CD4+ cells were not necessary for tumour rejection.

Alternative approaches with combination studies aimed to increase direct killing of tumour cells through ADCC and direct apoptotic signalling. ADCC assays demonstrated synergy between anti-CD40 mAb (SGN-40) and rituximab showing an additive anti-tumour response with combination therapy (Lewis et al. 2008a, b). SGN-40 appears to chemosensitise lymphoma cells to augment enhanced ADCC with improved efficacy in combination with multi-agent cytotoxic chemotherapy regimens such as ICE (ifosfamide, carboplatin, and etoposide) and CHOP (cyclophosphamide, doxorubicin, vincristine, and prednisolone), both with and without rituximab (Lewis et al. 2007). In vitro and xenograft models combining SGN-40 and rituximab demonstrated a synergistic effect in tumour cell apoptosis; however, SGN-40 did not potentiate rituximab-induced ADCC activity (Lewis et al. 2011). Both agents activated MAP kinase signalling with the oncoprotein BCL-6 being strongly downregulated by SGN-40 in each cell line, whilst this downregulation was cell line-specific with rituximab. SGN-40 alone induced expression of the pro-apoptotic proteins Fas and Tap63 (p53 family member) and rituximab partially blocked SGN-40-mediated induction of prosurvival BCL-xL expression.

An international phase IIb of 151 patients with refractory DLBCL was randomised to receive 3 cycles of R-ICE (rituximab, ifosfamide, cyclophosphamide, etoposide) + dacetuzumab (SGN-40) (8 mg/kg) versus R-ICE + placebo (Table 4) (Fayad et al. 2011). A futility analysis conducted after 112 patients were treated revealed a similar CR (36 % dacetuzumab vs. 42 % placebo) and ORR (64 vs. 68 %), and as a result, further enrolment was stopped. After approximately 1-year follow-up, there was a trend towards improved failure-free survival (FFS) (hazard ratio [HR] = 0.789) and OS (HR = 0.714) for dacetuzumab patients. There was a survival advantage in dacetuzumab patients who went on to receive subsequent autologous stem cell transplant (ASCT) (HR = 0.167, $p = 0.008$) with a 14 % reduction in death due to disease progression (25 % dacetuzumab vs. 39 % placebo). These data are based on results presented at the international conference of malignant lymphoma (ICML), Switzerland, which suggest a potential survival advantage with agonistic anti-CD40 mAb combination therapy despite no improvement in objective tumour response.

A phase I study investigated the role of CP-870,893 in combination with conventional gemcitabine in 22 patients with chemotherapy-naive advanced pancreatic ductal adenocarcinoma (Beatty et al. 2013). CP-870,893 with gemcitabine was well tolerated and associated with early evidence of efficacy with 4 PRs (ORR of 19 %). This is significant when compared to an ORR of just 5.4 % with gemcitabine monotherapy, and 1-year OS of 18 versus 28.6 % with combination therapy (Burris et al. 1997). Pancreatic cancers carry a particularly poor prognosis due to intrinsic chemotherapy resistance and a hostile tumour microenvironment characterised by the presence of tumour-associated macrophages and poor vascularity. Preliminary studies had demonstrated that the use of agonistic anti-CD40 mAb caused CD40-activated tumouricidal macrophages to rapidly infiltrate pancreatic tumours, causing targeted depletion of the tumour stroma (Beatty et al. 2011). Within the trial, combination therapy produced immune stimulation with transient depletion of B cells, increased inflammatory cytokines (IL-6, IL-8, IL-10) and increased B cell costimulatory molecules (CD86 and MHC class II receptor HLA-DR). This immune activation was transient and did not represent a biomarker of response. PET imaging demonstrated metabolic responses within the primary tumour in the majority of patients imaged; however, some patients developed concurrent disease progression of metastatic deposits, highlighting the heterogeneity of tumour response. Large studies are required to better assess anti-tumour efficacy with combination strategies in pancreatic cancer.

A phase I study investigated the role of CP-870,893 when combined with two chemotherapy agents, paclitaxel and carboplatin, in patients with advanced solid tumours (Vonderheide et al. 2013). CP-870,893 was either given on day 3 or 8 post chemotherapy. This scheduling was designed to establish the optimum time point after chemotherapy where released tumour-associated antigens were maximally present to provide an immunogenic stimulus. However, there was no significant difference in response or immune pharmacodynamics between the two schedules. The ORR was 20 % with best responses being PRs seen in patients with metastatic melanoma, renal cell carcinoma, prostate cancer, and ovarian cancer. Responses were observed in some patients who had previously progressed on platinum and taxane chemotherapy, highlighting that efficacy did not simply reflect chemotherapy activity. Toxicity analysis of the three drug combination was considered to be safe; however, one DLT was a fatal stroke occurring six days after the first CP-870,893 infusion. Immune pharmacodynamics analysis showed rapid depletion and activation of peripheral B cells and evidence of transient induction of melanoma-specific T cell responses in two patients tested. These findings were similar to those with CP-870,893 monotherapy leading to the conclusion that chemotherapy does not prevent immune activation. Encouragingly, the peripheral T cell depletion seen with weekly CP-870,893 dosing in the phase I study and preclinical study (Kedl et al. 2001; Ruter et al. 2010) was not observed with three weekly dosing alongside combination chemotherapy.

A phase Ib study investigated the combination of SGN-40, rituximab, and gemcitabine in 33 patients with relapsed/refractory DLBCL (Forero-Torres et al. 2013). The study population was described as predominantly elderly with a median age of 67 (range, 29–80). As mentioned earlier, preclinical studies had previously demonstrated synergy of anti-tumour activity with rituximab and SGN-40 in vivo (Lewis et al. 2008a, b, 2011). The combination of agents was generally well tolerated; however, a relationship between the one fatality and SGN-40 could not be excluded. The cause of the death was secondary to pneumonitis in a patient previously irradiated who received 20 infusions of SGN-40. The frequency of gemcitabine administration was reduced during the trial to overcome the development of thrombocytopenia. The ORR was 47 % with a CR of 20 %, median PFS of 25 weeks and median duration of response of over 6 months. All CRs had high CD40 expression levels (3+) whilst conversely CD40-negative expression was associated with non-response. There was no correlation between FcγRIIa and FcγRIIIa polymorphisms and objective response. The response rate observed was similar to an existing second line regimen with rituximab, gemcitabine, and oxaliplatin (R-GEMOX) (ORR 43 %) (Lopez et al. 2008); however, the CR rate was lower (20 vs. 34 %) and OS was not determined in the SGN-40 study to allow a comprehensive comparison. Long-term results of R-GEMOX demonstrated higher ORR of 57 and 37 % OS at 3.5 years as salvage therapy in transplant ineligible DLBCL patients (Corazzelli et al. 2009).

There are currently several ongoing combination trials involving anti-CD40 mAb with a mixture of chemotherapy and biological agents (Table 5). The study design and choice of agents to combine are based on preclinical studies to determine mechanisms of synergy between agents. For instance, two preclinical studies of SGN-40 and lenalidomide in CLL and MM have shown pretreatment with lenalidomide sensitised MM cells to SGN-40-induced cell death in vitro (Tai et al. 2005a, b; Lapalombella et al. 2009). The combination induced direct apoptosis in MM and CLL and markedly enhanced ADCC of autologous CD40-expressing MM cells and primary CLL B cells. Lenalidomide facilitated IL-2-mediated activation of NK cells and induced more potent mediators of ADCC against target tumour cells.

9 Currently Active Trials

See Table 5.

10 Conclusion

It remains a major scientific goal to address the unmet need for improved anti-cancer therapies to reduce the high burden of morbidity and mortality associated with the many incurable or poorly responsive tumour types. The goal of cancer immunotherapy is to activate the host immune system in a targeted way in order to increase recognition and eradication of malignant cells. The challenge is daunting given the vast hurdles needed to be overcome from initial target identification and validation to preclinical investigation, through to early 'proof of concept' clinical trials, late-phase efficacy, safety, and economic evaluation to final approval. Nonetheless, the last few decades of incremental scientific and clinical progress in this field are coming to fruition with the remarkable results from several approved and emerging immunostimulatory antibodies and immune checkpoint blockers, such as those that target CTLA-4 and PD-1.

The key reason that targeting CD40 to augment protective anti-tumour immunity remains attractive and offers significant therapeutic potential is that it exerts its effects by a plethora of different mechanisms. In broad terms, these include indirect modulation of host immune cells through boosting APC function, activating tumour-specific T cells, NK cells, and tumouricidal macrophages, or direct pro-apoptotic signalling and through the recruitment of innate immune effectors via ADCC/ADCP. Early clinical trials have shown modest clinical activity in the absence of troublesome toxicity. If developed through well-constructed clinical trials, which will most likely involve innovative combinations of agents, with careful attention to scheduling and exploiting multi-agent synergy, anti-CD40 mAb therapy could be harnessed to treat a broad range of lymphoid and solid malignancies. Equally, the development of new anti-CD40 agents that capitalise on the many strengths of existing agents but can be engineered to exploit the importance of engagement with the inhibitory FcγRIIb on neighbouring immune cells to facilitate antibody cross-linking will further potentiate immunostimulatory activity and thus clinical efficacy. The interactions between anti-CD40 mAb and FcγRs are dependent on the nature of the local immune environment and the anatomical location of the FcγRs. The realisation that coengagement with the inhibitory FcγRIIb is essential to the immunostimulatory activity of many anti-CD40 mAb has been a watershed development and stands in contrast to direct-targeting antibodies, which require activatory FcγR interactions to augment activity through cell deletion. The future of immunostimulatory antibody therapy is extremely bright and likely represents our greatest hopes of making a fundamental transformation to the natural course of the many currently incurable human cancers.

References

Advani R, Forero-Torres A, Furman RR, Rosenblatt JD, Younes A, Ren H, Harrop K, Whiting N, Drachman JG (2009) Phase I study of the humanized anti-CD40 monoclonal antibody dacetuzumab in refractory or recurrent non-Hodgkin's lymphoma. J Clin Oncol 27 (26):4371–4377

Ahonen C, Manning E, Erickson LD, O'Connor B, Lind EF, Pullen SS, Kehry MR, Noelle RJ (2002) The CD40-TRAF6 axis controls affinity maturation and the generation of long-lived plasma cells. Nat Immunol 3(5):451–456

Alderson MR, Armitage RJ, Tough TW, Strockbine L, Fanslow WC, Spriggs MK (1993) CD40 expression by human monocytes: regulation by cytokines and activation of monocytes by the ligand for CD40. J Exp Med 178(2):669–674

Armand P, Nagler A, Weller EA, Devine SM, Avigan DE, Chen YB, Kaminski MS, Holland HK, Winter JN, Mason JR, Fay JW, Rizzieri DA, Hosing CM, Ball ED, Uberti JP, Lazarus HM, Mapara MY, Gregory SA, Timmerman JM, Andorsky D, Or R, Waller EK, Rotem-Yehudar R, Gordon LI (2013) Disabling immune tolerance by programmed death-1 blockade with pidilizumab after autologous hematopoietic stem-cell transplantation for diffuse large B-cell lymphoma: results of an international phase II trial. J Clin Oncol 31(33):4199–4206

Armitage RJ, Fanslow WC, Strockbine L, Sato TA, Clifford KN, Macduff BM, Anderson DM, Gimpel SD, Davis-Smith T, Maliszewski CR et al (1992) Molecular and biological characterization of a murine ligand for CD40. Nature 357(6373):80–82

Arpin C, Dechanet J, Van Kooten C, Merville P, Grouard G, Briere F, Banchereau J, Liu YJ (1995) Generation of memory B cells and plasma cells in vitro. Science 268(5211):720–722

Beatty GL, Chiorean EG, Fishman MP, Saboury B, Teitelbaum UR, Sun W, Huhn RD, Song W, Li D, Sharp LL, Torigian DA, O'Dwyer PJ, Vonderheide RH (2011) CD40 agonists alter tumor stroma and show efficacy against pancreatic carcinoma in mice and humans. Science 331 (6024):1612–1616

Beatty GL, Torigian DA, Chiorean EG, Saboury B, Brothers A, Alavi A, Troxel AB, Sun W, Teitelbaum UR, Vonderheide RH, O'Dwyer PJ (2013) A phase I study of an agonist CD40 monoclonal antibody (CP-870,893) in combination with gemcitabine in patients with advanced pancreatic ductal adenocarcinoma. Clin Cancer Res 19(22):6286–6295

Bedian V, Donovan C, Garder J (2006) In vitro characterization and pre-clinical pharmacokinetics of CP-870,893, a human anti-CD40 agonist antibody. J Clin Oncol 24:109s, (suppl; abstr 2539)

Bensinger W, Maziarz RT, Jagannath S, Spencer A, Durrant S, Becker PS, Ewald B, Bilic S, Rediske J, Baeck J, Stadtmauer EA (2012) A phase 1 study of lucatumumab, a fully human anti-CD40 antagonist monoclonal antibody administered intravenously to patients with relapsed or refractory multiple myeloma. Br J Haematol 159(1):58–66

Berberich I, Shu G, Siebelt F, Woodgett JR, Kyriakis JM, Clark EA (1996) Cross-linking CD40 on B cells preferentially induces stress-activated protein kinases rather than mitogen-activated protein kinases. EMBO j 15(1):92–101

Berberich I, Shu GL, Clark EA (1994) Cross-linking CD40 on B cells rapidly activates nuclear factor-kappa B. J Immunol 153(10):4357–4366

Berner V, Liu H, Zhou Q, Alderson KL, Sun K, Weiss JM, Back TC, Longo DL, Blazar BR, Wiltrout RH, Welniak LA, Redelman D, Murphy WJ (2007) IFN-gamma mediates CD4+ T-cell loss and impairs secondary antitumor responses after successful initial immunotherapy. Nat Med 13(3):354–360

Bruhns P (2012) Properties of mouse and human IgG receptors and their contribution to disease models. Blood 119(24):5640–5649

Bruhns P, Iannascoli B, England P, Mancardi DA, Fernandez N, Jorieux S, Daeron M (2009) Specificity and affinity of human Fc gamma receptors and their polymorphic variants for human IgG subclasses. Blood 113(16):3716–3725

Buhtoiarov IN, Lum H, Berke G, Paulnock DM, Sondel PM, Rakhmilevich AL (2005) CD40 ligation activates murine macrophages via an IFN-gamma-dependent mechanism resulting in tumor cell destruction in vitro. J Immunol 174(10):6013–6022

Burington B, Yue P, Shi X, Advani R, Lau JT, Tan J, Stinson S, Stinson J, Januario T, de Vos S, Ansell S, Forero-Torres S, Fedorowicz G, Yang TT, Elkins K, Du C, Mohan S, Yu N, Modrusan Z, Seshagiri S, Yu SF, Pandita A, Koeppen H, French D, Polson AG, Offringa R, Whiting N, Ebens A, Dornan D (2011) CD40 pathway activation status predicts response to CD40 therapy in diffuse large B cell lymphoma. Sci Transl Med 3(74):74ra22

Burris HA 3rd, Moore MJ, Andersen J, Green MR, Rothenberg ML, Modiano MR, Cripps MC, Portenoy RK, Storniolo AM, Tarassoff P, Nelson R, Dorr FA, Stephens CD, Von Hoff DD (1997) Improvements in survival and clinical benefit with gemcitabine as first-line therapy for patients with advanced pancreas cancer: a randomized trial. J Clin Oncol 15(6):2403–2413

Byrd JC, Kipps TJ, Flinn IW, Cooper M, Odenike O, Bendiske J, Rediske J, Bilic S, Dey J, Baeck J, O'Brien S (2012) Phase I study of the anti-CD40 humanized monoclonal antibody lucatumumab (HCD122) in relapsed chronic lymphocytic leukemia. Leuk Lymphoma 53 (11):2136–2142

Carpenter EL, Mick R, Ruter J, Vonderheide RH (2009) Activation of human B cells by the agonist CD40 antibody CP-870,893 and augmentation with simultaneous toll-like receptor 9 stimulation. J Transl Med 7:93

Cartron G, Dacheux L, Salles G, Solal-Celigny P, Bardos P, Colombat P, Watier H (2002) Therapeutic activity of humanized anti-CD20 monoclonal antibody and polymorphism in IgG Fc receptor FcgammaRIIIa gene. Blood 99(3):754–758

Castillo R, Mascarenhas J, Telford W, Chadburn A, Friedman SM, Schattner EJ (2000) Proliferative response of mantle cell lymphoma cells stimulated by CD40 ligation and IL-4. Leukemia 14(2):292–298

Chen L, Ashe S, Brady WA, Hellstrom I, Hellstrom KE, Ledbetter JA, McGowan P, Linsley PS (1992) Costimulation of antitumor immunity by the B7 counterreceptor for the T lymphocyte molecules CD28 and CTLA-4. Cell 71(7):1093–1102

Chowdhury F, Johnson PW, Glennie MJ, Williams AP (2014) Ex vivo assays of dendritic cell activation and cytokine profiles as predictors of in vivo effects in an anti-human CD40 monoclonal antibody ChiLob 7/4 phase I trial. Cancer Immunol Res 2(3):229–240

Clark EA, Ledbetter JA (1986) Activation of human B cells mediated through two distinct cell surface differentiation antigens, Bp35 and Bp50. Proc Natl Acad Sci USA 83(12):4494–4498

Clynes RA, Towers TL, Presta LG, Ravetch JV (2000) Inhibitory Fc receptors modulate in vivo cytotoxicity against tumor targets. Nat Med 6(4):443–446

Cooke PW, James ND, Ganesan R, Wallace M, Burton A, Young LS (1999) CD40 expression in bladder cancer. J Pathol 188(1):38–43

Corazzelli G, Capobianco G, Arcamone M, Ballerini PF, Iannitto E, Russo F, Frigeri F, Becchimanzi C, Marcacci G, De Chiara A, Pinto A (2009) Long-term results of gemcitabine plus oxaliplatin with and without rituximab as salvage treatment for transplant-ineligible patients with refractory/relapsing B-cell lymphoma. Cancer Chemother Pharmacol 64(5):907–916

Costello RT, Gastaut JA, Olive D (1999) What is the real role of CD40 in cancer immunotherapy? Immunol Today 20(11):488–493

Dadgostar H, Zarnegar B, Hoffmann A, Qin XF, Truong U, Rao G, Baltimore D, Cheng G (2002) Cooperation of multiple signaling pathways in CD40-regulated gene expression in B lymphocytes. Proc Natl Acad Sci USA 99(3):1497–1502

Desjarlais JR, Lazar GA, Zhukovsky EA, Chu SY (2007) Optimizing engagement of the immune system by anti-tumor antibodies: an engineer's perspective. Drug Discov Today 12(21–22): 898–910

Eliopoulos AG, Davies C, Knox PG, Gallagher NJ, Afford SC, Adams DH, Young LS (2000) CD40 induces apoptosis in carcinoma cells through activation of cytotoxic ligands of the tumor necrosis factor superfamily. Mol Cell Biol 20(15):5503–5515

Falkson CI, Ibrahim J, Kirkwood JM, Coates AS, Atkins MB, Blum RH (1998) Phase III trial of dacarbazine versus dacarbazine with interferon alpha-2b versus dacarbazine with tamoxifen versus dacarbazine with interferon alpha-2b and tamoxifen in patients with metastatic malignant melanoma: an Eastern Cooperative Oncology Group study. J Clin Oncol 16(5):1743–1751

Fanale M, Assouline S, Kuruvilla J, Solal-Celigny P, Heo DS, Verhoef G, Corradini P, Abramson JS, Offner F, Engert A, Dyer MJ, Carreon D, Ewald B, Baeck J, Younes A, Freedman AS (2014) Phase IA/II, multicentre, open-label study of the CD40 antagonistic monoclonal antibody lucatumumab in adult patients with advanced non-Hodgkin or Hodgkin lymphoma. Br J Haematol 164(2):258–265

Fayad L, Ansell S, Advani R, Coiffier B, Bartlett NL, Stuart R, Forero-Torres A, Kuliczkowski K, Drachman JG (2011) A phase 2B trial comparing dacetuzumab + R-ICE vs placebo + R-ICE in patients with relapsed diffuse large B-cell lymphoma. Ann Oncol 22(Abstract Suppl. 4):145

Fluckiger AC, Durand I, Banchereau J (1994) Interleukin 10 induces apoptotic cell death of B-chronic lymphocytic leukemia cells. J Exp Med 179(1):91–99

Forero-Torres A, Bartlett N, Beaven A, Myint H, Nasta S, Northfelt DW, Whiting NC, Drachman JG, Lobuglio AF, Moskowitz CH (2013) Pilot study of dacetuzumab in combination with rituximab and gemcitabine for relapsed or refractory diffuse large B-cell lymphoma. Leuk Lymphoma 54(2):277–283

Francisco JA, Donaldson KL, Chace D, Siegall CB, Wahl AF (2000) Agonistic properties and in vivo antitumor activity of the anti-CD40 antibody SGN-14. Cancer Res 60(12):3225–3231

French RR, Chan HT, Tutt AL, Glennie MJ (1999) CD40 antibody evokes a cytotoxic T-cell response that eradicates lymphoma and bypasses T-cell help. Nat Med 5(5):548–553

Funakoshi S, Beckwith M, Fanslow W, Longo DL, Murphy WJ (1995) Epstein-Barr virus-induced human B-cell lymphoma arising in HuPBL-SCID chimeric mice: characterization and the role of CD40 stimulation in their treatment and prevention. Pathobiology 63(3):133–142

Funakoshi S, Longo DL, Beckwith M, Conley DK, Tsarfaty G, Tsarfaty I, Armitage RJ, Fanslow WC, Spriggs MK, Murphy WJ (1994) Inhibition of human B-cell lymphoma growth by CD40 stimulation. Blood 83(10):2787–2794

Funakoshi S, Longo DL, Murphy WJ (1996) Differential in vitro and in vivo antitumor effects mediated by anti-CD40 and anti-CD20 monoclonal antibodies against human B-cell lymphomas. J Immunother Emphasis Tumor Immunol 19(2):93–101

Furman RR, Forero-Torres A, Shustov A, Drachman JG (2010) A phase I study of dacetuzumab (SGN-40, a humanized anti-CD40 monoclonal antibody) in patients with chronic lymphocytic leukemia. Leuk Lymphoma 51(2):228–235

Gajewski TF, Meng Y, Blank C, Brown I, Kacha A, Kline J, Harlin H (2006) Immune resistance orchestrated by the tumor microenvironment. Immunol Rev 213:131–145

Gallagher NJ, Eliopoulos AG, Agathangelo A, Oates J, Crocker J, Young LS (2002) CD40 activation in epithelial ovarian carcinoma cells modulates growth, apoptosis, and cytokine secretion. Mol Pathol 55(2):110–120

Galy AH, Spits H (1992) CD40 is functionally expressed on human thymic epithelial cells. J Immunol 149(3):775–782

Ghamande S, Hylander BL, Oflazoglu E, Lele S, Fanslow W, Repasky EA (2001) Recombinant CD40 ligand therapy has significant antitumor effects on CD40-positive ovarian tumor xenografts grown in SCID mice and demonstrates an augmented effect with cisplatin. Cancer Res 61(20):7556–7562

Gladue R, Cole S, Donovan C (2006) In vivo efficacy of the CD40 agonist antibody CP-870,893 against a broad range of tumor types: Impact of tumor CD40 expression, dendritic cells, and chemotherapy. J Clin Oncol Abstract 24(103s):2514

Grewal IS, Flavell RA (1998) CD40 and CD154 in cell-mediated immunity. Annu Rev Immunol 16:111–135

Griffith TS, Wiley SR, Kubin MZ, Sedger LM, Maliszewski CR, Fanger NA (1999) Monocyte-mediated tumoricidal activity via the tumor necrosis factor-related cytokine, TRAIL. J Exp Med 189(8):1343–1354

Hamid O, Robert C, Daud A, Hodi FS, Hwu WJ, Kefford R, Wolchok JD, Hersey P, Joseph RW, Weber JS, Dronca R, Gangadhar TC, Patnaik A, Zarour H, Joshua AM, Gergich K, Elassaiss-Schaap J, Algazi A, Mateus C, Boasberg P, Tumeh PC, Chmielowski B, Ebbinghaus SW, Li XN, Kang SP, Ribas A (2013) Safety and tumor responses with lambrolizumab (anti-PD-1) in melanoma. N Engl J Med 369(2):134–144

Hart DN, McKenzie JL (1988) Isolation and characterization of human tonsil dendritic cells. J Exp Med 168(1):157–170

Heath WR, Carbone FR (1999) Cytotoxic T lymphocyte activation by cross-priming. Curr Opin Immunol 11(3):314–318

Hengartner MO (2000) The biochemistry of apoptosis. Nature 407(6805):770–776

Hill A, Chapel H (1993) X-linked immunodeficiency. The fruits of cooperation. Nature 361 (6412):494

Hirano A, Longo DL, Taub DD, Ferris DK, Young LS, Eliopoulos AG, Agathanggelou A, Cullen N, Macartney J, Fanslow WC, Murphy WJ (1999) Inhibition of human breast carcinoma growth by a soluble recombinant human CD40 ligand. Blood 93(9):2999–3007

Hodi FS, O'Day SJ, McDermott DF, Weber RW, Sosman JA, Haanen JB, Gonzalez R, Robert C, Schadendorf D, Hassel JC, Akerley W, van den Eertwegh AJ, Lutzky J, Lorigan P, Vaubel JM, Linette GP, Hogg D, Ottensmeier CH, Lebbe C, Peschel C, Quirt I, Clark JI, Wolchok JD, Weber JS, Tian J, Yellin MJ, Nichol GM, Hoos A, Urba WJ (2010) Improved survival with ipilimumab in patients with metastatic melanoma. N Engl J Med 363(8):711–723

Homig-Holzel C, Hojer C, Rastelli J, Casola S, Strobl LJ, Muller W, Quintanilla-Martinez L, Gewies A, Ruland J, Rajewsky K, Zimber-Strobl U (2008) Constitutive CD40 signaling in B cells selectively activates the noncanonical NF-kappaB pathway and promotes lymphomagenesis. J Exp Med 205(6):1317–1329

Horton HM, Bernett MJ, Peipp M, Pong E, Karki S, Chu SY, Richards JO, Chen H, Repp R, Desjarlais JR, Zhukovsky EA (2010) Fc-engineered anti-CD40 antibody enhances multiple effector functions and exhibits potent in vitro and in vivo antitumor activity against hematologic malignancies. Blood 116(16):3004–3012

Horton HM, Bernett MJ, Pong E, Peipp M, Karki S, Chu SY, Richards JO, Vostiar I, Joyce PF, Repp R, Desjarlais JR, Zhukovsky EA (2008) Potent in vitro and in vivo activity of an Fc-engineered anti-CD19 monoclonal antibody against lymphoma and leukemia. Cancer Res 68(19):8049–8057

Hu BT, Lee SC, Marin E, Ryan DH, Insel RA (1997) Telomerase is up-regulated in human germinal center B cells in vivo and can be re-expressed in memory B cells activated in vitro. J Immunol 159(3):1068–1071

Hussein M, Berenson JR, Niesvizky R, Munshi N, Matous J, Sobecks R, Harrop K, Drachman JG, Whiting N (2010) A phase I multidose study of dacetuzumab (SGN-40; humanized anti-CD40 monoclonal antibody) in patients with multiple myeloma. Haematologica 95(5):845–848

Jackaman C, Cornwall S, Graham PT, Nelson DJ (2011) CD40-activated B cells contribute to mesothelioma tumor regression. Immunol Cell Biol 89(2):255–267

Johnson PW, Challis R, Chowdhury F, Chan, Smith A, Steven NM, Edwards C, Ashton-Key M, Hodges E, Tutt AL, Ottensmeier CH, Williams A, Glennie M (2013) A trial of agonistic anti-CD40 antibody: biological effects in a cancer research UK phase I study. Presented at AACR 104th annual meeting 2013 on cancer research, vol 73 (Issue 8, Suppl 1), Washington, 6–10 Apr 2013

Johnson PW, Steven NM, Chowdhury F, Dobbyn J, Hall E, Ashton-Key M, Hodges E, Ottensmeier CH, Williams A, Glennie M (2010) A Cancer Research UK phase I study evaluating safety, tolerability, and biological effects of chimeric anti-CD40 monoclonal antibody (MAb), Chi Lob 7/4. J Clin Oncol 2010 ASCO Annu Meet (Abstract 2507) 28:15s
Kalbasi A, Fonsatti E, Natali PG, Altomonte M, Bertocci E, Cutaia O, Calabro L, Chiou M, Tap W, Chmielowski B, Maio M, Ribas A (2010) CD40 expression by human melanocytic lesions and melanoma cell lines and direct CD40 targeting with the therapeutic anti-CD40 antibody CP-870,893. J Immunother 33(8):810–816
Kawabe T, Naka T, Yoshida K, Tanaka T, Fujiwara H, Suematsu S, Yoshida N, Kishimoto T, Kikutani H (1994) The immune responses in CD40-deficient mice: impaired immunoglobulin class switching and germinal center formation. Immunity 1(3):167–178
Kedl RM, Jordan M, Potter T, Kappler J, Marrack P, Dow S (2001) CD40 stimulation accelerates deletion of tumor-specific CD8(+) T cells in the absence of tumor-antigen vaccination. Proc Natl Acad Sci USA 98(19):10811–10816
Klaus SJ, Berberich I, Shu G, Clark EA (1994) CD40 and its ligand in the regulation of humoral immunity. Semin Immunol 6(5):279–286
Klimp AH, de Vries EG, Scherphof GL, Daemen T (2002) A potential role of macrophage activation in the treatment of cancer. Crit Rev Oncol Hematol 44(2):143–161
Kurts C, Robinson BW, Knolle PA (2010) Cross-priming in health and disease. Nat Rev Immunol 10(6):403–414
Kusam S, Munugalavadla V, Sawant D, Dent A (2009) BCL6 cooperates with CD40 stimulation and loss of p53 function to rapidly transform primary B cells. Int J Cancer 125(4):977–981
Lake RA, Robinson BW (2005) Immunotherapy and chemotherapy–a practical partnership. Nat Rev Cancer 5(5):397–405
Lapalombella R, Gowda A, Joshi T, Mehter N, Cheney C, Lehman A, Chen CS, Johnson AJ, Caligiuri MA, Tridandapani S, Muthusamy N, Byrd JC (2009) The humanized CD40 antibody SGN-40 demonstrates pre-clinical activity that is enhanced by lenalidomide in chronic lymphocytic leukaemia. Br J Haematol 144(6):848–855
Law CL, Gordon KA, Collier J, Klussman K, McEarchern JA, Cerveny CG, Mixan BJ, Lee WP, Lin Z, Valdez P, Wahl AF, Grewal IS (2005) Preclinical antilymphoma activity of a humanized anti-CD40 monoclonal antibody, SGN-40. Cancer Res 65(18):8331–8338
Lazar GA, Dang W, Karki S, Vafa O, Peng JS, Hyun L, Chan C, Chung HS, Eivazi A, Yoder SC, Vielmetter J, Carmichael DF, Hayes RJ, Dahiyat BI (2006) Engineered antibody Fc variants with enhanced effector function. Proc Natl Acad Sci USA 103(11):4005–4010
Lee CS, Cragg M, Glennie M, Johnson P (2013) Novel antibodies targeting immune regulatory checkpoints for cancer therapy. Br J Clin Pharmacol 76(2):233–247
Lewis TS, McCormick RS, McEarchern JA et al (2008a) Preclinical analysis of the combined activity of SGN-40, anti-CD40 monoclonal antibody, with rituximab in non-Hodgkin lymphoma. Blood (Abstract 1583) 112:561–562
Lewis TS, McCormick RS, Emmerton K, Lau JT, Yu SF, McEarchern JA, Grewal IS, Law CL (2011) Distinct apoptotic signaling characteristics of the anti-CD40 monoclonal antibody dacetuzumab and rituximab produce enhanced antitumor activity in non-Hodgkin lymphoma. Clin Cancer Res 17(14):4672–4681
Lewis TS, McCormick RS, Kissler K, Stone IJ, Jonas M, Sutherland MSK, Gerber H-P, Drachman JG, Grewal IS, Law C-L (2007) The humanized anti-cd40 monoclonal antibody, SGN-40, potentiates chemotherapy regimens in NHL xenograft models via pro-apoptotic signaling. ASH Annu Meet Abs 110(11):2342
Lewis TS, McCormick RS, McEarchern JA, Kissler K, Stone IJ, Gerber H-P, Drachman JG, Grewal I, Law C-L (2008b) Preclinical analysis of the combined activity of SGN-40, anti-CD40 monoclonal antibody, with rituximab in non-hodgkin lymphoma. ASH Annu Meet Abs 112(11):1583
Li F, Ravetch JV (2011) Inhibitory Fcgamma receptor engagement drives adjuvant and anti-tumor activities of agonistic CD40 antibodies. Science 333(6045):1030–1034

Li F, Ravetch JV (2012) Apoptotic and antitumor activity of death receptor antibodies require inhibitory Fcgamma receptor engagement. Proc Natl Acad Sci USA 109(27):10966–10971

Li F, Ravetch JV (2013) Antitumor activities of agonistic anti-TNFR antibodies require differential FcgammaRIIB coengagement in vivo. Proc Natl Acad Sci USA 110(48):19501–19506

Li YY, Baccam M, Waters SB, Pessin JE, Bishop GA, Koretzky GA (1996) CD40 ligation results in protein kinase C-independent activation of ERK and JNK in resting murine splenic B cells. J Immunol 157(4):1440–1447

Long L, Tong X, Patawaran M, Aukerman SL, Jallal B, Luqman M (2005) Antagonist anti-CD40 antibody, CHIR-12.12, induces ADCC, inhibits tumor growth, and prolongs survival in a human multiple myeloma xenograft model. ASH Annu Meet Abs 106(11):3470

Lopez A, Gutierrez A, Palacios A, Blancas I, Navarrete M, Morey M, Perello A, Alarcon J, Martinez J, Rodriguez J (2008) GEMOX-R regimen is a highly effective salvage regimen in patients with refractory/relapsing diffuse large-cell lymphoma: a phase II study. Eur J Haematol 80(2):127–132

Luqman M, Klabunde S, Lin K, Georgakis GV, Cherukuri A, Holash J, Goldbeck C, Xu X, Kadel EE 3rd, Lee SH, Aukerman SL, Jallal B, Aziz N, Weng WK, Wierda W, O'Brien S, Younes A (2008) The antileukemia activity of a human anti-CD40 antagonist antibody, HCD122, on human chronic lymphocytic leukemia cells. Blood 112(3):711–720

Mauri C, Mars LT, Londei M (2000) Therapeutic activity of agonistic monoclonal antibodies against CD40 in a chronic autoimmune inflammatory process. Nat Med 6(6):673–679

McWhirter SM, Pullen SS, Holton JM, Crute JJ, Kehry MR, Alber T (1999) Crystallographic analysis of CD40 recognition and signaling by human TRAF2. Proc Natl Acad Sci USA 96 (15):8408–8413

Melero I, Hervas-Stubbs S, Glennie M, Pardoll DM, Chen L (2007) Immunostimulatory monoclonal antibodies for cancer therapy. Nat Rev Cancer 7(2):95–106

Middleton MR, Grob JJ, Aaronson N, Fierlbeck G, Tilgen W, Seiter S, Gore M, Aamdal S, Cebon J, Coates A, Dreno B, Henz M, Schadendorf D, Kapp A, Weiss J, Fraass U, Statkevich P, Muller M, Thatcher N (2000) Randomized phase III study of temozolomide versus dacarbazine in the treatment of patients with advanced metastatic malignant melanoma. J Clin Oncol 18 (1):158–166

Miga AJ, Masters SR, Durell BG, Gonzalez M, Jenkins MK, Maliszewski C, Kikutani H, Wade WF, Noelle RJ (2001) Dendritic cell longevity and T cell persistence is controlled by CD154-CD40 interactions. Eur J Immunol 31(3):959–965

Murphy WJ, Funakoshi S, Fanslow WC, Rager HC, Taub DD, Longo DL (1999) CD40 stimulation promotes human secondary immunoglobulin responses in HuPBL-SCID chimeras. Clin Immunol 90(1):22–27

Nimmerjahn F, Ravetch JV (2005) Divergent immunoglobulin g subclass activity through selective Fc receptor binding. Science 310(5753):1510–1512

Nimmerjahn F, Ravetch JV (2006) Fcgamma receptors: old friends and new family members. Immunity 24(1):19–28

Nimmerjahn F, Ravetch JV (2008) Fcgamma receptors as regulators of immune responses. Nat Rev Immunol 8(1):34–47

Noelle RJ, Roy M, Shepherd DM, Stamenkovic I, Ledbetter JA, Aruffo A (1992) A 39-kDa protein on activated helper T cells binds CD40 and transduces the signal for cognate activation of B cells. Proc Natl Acad Sci USA 89(14):6550–6554

Nowak AK, Robinson BW, Lake RA (2003) Synergy between chemotherapy and immunotherapy in the treatment of established murine solid tumors. Cancer Res 63(15):4490–4496

Oflazoglu E, Stone IJ, Brown L, Gordon KA, van Rooijen N, Jonas M, Law CL, Grewal IS, Gerber HP (2009) Macrophages and Fc-receptor interactions contribute to the antitumour activities of the anti-CD40 antibody SGN-40. Br J Cancer 100(1):113–117

Paulie S, Ehlin-Henriksson B, Mellstedt H, Koho H, Ben-Aissa H, Perlmann P (1985) A p50 surface antigen restricted to human urinary bladder carcinomas and B lymphocytes. Cancer Immunol Immunother 20(1):23–28

Pellat-Deceunynck C, Amiot M, Robillard N, Wijdenes J, Bataille R (1996) CD11a-CD18 and CD102 interactions mediate human myeloma cell growth arrest induced by CD40 stimulation. Cancer Res 56(8):1909–1916

Pellat-Deceunynck C, Bataille R, Robillard N, Harousseau JL, Rapp MJ, Juge-Morineau N, Wijdenes J, Amiot M (1994) Expression of CD28 and CD40 in human myeloma cells: a comparative study with normal plasma cells. Blood 84(8):2597–2603

Pham LV, Tamayo AT, Yoshimura LC, Lo P, Terry N, Reid PS, Ford RJ (2002) A CD40 Signalosome anchored in lipid rafts leads to constitutive activation of NF-kappaB and autonomous cell growth in B cell lymphomas. Immunity 16(1):37–50

Planken EV, Dijkstra NH, Willemze R, Kluin-Nelemans JC (1996) Proliferation of B cell malignancies in all stages of differentiation upon stimulation in the 'CD40 system'. Leukemia 10(3):488–493

Quezada SA, Jarvinen LZ, Lind EF, Noelle RJ (2004) CD40/CD154 interactions at the interface of tolerance and immunity. Annu Rev Immunol 22:307–328

Rakhmilevich AL, Alderson KL, Sondel PM (2012) T-cell-independent antitumor effects of CD40 ligation. Int Rev Immunol 31(4):267–278

Ren CL, Morio T, Fu SM, Geha RS (1994) Signal transduction via CD40 involves activation of lyn kinase and phosphatidylinositol-3-kinase, and phosphorylation of phospholipase C gamma 2. J Exp Med 179(2):673–680

Restifo NP, Kawakami Y, Marincola F, Shamamian P, Taggarse A, Esquivel F, Rosenberg SA (1993) Molecular mechanisms used by tumors to escape immune recognition: immunogenetherapy and the cell biology of major histocompatibility complex class I. J Immunother Emphasis Tumor Immunol 14(3):182–190

Richman LP, Vonderheide RH (2014) Role of crosslinking for agonistic CD40 monoclonal antibodies as immune therapy of cancer. Cancer Immunol Res 2(1):19–26

Ridge JP, Di Rosa F, Matzinger P (1998) A conditioned dendritic cell can be a temporal bridge between a CD4+ T-helper and a T-killer cell. Nature 393(6684):474–478

Robert C, Thomas L, Bondarenko I, O'Day S, Weber J, Garbe C, Lebbe C, Baurain JF, Testori A, Grob JJ, Davidson N, Richards J, Maio M, Hauschild A, Miller WH Jr, Gascon P, Lotem M, Harmankaya K, Ibrahim R, Francis S, Chen TT, Humphrey R, Hoos A, Wolchok JD (2011) Ipilimumab plus dacarbazine for previously untreated metastatic melanoma. N Engl J Med 364 (26):2517–2526

Ruter J, Antonia SJ, Burris HA, Huhn RD, Vonderheide RH (2010) Immune modulation with weekly dosing of an agonist CD40 antibody in a phase I study of patients with advanced solid tumors. Cancer Biol Ther 10(10):983–993

Sabel MS, Yamada M, Kawaguchi Y, Chen FA, Takita H, Bankert RB (2000) CD40 expression on human lung cancer correlates with metastatic spread. Cancer Immunol Immunother 49 (2):101–108

Schoenberger SP, Toes RE, van der Voort EI, Offringa R, Melief CJ (1998) T-cell help for cytotoxic T lymphocytes is mediated by CD40-CD40L interactions. Nature 393(6684):480–483

Schriever F, Freedman AS, Freeman G, Messner E, Lee G, Daley J, Nadler LM (1989) Isolated human follicular dendritic cells display a unique antigenic phenotype. J Exp Med 169 (6):2043–2058

Shi X, Dornan D (2012) To respond or not to respond to CD40 agonism: that is the prediction. Oncoimmunology 1(1):83–85

Slobodova Z, Ehrmann J, Krejci V, Zapletalova J, Melichar B (2011) Analysis of CD40 expression in breast cancer and its relation to clinicopathological characteristics. Neoplasma 58 (3):189–197

Smith CA, Farrah T, Goodwin RG (1994) The TNF receptor superfamily of cellular and viral proteins: activation, costimulation, and death. Cell 76(6):959–962

Stavenhagen JB, Gorlatov S, Tuaillon N, Rankin CT, Li H, Burke S, Huang L, Vijh S, Johnson S, Bonvini E, Koenig S (2007) Fc optimization of therapeutic antibodies enhances their ability to kill tumor cells in vitro and controls tumor expansion in vivo via low-affinity activating Fcgamma receptors. Cancer Res 67(18):8882–8890

Sznol M, Kluger HM, Wolchok JD (2014) Survival, response duration, and activity by BRAF mutation (MT) status of nivolumab (NIVO, anti-PD-1, BMS-936558, ONO-4538) and ipilimumab (IPI) concurrent therapy in advanced melanoma (MEL). J Clin Oncol 2014 ASCO Annu Meet (LBA9003^) 32:35s

Szocinski JL, Khaled AR, Hixon J, Halverson D, Funakoshi S, Fanslow WC, Boyd A, Taub DD, Durum SK, Siegall CB, Longo DL, Murphy WJ (2002) Activation-induced cell death of aggressive histology lymphomas by CD40 stimulation: induction of bax. Blood 100(1):217–223

Tai YT, Catley LP, Mitsiades CS, Burger R, Podar K, Shringpaure R, Hideshima T, Chauhan D, Hamasaki M, Ishitsuka K, Richardson P, Treon SP, Munshi NC, Anderson KC (2004) Mechanisms by which SGN-40, a humanized anti-CD40 antibody, induces cytotoxicity in human multiple myeloma cells: clinical implications. Cancer Res 64(8):2846–2852

Tai YT, Li X, Tong X, Santos D, Otsuki T, Catley L, Tournilhac O, Podar K, Hideshima T, Schlossman R, Richardson P, Munshi NC, Luqman M, Anderson KC (2005a) Human anti-CD40 antagonist antibody triggers significant antitumor activity against human multiple myeloma. Cancer Res 65(13):5898–5906

Tai YT, Li XF, Catley L, Coffey R, Breitkreutz I, Bae J, Song W, Podar K, Hideshima T, Chauhan D, Schlossman R, Richardson P, Treon SP, Grewal IS, Munshi NC, Anderson KC (2005b) Immunomodulatory drug lenalidomide (CC-5013, IMiD3) augments anti-CD40 SGN-40-induced cytotoxicity in human multiple myeloma: clinical implications. Cancer Res 65 (24):11712–11720

Teoh G, Tai YT, Urashima M, Shirahama S, Matsuzaki M, Chauhan D, Treon SP, Raje N, Hideshima T, Shima Y, Anderson KC (2000) CD40 activation mediates p53-dependent cell cycle regulation in human multiple myeloma cell lines. Blood 95(3):1039–1046

Thomas WD, Smith MJ, Si Z, Hersey P (1996) Expression of the co-stimulatory molecule CD40 on melanoma cells. Int J Cancer 68(6):795–801

Tobinai K, Takahashi T, Akinaga S (2012) Targeting chemokine receptor CCR4 in adult T-cell leukemia-lymphoma and other T-cell lymphomas. Curr Hematol Malig Rep 7(3):235–240

Todryk SM, Tutt AL, Green MH, Smallwood JA, Halanek N, Dalgleish AG, Glennie MJ (2001) CD40 ligation for immunotherapy of solid tumours. J Immunol Methods 248(1–2):139–147

Topalian SL, Sznol M, McDermott DF, Kluger HM, Carvajal RD, Sharfman WH, Brahmer JR, Lawrence DP, Atkins MB, Powderly JD, Leming PD, Lipson EJ, Puzanov I, Smith DC, Taube JM, Wigginton JM, Kollia GD, Gupta A, Pardoll DM, Sosman JA, Hodi FS (2014) Survival, durable tumor remission, and long-term safety in patients with advanced melanoma receiving nivolumab. J Clin Oncol 32(10):1020–1030

Tsubata T, Wu J, Honjo T (1993) B-cell apoptosis induced by antigen receptor crosslinking is blocked by a T-cell signal through CD40. Nature 364(6438):645–648

Turner JG, Rakhmilevich AL, Burdelya L, Neal Z, Imboden M, Sondel PM, Yu H (2001) Anti-CD40 antibody induces antitumor and antimetastatic effects: the role of NK cells. J Immunol 166(1):89–94

Tutt AL, O'Brien L, Hussain A, Crowther GR, French RR, Glennie MJ (2002) T cell immunity to lymphoma following treatment with anti-CD40 monoclonal antibody. J Immunol 168 (6):2720–2728

Urashima M, Chauhan D, Uchiyama H, Freeman GJ, Anderson KC (1995) CD40 ligand triggered interleukin-6 secretion in multiple myeloma. Blood 85(7):1903–1912

van Kooten C, Banchereau J (1997) Functions of CD40 on B cells, dendritic cells and other cells. Curr Opin Immunol 9(3):330–337

van Kooten C, Banchereau J (2000) CD40-CD40 ligand. J Leukoc Biol 67(1):2–17

van Mierlo GJ, den Boer AT, Medema JP, van der Voort EI, Fransen MF, Offringa R, Melief CJ, Toes RE (2002) CD40 stimulation leads to effective therapy of CD40(-) tumors through induction of strong systemic cytotoxic T lymphocyte immunity. Proc Natl Acad Sci U S A 99 (8):5561–5566

von Leoprechting A, van der Bruggen P, Pahl HL, Aruffo A, Simon JC (1999) Stimulation of CD40 on immunogenic human malignant melanomas augments their cytotoxic T lymphocyte-mediated lysis and induces apoptosis. Cancer Res 59(6):1287–1294

Vonderheide RH (2007) Prospect of targeting the CD40 pathway for cancer therapy. Clin Cancer Res 13(4):1083–1088

Vonderheide RH, Burg JM, Mick R, Trosko JA, Li D, Shaik MN, Tolcher AW, Hamid O (2013) Phase I study of the CD40 agonist antibody CP-870,893 combined with carboplatin and paclitaxel in patients with advanced solid tumors. Oncoimmunology 2(1):e23033

Vonderheide RH, Flaherty KT, Khalil M, Stumacher MS, Bajor DL, Hutnick NA, Sullivan P, Mahany JJ, Gallagher M, Kramer A, Green SJ, O'Dwyer PJ, Running KL, Huhn RD, Antonia SJ (2007) Clinical activity and immune modulation in cancer patients treated with CP-870,893, a novel CD40 agonist monoclonal antibody. J Clin Oncol 25(7):876–883

Vonderheide RH, Glennie MJ (2013) Agonistic CD40 antibodies and cancer therapy. Clin Cancer Res 19(5):1035–1043

Voorzanger-Rousselot N, Favrot M, Blay JY (1998) Resistance to cytotoxic chemotherapy induced by CD40 ligand in lymphoma cells. Blood 92(9):3381–3387

Vosters O, Beuneu C, Nagy N, Movahedi B, Aksoy E, Salmon I, Pipeleers D, Goldman M, Verhasselt V (2004) CD40 expression on human pancreatic duct cells: role in nuclear factor-kappa B activation and production of pro-inflammatory cytokines. Diabetologia 47(4):660–668

Wang D, Freeman GJ, Levine H, Ritz J, Robertson MJ (1997) Role of the CD40 and CD95 (APO-1/Fas) antigens in the apoptosis of human B-cell malignancies. Br J Haematol 97(2):409–417

White AL, Chan HT, Roghanian A, French RR, Mockridge CI, Tutt AL, Dixon SV, Ajona D, Verbeek JS, Al-Shamkhani A, Cragg MS, Beers SA, Glennie MJ (2011) Interaction with FcgammaRIIB is critical for the agonistic activity of anti-CD40 monoclonal antibody. J Immunol 187(4):1754–1763

White AL, Dou L, Chan HT, Field VL, Mockridge CI, Moss K, Williams EL, Booth SG, French RR, Potter EA, Butts C, Al-Shamkhani A, Cragg MS, Verbeek JS, Johnson PW, Glennie MJ, Beers SA (2014) Fcgamma receptor dependency of agonistic CD40 antibody in lymphoma therapy can be overcome through antibody multimerization. J Immunol 193(4):1828–1835

Williams EL, Tutt AL, Beers SA, French RR, Chan CH, Cox KL, Roghanian A, Penfold CA, Butts CL, Boross P, Verbeek JS, Cragg MS, Glennie MJ (2013) Immunotherapy targeting inhibitory Fcgamma receptor IIB (CD32b) in the mouse is limited by monoclonal antibody consumption and receptor internalization. J Immunol 191(8):4130–4140

Williams EL, Tutt AL, French RR, Chan HT, Lau B, Penfold CA, Mockridge CI, Roghanian A, Cox KL, Verbeek JS, Glennie MJ, Cragg MS (2012) Development and characterisation of monoclonal antibodies specific for the murine inhibitory FcgammaRIIB (CD32B). Eur J Immunol 42(8):2109–2120

Wingett DG, Vestal RE, Forcier K, Hadjokas N, Nielson CP (1998) CD40 is functionally expressed on human breast carcinomas: variable inducibility by cytokines and enhancement of Fas-mediated apoptosis. Breast Cancer Res Treat 50(1):27–36

Wolchok JD, Kluger H, Callahan MK, Postow MA, Rizvi NA, Lesokhin AM, Segal NH, Ariyan CE, Gordon RA, Reed K, Burke MM, Caldwell A, Kronenberg SA, Agunwamba BU, Zhang X, Lowy I, Inzunza HD, Feely W, Horak CE, Hong Q, Korman AJ, Wigginton JM, Gupta A, Sznol M (2013) Nivolumab plus ipilimumab in advanced melanoma. N Engl J Med 369 (2):122–133

Xu J, Foy TM, Laman JD, Elliott EA, Dunn JJ, Waldschmidt TJ, Elsemore J, Noelle RJ, Flavell RA (1994) Mice deficient for the CD40 ligand. Immunity 1(5):423–431

Yellin MJ, Brett J, Baum D, Matsushima A, Szabolcs M, Stern D, Chess L (1995) Functional interactions of T cells with endothelial cells: the role of CD40L-CD40-mediated signals. J Exp Med 182(6):1857–1864

Ziebold JL, Hixon J, Boyd A, Murphy WJ (2000) Differential effects of CD40 stimulation on normal and neoplastic cell growth. Arch Immunol Ther Exp (Warsz) 48(4):225–233

Index

Current Topics in Microbiology and Immunology (2017) 405:209–210
DOI 10.1007/978-3-319-23910-1

CPI Antony Rowe
Chippenham, UK
2018-05-08 11:04